DSM-III-R Classification
Axes I and II Categories and Codes
© Copyright 1987, American Psychiatric Association

All official DSM-III-R codes are included in ICD-9-CM. Codes followed by a * are used for more than one DSM-III-R diagnosis or subtype in order to maintain compatibility with ICD-9-CM.

A long dash following a diagnostic term indicates the need for a fifth digit subtype or other qualifying term.

The term specify *following the name of some diagnostic categories indicates qualifying terms that clinicians may wish to add in parentheses after the name of the disorder.*

NOS = Not Otherwise Specified

The current severity of a disorder may be specified after the diagnosis as:

mild   currently
moderate   meets
severe   diagnostic
           criteria

*in partial remission
(or residual state)
in complete remission*

DISORDERS USUALLY FIRST EVIDENT IN INFANCY, CHILDHOOD, OR ADOLESCENCE

DEVELOPMENTAL DISORDERS
Note: These are coded on Axis II.

Mental Retardation
- 317.00   Mild mental retardation
- 318.00   Moderate mental retardation
- 318.10   Severe mental retardation
- 318.20   Profound mental retardation
- 319.00   Unspecified mental retardation

Pervasive Developmental Disorders
- 299.00   Autistic disorder
  Specify if childhood onset
- 299.80   Pervasive developmental disorder NOS

Specific Developmental Disorders
Academic skills disorders
- 315.10   Developmental arithmetic disorder
- 315.80   Developmental expressive writing disorder
- 315.00   Developmental reading disorder

Language and speech disorders
- 315.39   Developmental articulation disorder
- 315.31*   Developmental expressive language disorder
- 315.31*   Developmental receptive language disorder

Motor skills disorder
- 315.40   Developmental coordination disorder
- 315.90*   Specific developmental disorder NOS

Other Developmental Disorders
- 315.90*   Developmental disorder NOS

Disruptive Behavior Disorders
- 314.01   Attention-deficit hyperactivity disorder

Conduct disorder
- 312.20   group type
- 312.00   solitary aggressive type
- 312.90   undifferentiated type
- 313.81   Oppositional defiant disorder

Anxiety Disorders of Childhood or Adolescence
- 309.21   Separation anxiety disorder
- 313.21   Avoidant disorder of childhood or adolescence
- 313.00   Overanxious disorder

Eating Disorders
- 307.10   Anorexia nervosa
- 307.51   Bulimia nervosa
- 307.52   Pica
- 307.53   Rumination disorder of infancy
- 307.50   Eating disorder NOS

Gender Identity Disorders
- 302.60   Gender identity disorder of childhood
- 302.50   Transsexualism
  Specify sexual history: asexual, homosexual, heterosexual, unspecified
- 302.85*   Gender identity disorder of adolescence or adulthood, nontranssexual type
  Specify sexual history: asexual, homosexual, heterosexual, unspecified
- 302.85*   Gender identity disorder NOS

Tic Disorders
- 307.23   Tourette's disorder
- 307.22   Chronic motor or vocal tic disorder
- 307.21   Transient tic disorder
  Specify: single episode or recurrent
- 307.20   Tic disorder NOS

Elimination Disorders
- 307.70   Functional encopresis
  Specify: primary or secondary type
- 307.60   Functional enuresis
  Specify: primary or secondary type
  Specify: nocturnal only, diurnal only, nocturnal and diurnal

Speech Disorders Not Elsewhere Classified
- 307.00*   Cluttering
- 307.00*   Stuttering

Other Disorders of Infancy, Childhood, or Adolescence
- 313.23   Elective mutism
- 313.82   Identity disorder
- 313.89   Reactive attachment disorder of infancy or early childhood
- 307.30   Stereotypy/habit disorder
- 314.00   Undifferentiated attention-deficit disorder

ORGANIC MENTAL DISORDERS
Dementias Arising in the Senium and Presenium
Primary degenerative dementia of the Alzheimer type, senile onset,
- 290.30   with delirium

290.20	with delusions
290.21	with depression
290.00*	uncomplicated
	(Note: code 331.00
	Alzheimer's disease on
	Axis III)

Code in fifth digit:
1 = with delirium, 2 = with
delusions, 3 = with depression,
0* = uncomplicated.

290.1x	Primary degenerative
	dementia of the
	Alzheimer type,
	presenile onset, _____
	(Note: code 331.00
	Alzheimer's disease on
	Axis III)
290.4x	Multi-infarct dementia, _
290.00*	Senile dementia NOS
	Specify etiology on
	Axis III if known
290.10*	Presenile dementia NOS
	Specify etiology on
	Axis III if known (e.g.,
	Pick's disease, Jakob-
	Creutzfeldt disease)

**Psychoactive Substance-
Induced Organic Mental
Disorders**

Alcohol
303.00	intoxication
291.40	idiosyncratic
	intoxication
291.80	uncomplicated alcohol
	withdrawal
291.00	withdrawal delirium
291.30	hallucinosis
291.10	amnestic disorder
291.20	dementia associated
	with alcoholism

Amphetamine or
similarly acting
sympathomimetic
305.70*	intoxication
292.00*	withdrawal
292.81*	delirium
292.11*	delusional disorder

Caffeine
| 305.90* | intoxication |

Cannabis
| 305.20* | intoxication |
| 292.11* | delusional disorder |

Cocaine
305.60*	intoxication
292.00*	withdrawal
292.81*	delirium
292.11*	delusional disorder

Hallucinogen
305.30*	hallucinosis
292.11*	delusional disorder
292.84*	mood disorder
292.89*	posthallucinogen
	perception disorder

Inhalant
| 305.90* | intoxication |

Nicotine
| 292.00* | withdrawal |

Opioid
| 305.50* | intoxication |
| 292.00* | withdrawal |

Phencyclidine (PCP) or
similarly acting
arylcyclohexylamine
305.90*	intoxication
292.81*	delirium
292.11*	delusional disorder
292.84*	mood disorder
292.90*	organic mental
	disorder NOS

Sedative, hypnotic, or
anxiolytic
305.40*	intoxication
292.00*	uncomplicated
	sedative, hypnotic, or
	anxiolytic withdrawal
292.00*	withdrawal delirium
292.83*	amnestic disorder

Other or unspecified
psychoactive substance
305.90*	intoxication
292.00*	withdrawal
292.81*	delirium
292.82*	dementia
292.83*	amnestic disorder
292.11*	delusional disorder
292.12	hallucinosis
292.84*	mood disorder
292.89*	anxiety disorder
292.89*	personality disorder
292.90*	organic mental
	disorder NOS

**Organic Mental Disorders
associated with Axis III
physical disorders or
conditions, or whose etiology
is unknown.**
293.00	Delirium
294.10	Dementia
294.00	Amnestic disorder
293.81	Organic delusional
	disorder
293.82	Organic hallucinosis
293.83	Organic mood disorder
	Specify: manic,
	depressed, mixed
294.80*	Organic anxiety disorder
310.10	Organic personality
	disorder
	Specify if explosive
	type
294.80*	Organic mental disorder
	NOS

**PSYCHOACTIVE SUBSTANCE
USE DISORDERS**

Alcohol
| 303.90 | dependence |
| 305.00 | abuse |

Amphetamine or
similarly acting
sympathomimetic

| 304.40 | dependence |
| 305.70* | abuse |

Cannabis
| 304.30 | dependence |
| 305.20* | abuse |

Cocaine
| 304.20 | dependence |
| 305.60* | abuse |

Hallucinogen
| 304.50* | dependence |
| 305.30* | abuse |

Inhalant
| 304.60 | dependence |
| 305.90* | abuse |

Nicotine
| 305.10 | dependence |

Opioid
| 304.00 | dependence |
| 305.50* | abuse |

Phencyclidine (PCP) or
similarly acting
arylcyclohexylamine
| 304.50* | dependence |
| 305.90* | abuse |

Sedative, hypnotic, or
anxiolytic
304.10	dependence
305.40*	abuse
304.90*	Polysubstance
	dependence
304.90*	Psychoactive substance
	dependence NOS
305.90*	Psychoactive substance
	abuse NOS

SCHIZOPHRENIA
Code in fifth digit:
1 = subchronic, 2 = chronic,
3 = subchronic with acute
exacerbation, 4 = chronic with
acute exacerbation,
5 = remission, 0 = unspecified.

Schizophrenia
295.2x	catatonic, _____
295.1x	disorganized, _____
295.3x	paranoid, _____
	Specify if stable type
295.9x	undifferentiated, _____
295.6x	residual, _____
	Specify if late onset

**DELUSIONAL (PARANOID)
DISORDER)**
297.10	Delusional (Paranoid)
	disorder
	Specify type:
	erotomanic
	grandiose
	jealous
	persecutory
	somatic
	unspecified

(*continued on last page*)

Psychotherapeutic Drug Identification Guide

This guide contains actual size, color reproductions of some commonly prescribed major psychotherapeutic drugs. This guide mainly illustrates tablets and capsules. A † symbol preceding the name of the drug indicates that other doses are available. Check directly with the manufacturer. *(While the the photos are intended as accurate reproductions of the drugs, the guide should be used only as a quick identification aid).*

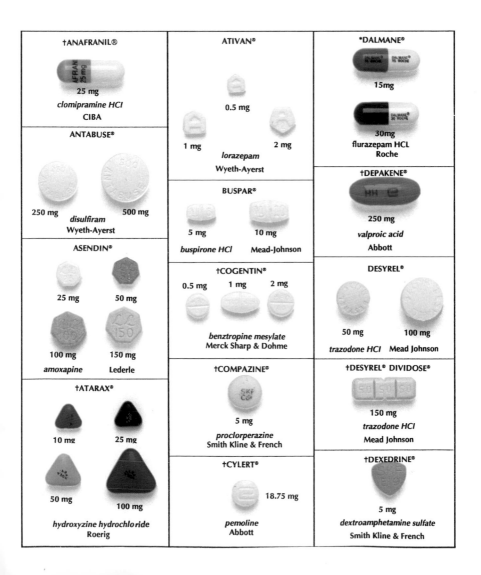

†ANAFRANIL®

25 mg

clomipramine HCl
CIBA

ANTABUSE®

250 mg 500 mg
disulfiram
Wyeth-Ayerst

ASENDIN®

25 mg 50 mg

100 mg 150 mg
amoxapine Lederle

†ATARAX®

10 mg 25 mg

50 mg 100 mg

hydroxyzine hydrochloride
Roerig

ATIVAN®

0.5 mg

1 mg 2 mg
lorazepam
Wyeth-Ayerst

BUSPAR®

5 mg 10 mg
buspirone HCl Mead-Johnson

†COGENTIN®

0.5 mg 1 mg 2 mg

benztropine mesylate
Merck Sharp & Dohme

†COMPAZINE®

5 mg
prochlorperazine
Smith Kline & French

†CYLERT®

18.75 mg

pemoline
Abbott

*DALMANE®

15mg

30mg
flurazepam HCL
Roche

†DEPAKENE®

250 mg
valproic acid
Abbott

DESYREL®

50 mg 100 mg
trazodone HCl Mead Johnson

†DESYREL® DIVIDOSE®

150 mg
trazodone HCl
Mead Johnson

†DEXEDRINE®

5 mg
dextroamphetamine sulfate
Smith Kline & French

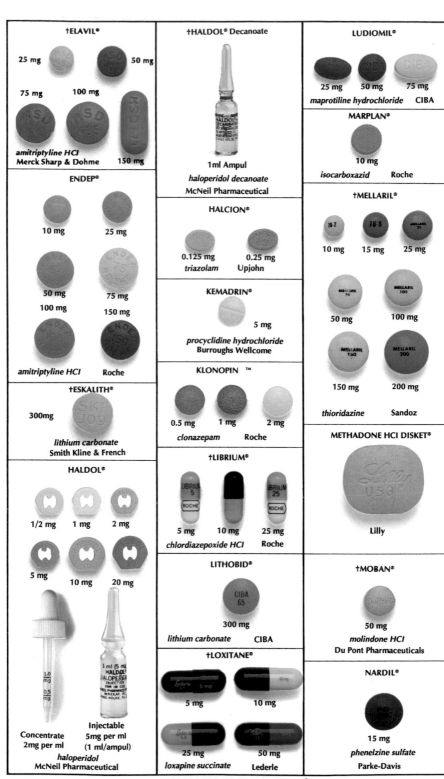

†ELAVIL®

25 mg 50 mg
75 mg 100 mg
150 mg

amitriptyline HCl
Merck Sharp & Dohme

ENDEP®

10 mg 25 mg
50 mg 75 mg
100 mg 150 mg

amitriptyline HCl Roche

†ESKALITH®

300mg

lithium carbonate
Smith Kline & French

HALDOL®

1/2 mg 1 mg 2 mg
5 mg 10 mg 20 mg

Concentrate
2mg per ml

Injectable
5mg per ml
(1 ml/ampul)

haloperidol
McNeil Pharmaceutical

†HALDOL® Decanoate

1ml Ampul

haloperidol decanoate
McNeil Pharmaceutical

HALCION®

0.125 mg 0.25 mg
triazolam Upjohn

KEMADRIN®

5 mg

procyclidine hydrochloride
Burroughs Wellcome

KLONOPIN ™

0.5 mg 1 mg 2 mg

clonazepam Roche

†LIBRIUM®

5 mg 10 mg 25 mg
chlordiazepoxide HCl Roche

LITHOBID®

300 mg

lithium carbonate CIBA

†LOXITANE®

5 mg 10 mg
25 mg 50 mg
loxapine succinate Lederle

LUDIOMIL®

25 mg 50 mg 75 mg

maprotiline hydrochloride CIBA

MARPLAN®

10 mg

isocarboxazid Roche

†MELLARIL®

10 mg 15 mg 25 mg
50 mg 100 mg
150 mg 200 mg

thioridazine Sandoz

METHADONE HCl DISKET®

Lilly

†MOBAN®

50 mg

molindone HCl
Du Pont Pharmaceuticals

NARDIL®

15 mg

phenelzine sulfate
Parke-Davis

WILLIAMS AND WILKINS ©

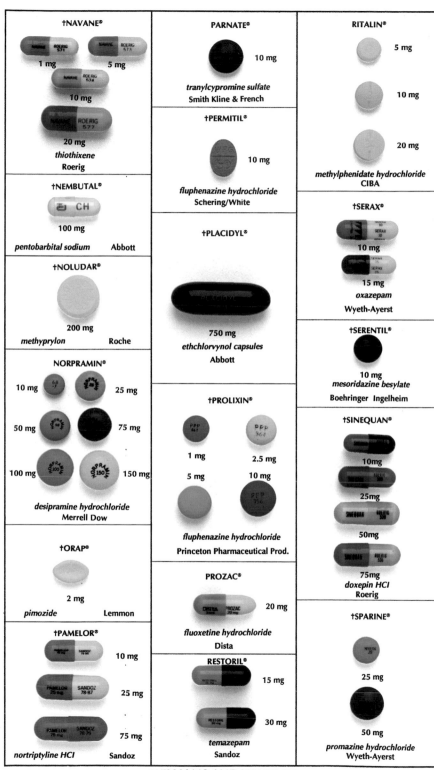

†NAVANE®

1 mg   5 mg

10 mg

20 mg

thiothixene
Roerig

†NEMBUTAL®

100 mg

pentobarbital sodium   Abbott

†NOLUDAR®

200 mg

methyprylon   Roche

NORPRAMIN®

10 mg   25 mg

50 mg   75 mg

100 mg   150 mg

desipramine hydrochloride
Merrell Dow

†ORAP®

2 mg

pimozide   Lemmon

†PAMELOR®

10 mg

25 mg

75 mg

nortriptyline HCl   Sandoz

PARNATE®

10 mg

tranylcypromine sulfate
Smith Kline & French

†PERMITIL®

10 mg

fluphenazine hydrochloride
Schering/White

†PLACIDYL®

750 mg
ethchlorvynol capsules
Abbott

†PROLIXIN®

1 mg   2.5 mg

5 mg   10 mg

fluphenazine hydrochloride
Princeton Pharmaceutical Prod.

PROZAC®

20 mg

fluoxetine hydrochloride
Dista

RESTORIL®

15 mg

30 mg

temazepam
Sandoz

RITALIN®

5 mg

10 mg

20 mg

methylphenidate hydrochloride
CIBA

†SERAX®

10 mg

15 mg

oxazepam
Wyeth-Ayerst

†SERENTIL®

10 mg
mesoridazine besylate
Boehringer Ingelheim

†SINEQUAN®

10mg

25mg

50mg

75mg
doxepin HCl
Roerig

†SPARINE®

25 mg

50 mg

promazine hydrochloride
Wyeth-Ayerst

WILLIAMS AND WILKINS ©

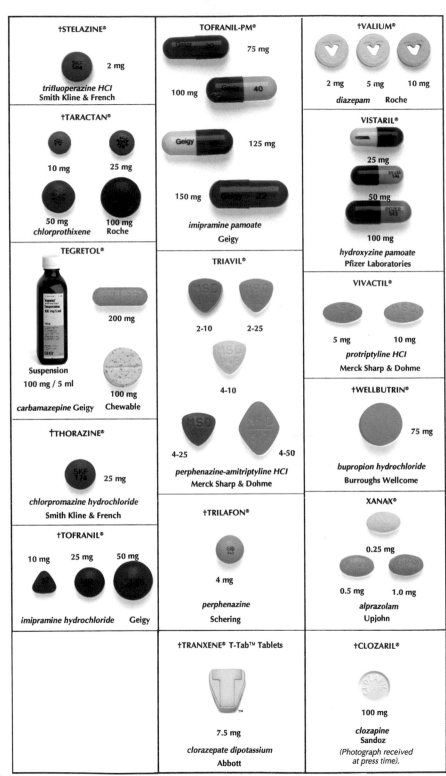

†STELAZINE®	**TOFRANIL-PM®**	**†VALIUM®**
2 mg	75 mg	2 mg 5 mg 10 mg
trifluoperazine HCI Smith Kline & French	100 mg 40	*diazepam* Roche
†TARACTAN®	125 mg Geigy	**VISTARIL®**
10 mg 25 mg	150 mg	25 mg
50 mg 100 mg *chlorprothixene* Roche	*imipramine pamoate* Geigy	50 mg
TEGRETOL®	**TRIAVIL®**	100 mg *hydroxyzine pamoate* Pfizer Laboratories
200 mg	2-10 2-25	**VIVACTIL®**
Suspension 100 mg / 5 ml 100 mg Chewable	4-10	5 mg 10 mg *protriptyline HCI* Merck Sharp & Dohme
carbamazepine Geigy	4-25 4-50 *perphenazine-amitriptyline HCI* Merck Sharp & Dohme	**†WELLBUTRIN®**
†THORAZINE®		75 mg
25 mg	**†TRILAFON®**	*bupropion hydrochloride* Burroughs Wellcome
chlorpromazine hydrochloride Smith Kline & French	4 mg *perphenazine* Schering	**XANAX®**
†TOFRANIL®		0.25 mg
10 mg 25 mg 50 mg		0.5 mg 1.0 mg *alprazolam* Upjohn
imipramine hydrochloride Geigy	**†TRANXENE® T-Tab™ Tablets**	**†CLOZARIL®**
	7.5 mg *clorazepate dipotassium* Abbott	100 mg *clozapine* Sandoz *(Photograph received at press time).*

WILLIAMS AND WILKINS ©

POCKET HANDBOOK OF CLINICAL PSYCHIATRY

SENIOR CONTRIBUTING EDITOR

Robert Cancro, M.D., MED.D.Sc.

Professor and Chairman, Department of Psychiatry,
New York University School of Medicine;
Director, Department of Psychiatry, Tisch Hospital, the University
Hospital of New York University Medical Center;
Director, Nathan S. Kline Institute for
Psychiatric Research, Orangeburg, New York

POCKET
HANDBOOK
OF
CLINICAL
PSYCHIATRY

Harold I. Kaplan, M.D.

Professor of Psychiatry, New York University School of Medicine
Attending Psychiatrist, Tisch Hospital, the University
Hospital of New York University Medical Center
Attending Psychiatrist, Bellevue Hospital
New York, New York

Benjamin J. Sadock, M.D.

Professor and Vice Chairman, Department of Psychiatry,
New York University School of Medicine,
Attending Psychiatrist, Tisch Hospital, the University
Hospital of New York University Medical Center
Attending Psychiatrist, Bellevue Hospital
New York, New York

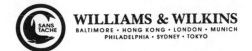

WILLIAMS & WILKINS
BALTIMORE • HONG KONG • LONDON • MUNICH
PHILADELPHIA • SYDNEY • TOKYO

**Williams
& Wilkins**

Editor: Michael G. Fisher
Associate Editor: Carol Eckhart
Copy Editor: Jennifer Conway
Designer: Norman W. Och
Illustration Planner: Bob Och
Production Coordinator: Charles E. Zeller
Cover Designer: Dan Pfisterer
Project Editor: Lynda Abrams

Copyright © 1990
Williams & Wilkins
428 East Preston Street
Baltimore, Maryland 21202, USA

Notice. The indications and dosages of all drugs in this book have been recommended in the medical literature and conform to the practices of the general medical community. The medications described do not necessarily have specific approval by the Food and Drug Administration for use in the diseases and dosages for which they are recommended. The package insert for each drug should be consulted for use and dosage as approved by the FDA. Because standards for usage change, it is advisable to keep abreast of revised recommendations, particularly those concerning new drugs.

Printed in the United States of America

Library of Congress Cataloging in Publication Data

Kaplan, Harold I., 1927–
    Pocket handbook of clinical psychiatry / Harold I. Kaplan, Benjamin J. Sadock.
      p.   cm.
    ISBN 0-683-04523-7
    1. Psychiatry—Handbooks, manuals, etc.   I. Sadock, Benjamin J.   II. Title.
    [DNLM: 1. Mental Disorders—handbooks.   WM 34 K17p]
RC456.K36   1990
616.89—dc20
DNLM/DLC
for Library of Congress   90-11962
                                                                                 CIP

                                                                    92   93   94
                                                      5   6   7   8   9   10

*Dedicated
to our wives,
Nancy Barrett Kaplan
and
Virginia Alcott Sadock
without whose help and sacrifice
this book would not have been possible*

Preface

The *Pocket Handbook of Clinical Psychiatry* has been written for the medical student, psychiatric resident, and practicing psychiatrist, who require a ready reference to diagnose and treat the full range of psychiatric disorders in adults and children. The nonpsychiatric physician who encounters and treats many patients with emotional disturbances also will find it useful.

With the aid of this compact guide, management of psychiatric illness can readily be commenced, aspects of both psychologic and pharmacologic treatments can be implemented, and dose ranges and available preparations of various psychotropic medications can easily be determined. All diagnoses conform to the criteria listed in the revised 3rd edition of the American Psychiatric Association's *Diagnostic and Statistical Manual of Mental Disorders* (DSM-III-R).

The *Pocket Handbook* is the digest companion to our much larger and more encyclopedic 5th edition of the *Comprehensive Textbook of Psychiatry*, for which we served as editors. The *Pocket Handbook* represents a distillation in that it provides brief summaries of psychiatric disorders, which include key aspects of their etiology, epidemiology, and treatment. Psychopharmacologic principles and prescribing methods are discussed briefly but thoroughly. Each chapter ends with references to the more detailed relevant sections in the 5th edition of the *Comprehensive Textbook of Psychiatry*. A unique aspect of this book are the colored illustrations of all the major psychotropic drugs, indicating both the forms in which they are commercially available and their dose ranges to help in conveniently recognizing and prescribing the medications.

The *Pocket Handbook* cannot substitute for a major textbook of psychiatry, such as Kaplan and Sadock's *Comprehensive Textbook of Psychiatry* or its companion, *Synopsis of Psychiatry*. It is meant instead to be used as an easily accessible reference by the busy doctor-in-training or clinical practitioner.

We wish to thank several persons who helped in the preparation of this book: Lynda Abrams, M.A., Educational Coordinator of the Department of Psychiatry at NYU Medical Center who was project editor; Judith Miller; Peter Kaplan, M.D., Philip Kaplan, M.D., James Sadock, and Victoria Sadock offered helpful suggestions.

We especially wish to thank our collaborators, each of whom contributed his or her share to the entire work. All are members of the psychiatric faculty at the NYU Medical Center, and it was a pleasure to work with them in this task. Finally, the authors wish to thank Robert Cancro, M.D., Professor and Chairman of the Department of Psychiatry at NYU Medical Center, who served as Senior Contributing Editor. The authors are deeply grateful for his unwavering support and for the inspiration and leadership he provides to the entire NYU Department of Psychiatry.

Harold I. Kaplan, M.D.
Benjamin J. Sadock, M.D.

July 1990
New York University Medical Center

In Collaboration With

James C.-Y. Chou, M.D.
Research Assistant Professor of Psychiatry, New York University School of Medicine, New York, New York

Rebecca M. Jones, M.D.
Research Assistant Professor of Psychiatry, New York University School of Medicine, New York, New York

Richard Perry, M.D.
Clinical Associate Professor of Psychiatry, New York University School of Medicine, New York, New York

Barry Reisberg, M.D.
Professor of Psychiatry, New York University School of Medicine, New York, New York

Virginia A. Sadock, M.D.
Clinical Professor of Psychiatry, New York University School of Medicine, New York, New York

Matthew B. Smith, M.D.
Clinical Instructor of Psychiatry, New York University School of Medicine, New York, New York

Norman Sussman, M.D.
Clinical Associate Professor of Psychiatry, New York University School of Medicine, New York, New York

Henry Weinstein, M.D.
Clinical Associate Professor of Psychiatry, New York University School of Medicine, New York, New York

Contents

1

Diagnosis and Classification in Psychiatry

I. General introduction

A mental disorder is an illness with psychologic or behavioral manifestations associated with impairment in functioning due to biologic, social, psychologic, genetic, physical, or chemical disturbance. Each illness has characteristic signs and symptoms.

Psychiatric disorders are classified according to the revised third edition of the American Psychiatric Association's *Diagnostic and Statistical Manual of Mental Disorders* (DSM-III-R). Over 200 types of illnesses are so classified. The official DSM-III-R chart and code numbers (which are used on insurance forms) are printed on front and back pages of this handbook.

The DSM-III-R diagnostic system attempts to be reliable (get same results with different observers) and valid (measure what it is supposed to, e.g., are diagnosed schizophrenics really schizophrenic?). DSM-III-R uses a descriptive approach, and the characteristic signs and symptoms of each disorder should be present before diagnosis is made.

In addition to the DSM-III-R classification, mental disorders are broadly described as psychotic, neurotic, functional, and organic.

1. Psychotic — loss of reality testing with delusions and hallucinations, e.g., schizophrenia.

2. Neurotic — no loss of reality testing; based on mainly intrapsychic conflicts that cause anxiety, e.g., phobic neurosis (phobic disorder).

3. Functional — no known structural damage or clear-cut etiologic factor to account for impairment, e.g., multiple personality disorder.

4. Organic — illness caused by a specific agent that causes structural change; usually associated with cognitive impairment, e.g., Pick's disease.

II. Classification of disorders

Eighteen major categories of mental disorders are listed in DSM-III-R; they are defined and classified below.

A. Disorders usually first evident in infancy, childhood, or adolescence

1. Mental retardation. Abnormal intellectual functioning; onset during developmental period; associated with impaired maturation, learning, and social maladjustment; classified as **mild (50–55 to 70), moderate (35–40 to 50–55), severe (20–25 to 35–40),** or **profound (below 20–25).**

2. Pervasive developmental disorders. Characterized by autistic, atypical withdrawn behavior, gross immaturity, inadequate development, and failure to develop separate identity from mother; classified into **autistic disorder** and a **not otherwise specified (NOS)** type.

3. Specific developmental disorders. Maturational deficits in development associated with difficulty in acquiring specific skills in one or more of the following areas: (1) academic—**arithmetic, expressive writing, reading**; (2) language and speech—**articulation, language (expressive and receptive)**; and (3) motor—**coordination**.

4. **Disruptive behavior disorders.** Characterized by inattention, overaggressiveness, delinquency, destructiveness, hostility, feelings of rejection, negativism, or impulsiveness. Patients usually have no consistent parental discipline or acceptance. Divided into **attention-deficit hyperactivity disorder** (poor attention span, impulsiveness), **conduct disorder** (delinquency), and **oppositional defiant disorder** (negativism).

5. **Anxiety disorders of childhood or adolescence.** Characterized by chronic anxiety, unrealistic fears, hypersensitive autonomic responses, or fear of leaving home. Patients are usually immature, inhibited, timid, approval-seeking, and apprehensive in new situations or places. Divided into **separation anxiety disorder, avoidant disorder of childhood or adolescence**, and **overanxious disorder**.

6. **Eating disorders.** Characterized by disturbed or bizarre feeding and eating habits that usually begin in childhood or adolescence and may last into adulthood. Divided into **anorexia nervosa** (starvation), **bulimia nervosa** (gorging and vomiting), **pica** (eating nonnutritional substances), and **rumination disorder of infancy** (regurgitation).

7. **Gender identity disorders.** Persons who are unsure of their gender or who believe they are a member of the opposite sex. Included here are **gender identity disorder of childhood, adolescence, or adulthood**, in which patients dress in clothes of the opposite sex in fantasy or reality, and **transsexualism**, in which the person wants the genitals of the opposite sex and may seek sex reassignment surgery.

8. **Tic disorders.** Characterized by sudden involuntary, recurrent, stereotyped motor movement or vocal sounds. Divided into **Tourette's disorder** (vocal tic and coprolalia), **chronic motor or vocal tic disorder**, and **transient tic disorder**.

9. **Elimination disorders.** Inability to maintain bowel control (**functional encopresis**) or bladder control (**functional enuresis**) as a result of physiologic or psychologic immaturity.

10. **Speech disorders not elsewhere classified.** Children who have problems of speech, e.g., rate, rhythm, intelligibility, resulting from faulty learning or neurologic impairment. Divided into **stuttering** (repetitive, prolonged sounds) and **cluttering** (dysrhythmic speech).

11. **Other disorders of infancy, childhood, or adolescence.** **Elective mutism** (voluntary refusal to speak); **identity disorder** (lack of social or vocational sense of self); **reactive attachment disorder of infancy or early childhood** (severe impairment of ability to relate, beginning before age 5); **stereotypy/habit disorder** (thumb sucking, nail biting, skin picking).

B. **Organic mental disorders (OMD).** Disorders characterized by changes in brain tissue function, resulting in impaired learning, orientation, judgment, and intellectual functions. **Primary degenerative dementia of the Alzheimer type, senile onset**—occurs in persons over age 65, is manifested by progressive intellectual disorientation and delirium, delusions, or depression;

presenile onset—age 65 or below; **multi-infarct dementia**—OMD is caused by vessel thrombosis/hemorrhage; **presenile** or **senile dementia NOS**—includes miscellaneous group, e.g., Pick's disease, Jakob-Creutzfeldt disease, is caused by slow-growing transmittable virus.

  1. Psychoactive substance-induced OMD. Subclass of OMD caused by psychoactive drugs, i.e., **alcohol; amphetamine or similarly acting sympathomimetic; caffeine; cannabis; cocaine; hallucinogen; inhalant; nicotine; opioid; phencyclidine (PCP) or similarly acting arylcyclohexylamine; or sedative, hypnotic, or anxiolytic.** Each may produce intoxication; withdrawal; delirium; dementia; amnesia; delusions; hallucinosis; or mood, anxiety, or personality disorder in addition to the OMD.

    a. **Alcohol-induced OMD** — subclass that includes **alcohol intoxication** (simple drunkenness), **idiosyncratic intoxication** (pathologic intoxication), **uncomplicated alcohol withdrawal, withdrawal delirium** (delirium tremens [DTs]), **alcohol hallucinosis** (differentiated from DTs by clear sensorium), **alcohol amnestic disorder** (Korsakoff's syndrome), and **alcohol dementia** (Wernicke's syndrome—ataxia, ophthalmoplegia, and confusion); severe cases may have combined Wernicke-Korsakoff syndrome.

  2. OMD associated with physical disorders or conditions. Includes syphilis, encephalitis, abscess, cardiovascular disease or trauma, epilepsy, intracranial neoplasm, endocrine disorders, pellegra, avitaminosis, systemic infection, e.g., typhoid, malaria, and degenerative central nervous system (CNS) diseases, e.g., multiple sclerosis. May produce delirium, dementia, amnesia, delusions, hallucinations, mood changes, anxiety, and personality disorders in addition to signs of OMD.

C. Psychoactive substance use disorders. Dependence on or abuse of any psychoactive drug (previously called drug addiction). Covers patients addicted to or dependent on such drugs as alcohol, nicotine (tobacco), or caffeine. Patient may be dependent on opium, opium alkaloids, and their derivatives; synthetic analgesics with morphine-like effects, such as PCP; barbiturates; other hypnotics, sedatives, or tranquilizers; cocaine; inhalants; *Cannabis sativa* (hashish and marijuana); other psychostimulants, such as amphetamines; and hallucinogens.

D. Schizophrenia. Covers disorders manifested by disturbances of thinking (alterations of concept formation that may lead to misinterpretation of reality and to delusions and hallucinations), affect (ambivalent, constricted, and inappropriate responsiveness and loss of empathy with others), and behavior (withdrawn, regressive, and bizarre). **Disorganized (hebephrenic) type**—disorganized thinking, giggling, shallow and inappropriate affect, silly and regressive behavior and mannerisms, frequent somatic complaints, and, occasionally, transient and unorganized delusions and hallucinations. **Catatonic type**—the excited subtype is characterized by excessive and sometimes violent motor activity; the withdrawn subtype is characterized by generalized inhibition, stupor, mutism, negativism, waxy flexibility, or, in some cases, a vegetative state. **Paranoid type**—schizophrenia characterized by persecutory or grandiose delusions and sometimes by hallucinations or excessive religiosity; the patient is often hostile and aggressive. **Undifferentiated type**—

disorganized behavior with prominent delusions and hallucinations. **Residual type**—patients with signs of schizophrenia, after a psychotic schizophrenic episode, who are no longer psychotic.

E. **Delusional (paranoid) disorder.** Psychotic disorder in which there are persistent delusions, e.g., **erotomanic, grandiose, jealous, persecutory, somatic,** and **unspecified.** Paranoia is a rare condition characterized by the gradual development of an elaborate delusional system with grandiose ideas; has chronic course; rest of personality remains intact.

F. **Psychotic disorders not elsewhere classified.** Brief reactive psychosis—psychotic disorder of less than 4 weeks' duration brought on by external stressor; **schizophreniform disorder**—similar to schizophrenia with delusions, hallucinations, and incoherence but lasts less than 6 months; **schizoaffective disorder**—covers patients with a mixture of schizophrenic symptoms and pronounced elation **(bipolar subtype)** or depression **(depressive subtype).** Induced psychotic disorder—same delusion occurs in two persons (shared paranoid disorder, *folie à deux*); **psychotic disorder NOS** (atypical psychosis)—psychotic features that are related to (1) a specific culture (koro—among Asians, fear of shrinking penis), (2) a certain time or event (postpartum psychosis—48–72 hours after childbirth), or (3) a unique symptomatology (Capgras' syndrome—patients think they have a double).

G. **Mood disorders.** Characterized by a single disorder of mood, i.e., extreme depression or elation that dominates the patient's mental life and is responsible for diminished function (previously called affective disorders).

Bipolar disorder. Marked by severe mood swings between depression and elation and by remission and recurrence; **cyclothymia**—less severe type of bipolar disorder. **Major depression**—severely depressed mood, mental and motor retardation, apprehension, uneasiness, perplexity, agitation, guilt feelings, suicidal ideation; usually recurrent. **Dysthymia**—less severe form of depression usually caused by identifiable event or loss (also called depressive neurosis). Researchers use terms bipolar I (full expression of mania) and bipolar II (hypomania with depression).

H. **Anxiety disorders (anxiety and phobic neuroses).** Characterized by massive anxiety **(generalized anxiety disorder)** often to the point of panic **(panic disorder)** and fears of going outside the home **(agoraphobia)**; fear of specific situations or objects **(simple phobia)** or of performance, public speaking **(social phobia)**; involuntary and persistent intrusions of thoughts, desires, urges, or actions **(obsessive-compulsive disorder)**; **post-traumatic stress disorder**—follows extraordinary life stress (war, catastrophe) and is characterized by anxiety, nightmares, agitation, and sometimes depression.

I. **Somatoform disorders.** Marked by preoccupation with the body and fears of disease. Classified into **somatization disorder**—multiple somatic complaints without organic pathology; **conversion disorder** (hysterical neurosis, conversion type)—disorder in which the special senses or voluntary nervous system is affected, causing blindness, deafness, anosmia, anesthesias, parasthesias, paralyses, ataxias, akinesias, or dyskinesias; patients often show inappropriate lack of concern and may derive some benefits from their actions. **Hypochondriasis** (hypochondriacal neurosis)—condition marked by preoccupation with the body and persistent fears of presumed disease; **somatoform pain disorder**—preoccupation with pain for at least 6 months without cause; **body dysmorphic disorder**—unrealistic concern that part of body is deformed.

J. **Dissociative disorders (hysterical neuroses, dissociative type).** Characterized by sudden, temporary change in consciousness or identity. **Psychogenic amnesia**—loss of memory without organic cause; **psychogenic fugue**—unexpected wandering from home; **multiple personality disorder**—person has two or more separate identities; **depersonalization disorder**—feeling that things are unreal.

K. **Sexual disorders.** Divided into paraphilias and sexual dysfunctions. Paraphilias cover persons whose sexual interests are primarily directed toward objects other than people, toward sexual acts not usually associated with coitus, or toward coitus performed under bizarre circumstances. Included are **exhibitionism, fetishism, frotteurism, pedophilia, sexual masochism, sexual sadism, transvestic fetishism** (cross-dressing), and **voyeurism**. Sexual dysfunctions cover disorders of **desire, arousal, orgasm,** and **sexual pain** in which the person is unable or unwilling to perform sex or to experience pleasure.

L. **Sleep disorders.** Cover (1) **dyssomnias** in which the person has sleep problems, cannot fall asleep (**insomnia**), sleeps too much (**hypersomnia**), or has a **sleep-wake schedule disorder**, and (2) **parasomnias,** such as **dream anxiety disorder (nightmares), sleepwalking**, or **sleep terror disorder** (person wakes up in immobilized state of terror).

M. **Factitious disorders.** Characterized by the intentional production or feigning of either psychologic or physical symptoms, or both, to assume sick role (also called Munchausen's syndrome).

N. **Impulse control disorders (not elsewhere classified).** Persons who cannot control impulses and who act out. Subtypes include **intermittent explosive disorder** (aggression), **kleptomania** (stealing), **pyromania** (fire setting), **trichotillomania** (hair pulling), and **pathological gambling**.

O. **Adjustment disorder.** Maladaptive reaction to a clearly defined life stress. Divided into subtypes depending on symptoms—**anxious mood, depressed mood, conduct disturbance, withdrawal, work or academic inhibition, physical complaints, mixed emotional features**, and **mixed disturbance of emotions and conduct**.

P. **Psychological factors affecting physical condition.** Disorders characterized by physical symptoms caused or affected by emotional factors; usually involve a single organ system with autonomic nervous system control or input. Examples include atopic dermatitis, backache, bronchial asthma, hypertension, migraine, ulcer, irritable colon, and colitis.

Q. **Personality disorders.** Disorders characterized by deeply ingrained, generally lifelong maladaptive patterns of behavior that are usually recognizable at adolescence or earlier.

   1. **Paranoid personality.** Characterized by unwarranted suspicion, hypersensitivity, jealousy, envy, rigidity, excessive self-importance, and a tendency to blame and ascribe evil motives to others.

   2. **Schizoid personality.** Characterized by shyness, oversensitivity, seclusiveness, avoidance of close or competitive relationships, eccentricity,

no loss of capacity to recognize reality, daydreaming, and an inability to express hostility and aggression.

3. **Schizotypal personality.** Similar to schizoid, but the person exhibits slight losses of reality testing, odd beliefs, illusions, and autistic thinking and is aloof and withdrawn.

4. **Obsessive-compulsive personality.** Characterized by excessive concern with conformity and standards of conscience; patient may be rigid, overconscientious, overdutiful, overinhibited, and unable to relax.

5. **Histrionic personality.** Characterized by emotional instability, excitability, overreactivity, vanity, immaturity, dependency, and self-dramatization that is attention-seeking and seductive.

6. **Avoidant personality.** Characterized by low energy, easy fatigability, lack of enthusiasm, inability to enjoy life, and oversensitivity to stress.

7. **Antisocial personality.** Covers unsocialized persons in conflict with society. Persons are incapable of loyalty; are selfish, callous, irresponsible, impulsive, and unable to feel guilt or learn from experience; have a low level of frustration tolerance; and have a tendency to blame others.

8. **Passive-aggressive personality.** Characterized by both passivity and aggressiveness, often expressed by obstructionism, pouting, procrastination, inefficiency, and stubbornness.

9. **Narcissistic personality.** Characterized by grandiose feelings, sense of entitlement, lack of empathy, envy, manipulativeness, and need for attention and admiration.

10. **Borderline personality.** Characterized by instability, impulsiveness, chaotic sexuality, suicidal acts, self-mutilation, identity problems, and feelings of emptiness/boredom.

11. **Dependent personality.** Characterized by passive and submissive behavior; person is unsure of himself/herself and becomes entirely dependent on others.

12. **Self-defeating personality.** Person is drawn to situations that produce personal suffering or failure.

13. **Sadistic personality.** Person uses physical or mental cruelty toward others.

R. **Conditions not attributable to a mental disorder.** Persons who have problems not severe enough to warrant a psychiatric diagnosis but that interfere with functioning. Classified into **antisocial behavior** (repeated criminal acts); **borderline intellectual functioning** (I.Q. 71–84); **malingering** (voluntary production of symptoms); **marital problems; noncompliance with medical treatment; occupational/academic/parent-child problems**; and **phase of life or other life circumstance problem** (parenthood, unemployment), and **uncomplicated bereavement**.

For more detailed discussion of this topic, see Akiskal HS: The Classification of Mental Disorders, Chap. 11, pp 583–598 in *CTP/V*.

2

Psychiatric Examination: History, Mental Status, and Clinical Signs and Symptoms

I. General introduction

Patient interviewing is the core skill in medicine and psychiatry, and communication between doctor and patient is the basis of good medical practice. Purpose of interview is to (1) obtain historical perspective of patient's life, (2) establish rapport and a therapeutic alliance, (3) develop mutual trust and confidence, (4) understand present functioning, (5) make a diagnosis, and (6) establish a treatment plan.

II. Clinical interview techniques

Arrange a comfortable setting with privacy.

Introduce yourself, greet patient by name, tell purpose of interview.

Put patient at ease, establish rapport by showing personal qualities of empathy and sensitivity.

Do not make value judgments.

Carefully observe patient's nonverbal behavior, posture, mannerisms, and physical appearance.

Avoid excessive note-taking.

Keep interview active. Do not argue or get angry.

Use language commensurate with patient's intelligence.

Length of interview: 15–90 minutes depending on patient's status (average time, 45–60 minutes); less time with delirious or uncooperative patients; more time with verbal, cooperative patients.

Open-ended questions for neurotic, verbal, high intelligence quotient (I.Q.) patients, e.g., "Tell me more about that." Structured and closed-ended questions used in limited-time interview, psychosis, delirium, dementia (closed-ended questions usually require yes or no answer). Avoid suggesting answers, e.g., "You feel depressed, don't you?" (Table 2-1). Special types of interviews are needed depending on the situation (Table 2-2).

The psychiatric examination consists of two parts: the history and the mental status. An outline of the psychiatric history and mental status follows. Sample questions and suggestions about the findings are given. To provide a systematic approach, all topics should eventually be covered, although the order should not be followed rigidly.

III. Psychiatric history

The psychiatric history is the chronologic story of the patient's life from birth to present (also called anamnesis).

Topics	Questions/Comments
Identifying data: Name, age, race, sex, marital status, religion, education, ad-	This may be recorded while writing up the interview.

dress, phone number, occupation, source of referral, and source of information if patient cannot cooperate.

Chief complaint (CC): Brief statement in *patient's own words* of why patient is in hospital or is being seen in consultation.

"Why are you coming to see a psychiatrist?" "What brought you to the hospital?" "What seems to be the problem?" Record answers verbatim.

History of present illness (HPI): Development of symptoms from time of onset to present; relationship of life events, conflicts, stressors; drugs; change from previous level of functioning.

Record in patient's own words as much as possible. Get history of previous hospitalizations and treatment.

Previous psychiatric/medical illness: Psychiatric disorders; psychosomatic, medical, neurologic illness (craniocerebral trauma, convulsions).

Ascertain extent of illness, treatment, medications, outcomes, hospitals, doctors. Evaluate if illness serves some additional purpose (secondary gain).

Past personal history:
  Birth and infancy

To the extent known by patient, ascertain mother's pregnancy and delivery, planned or unwanted pregnancy, developmental landmarks—standing, walking, talking, temperament.

  Childhood

Feeding habits, toilet training, personality (shy, outgoing), general conduct and behavior, relationship with parents or caregivers, peers. Separations, nightmares, bedwetting, fears.

  Adolescence

Peer and authority relationships, school history, grades, emotional problems, drug use, age of puberty.

  Adulthood

Work history, choice of career, marital history, children, education, finances, military history, religion.

Sexual history: Sexual development, masturbation, anorgasmia, impotence, premature ejaculation, paraphilia, sexual orientation, general attitudes and feelings.

"Are there or have there been any problems or concerns about your sex life?" "How did you learn about sex?"

Family history: Psychiatric/medical and genetic illness in mother, father, siblings; age of parents and occupations; if deceased, date and cause. Feelings about each family member, finances.

Get medication history of family (medications effective in family members for similar disorders may be effective in patient). ''Describe your living conditions.'' ''Did you have your own room?''

TABLE 2–1. **PROS AND CONS OF OPEN- AND CLOSED-ENDED QUESTIONS**[a]

Aspect	Broad, Open-Ended Questions	Narrow, Closed-Ended Questions
Genuineness	High They produce spontaneous formulations	Low They lead the patient
Reliability	Low They may lead to nonreproducible answers	High Narrow focus; but they may suggest answers
Precision	Low Intent of question is vague	High Intent of question is clear
Time efficiency	Low Circumstantial elaborations	High May invite yes/no answers
Completeness of diagnostic coverage	Low Patient selects the topic	High Interviewer selects the topic
Acceptance by patient	Varies Most patients prefer expressing themselves freely; others become guarded and feel insecure	Varies Some patients enjoy clear-cut checks; others hate to be pressed into a yes/no format

[a]Table from Othmer E, Othmer SC: *The Clinical Interview Using DSM-III-R*. American Psychiatric Press, Washington, DC, 1989, p 55, with permission.

TABLE 2–2. **SPECIAL TYPES OF INTERVIEWS**

Withdrawn patient	Be active, structure interview, Pay attention to nonverbal clues, body movements. Change subject if patient has difficulty discussing certain areas.
Family interview	Focus attention on identified patient's problem. Ask how each member reacts—angry, interested, frightened, anxious, who wants to help.
Depression	Elicit suicidal ideation if present; does patient have a plan? Try to raise self-esteem by commenting positively on accomplishments.
Aggressive patient	Do not be close in closed room. Sit near door for quick exit. Have security guard nearby or in room. Set limits. If patient seems too agitated, terminate interview immediately.
Psychosomatic patient	Do not discuss somatic symptoms as ''in your head.'' Assure patient that complaint is ''real.''
Delusional patient	Do not challenge delusions directly; you may tell patients that you do not agree with their thinking but that you understand their belief system.
Manic patient	Try to set limits. Tell patient you need specific information, e.g., who is in your family, and later you will talk about other areas. Be firm but not belligerent.
Amytal interview	10% sodium amytal intravenously at 1 mL/minute. After 150–500 mg, patient gets drowsy and is willing to answer queries. Used in catatonia, mutism, amnesia. Patient confusion is suggestive of organic condition. Benzodiazepines, e.g., diazepam (Valium), may also be used to induce narcosis.

IV. Mental status

The mental status is a cross-section of the patient's psychologic life and represents the sum total of the psychiatrist's observations and impressions *at the moment*. It also serves for future comparison to follow the progress of the patient.

Topics	Questions/Suggestions
General appearance: Note appearance, gait, dress, grooming (neat or unkempt), posture, gestures, facial expressions. Does patient appear older or younger than stated age?	Introduce yourself and direct patient to take a seat. In hospital, bring chair to bedside, do not sit on bed. Suggestions: Unkempt and disheveled in organic mental disorder (OMD); pinpoint pupils in narcotic addiction; withdrawal and stooped posture in depression.
Motoric behavior: Level of activity—psychomotor agitation or psychomotor retardation—tics, tremors, automatisms, mannerisms, grimacing, stereotypies, negativism, apraxia, echopraxia, waxy flexibility; emotional appearance—anxious, tense, panicky, bewildered, sad, unhappy; voice—faint, loud, hoarse; eye contact.	You may ask about obvious mannerisms, e.g., "I notice that your hand shakes; can you tell me about that?" Suggestions: Fixed posturing, odd behavior in schizophrenia. Hyperactive with stimulant (cocaine) abuse and in mania. Psychomotor retardation in depression; tremors with anxiety. Eye contact is normally made approximately half the time during the interview.
Attitude during interview: How patient relates to examiner—irritable, aggressive, seductive, guarded, defensive, indifferent, apathetic, cooperative, sarcastic.	Comment about attitude. "You seem irritated about something; is that an accurate observation?" Suggestions: Suspiciousness in paranoia; seductive in hysteria; apathetic in OMD.
Mood: Steady or sustained emotional state—gloomy, tense, hopeless, ecstatic, resentful, happy, bashful, sad, exultant, elated, euphoric, depressed, apathetic, anhedonic, fearful, suicidal, grandiose, nihilistic.	"How do you feel?" "How are your spirits?" "Do you have thoughts that life is not worth living or that you want to harm yourself?" "Do you have plans to take your own life?" "Do you want to die?" Suggestions: Suicidal ideas in 25% of depressives; elation in mania.
Affect: Feeling tone associated with idea—labile, blunt, appropriate to content, inappropriate, flat, *la belle indifférence*.	Observe nonverbal signs of emotion, body movement, facies, rhythm of voice (prosody). Suggestions: Changes in affect usual with schizophrenia; loss of prosody in OMD, catatonia.

Speech: Slow, fast, pressured, garrulous, spontaneous, taciturn, stammering, stuttering, slurring, staccato. Pitch, articulation, aphasia, coprolalia, echolalia, incoherent, logorrhea, mute, paucity, stilted.

Ask patient to say "Methodist Episcopalian" to test for dysarthria.
Suggestions: Manic patients show pressured speech; paucity of speech in depression; uneven or slurred speech in OMD.

Perceptual disorders: Hallucinations—olfactory, auditory, haptic (tactile), gustatory, visual; illusions; hypnopompic or hypnagogic experiences; feelings of unreality, *déjà vu*, *déjà entendu*, macroposia.

"Do you ever see things or hear voices?" "Do you have strange experiences as you fall asleep or upon awakening?" "Has the world changed in any way?"
Suggestions: Visual hallucinations suggest organicity. Auditory hallucinations suggest schizophrenia. Tactile hallucinations suggest OMD, cocainism, delirium tremens (DTs).

Thought content: Delusions—persecutory (paranoid), grandiose, infidelity, somatic, sensory, thought broadcasting, thought insertion, ideas of reference, ideas of unreality, phobias, obsessions, compulsions, ambivalence, autism, dereism, blocking, suicidal or homicidal preoccupation, conflicts, nihilistic ideas, hypochondriasis, depersonalization, derealization, flight of ideas, *idée fixe*, magical thinking, neologisms.

"Do you feel people want to harm you?" "Do you have special powers?" "Is anyone trying to influence you?" "Do you have strange body sensations?" "Are there thoughts that you can't get out of your mind?" "Do you think about the end of the world?" Ask about fantasies and dreams.
Suggestions: Are delusions congruent with mood (grandiose delusions with elated mood) or incongruent? Mood-incongruent delusions point to schizophrenia. Illusions are common in delirium.

Thought process: Goal-directed ideas, loosened associations, illogical, tangential, relevant, circumstantial, rambling, ability to abstract, flight of ideas, clang associations, perseveration.

Ask meaning of proverbs, to test abstraction, e.g., "People in glass houses should not throw stones." Concrete answer is, "Glass breaks." Abstract answers deal with projection, morality, criticism. Ask similarity between bird and butterfly (both alive), bread and cake (both food).
Suggestions: Loose associations point to schizophrenia; flight of ideas, to mania; inability to abstract, to schizophrenia, OMD.

Sensorium: Level of consciousness—alert, clear, confused, clouded, comatose, stuporous; orientation to time, place, person; cognition.

"What place is this?" "What is the date?" "Do you know who I am?" "Do you know who you are?"
Suggestions: OMD shows clouded or

wandering sensorium. Orientation to person remains intact longer than orientation to time or place.

Memory:
Remote memory (long-term memory)

"Where were you born?" "Where did you go to school?" "Date of marriage?" "Birthdays of children?" What were last week's newspaper headlines?"
Suggestions: Alzheimer's dementia patients retain remote memory longer than recent memory. Hypermnesia is seen in paranoid personality. Gap in memory may be localized or filled in with confabulatory details. Organic amnestic syndrome is associated with loss of both remote and recent memory.

Recent memory

"Where were you yesterday?" "What did you eat at your last meal?" In OMD, recent memory loss occurs before remote memory loss.

Immediate memory (short-term memory)

Ask patient to repeat six digits forward, then backward (normal response). Ask patient to try to remember three nonrelated items; test patient after 5 minutes.
Suggestions: Loss of memory occurs with organicity, dissociative disorder, conversion disorder. Anxiety can impair immediate retention and recent memory. Anterograde memory loss occurs after taking certain drugs, e.g., benzodiazepines; retrograde memory loss occurs after trauma.

Concentration and calculation: Ability to pay attention, distractibility, ability to do simple math.

Ask patient to count from 1 to 20 rapidly; do simple calculations (2×3, 4×9); do serial 7 test, i.e., subtract 7 from 100 and keep subtracting 7. "How many nickels in $1.35?"
Suggestions: Rule out OMD versus anxiety or depression (pseudodementia).

Information and intelligence: Use of vocabulary, level of education, fund of knowledge.

"Distance from New York City to Los Angeles." "Name some vegetables." "What is the largest river in the United States?"

Suggestions: Check educational level to judge results. Rule out mental retardation, borderline I.Q.

Judgment: Ability to understand relationship between facts and to draw conclusions; response in social situations.

"What is the thing to do if you find an envelope in the street that is sealed, stamped, and addressed?"
Suggestions: Impaired in OMD, schizophrenia, borderline I.Q., intoxication.

Insight level: Realizing that there is physical or mental problem; denial of illness, ascribing blame to outside factors; recognizing need for treatment.

"Do you think you have a problem?" "Do you need treatment?" "What are your plans for the future?"
Suggestions: Impaired in OMD, psychosis, borderline I.Q.

V. Medical and neurologic examination

Some psychiatric disorders may have an organic cause, e.g., depression secondary to meningioma. Neurologic and/or medical examination may be indicated in these situations. See Chapter 24 for laboratory tests used in psychiatry.

VI. How to record results of the history and the mental status

By end of examination, you must be able to judge (1) presence/absence of psychosis, (2) any organic defects, and (3) if patient is suicidal or homicidal in addition to diagnosis.

Record every case on an axis, which is a class of information. There are five axes in DSM-III-R. Assess and comment on each axis.

Axis I: Clinical syndromes

List the mental disorder here, e.g., schizophrenia, bipolar disorder. So-called V codes, which are conditions not attributable to a mental disorder that are a focus of attention or treatment, are also listed on Axis I. These problems are not sufficiently severe to warrant to a psychiatric diagnosis, e.g., marital problems.

Axis II: Developmental disorders and personality disorders

These disorders begin in childhood or adolescence and are listed here, e.g., attention-deficit hyperactivity disorder. A diagnosis on Axis I and Axis II can coexist. The Axis I or Axis II condition that is responsible for bringing the patient to the psychiatrist or hospital is called the principal or main diagnosis.

Axis III: Physical disorders or conditions

If the patient has a physical disorder, e.g., cirrhosis, list that here.

Axis IV: Severity of psychosocial stressor

Rate the severity of stress in the patient's life according to Table 2-3. Use the 12 months prior to the current evaluation as a reference. Use codes 1 (none) to 6 (catastrophic).

Axis V: Global assessment of functioning

Rate the highest level of functioning of the patient according to Table 2-4. Use the 12 months prior to the current evaluation as a reference point.

TABLE 2–3.   **DSM-III-R SEVERITY OF PSYCHOSOCIAL STRESSORS SCALE: ADULTS**

Code	Term	Examples of stressors	
		Acute events	**Enduring circumstances**
1	**None**	No acute events that may be relevant to the disorder	No enduring circumstances that may be relevant to the disorder
2	**Mild**	Broke up with boyfriend or girlfriend; started or graduated from school; child left home	Family arguments; job dissatisfaction; residence in high-crime neighborhood
3	**Moderate**	Marriage; marital separation; loss of job; retirement; miscarriage	Marital discord; serious financial problems; trouble with boss; being a single parent
4	**Severe**	Divorce; birth of first child	Unemployment; poverty
5	**Extreme**	Death of spouse; serious physical illness diagnosed; victim of rape	Serious chronic illness in self or child; ongoing physical or sexual abuse
6	**Catastrophic**	Death of child; suicide of spouse; devastating natural disaster	Captivity as hostage; concentration camp experience
0	**Inadequate information, or no change in condition**		

DSM-III-R SEVERITY OF PSYCHOSOCIAL STRESSORS SCALE: CHILDREN AND ADOLESCENTS

Code	Term	Examples of stressors	
		Acute events	**Enduring circumstances**
1	**None**	No acute events that may be relevant to the disorder	No enduring circumstances that may be relevant to the disorder
2	**Mild**	Broke up with boyfriend or girlfriend; change of school	Overcrowded living quarters; family arguments
3	**Moderate**	Expelled from school; birth of sibling	Chronic disabling illness in parent; chronic parental discord
4	**Severe**	Divorce of parents; unwanted pregnancy; arrest	Harsh or rejecting parents; chronic life-threatening illness in parent; multiple foster home placements
5	**Extreme**	Sexual or physical abuse; death of a parent	Recurrent sexual or physical abuse
6	**Catastrophic**	Death of both parents	Chronic life-threatening illness
0	**Inadequate information, or no change in condition**		

Used with permission, APA.

A sample DSM-III-R diagnosis could look like this:

Axis I	Schizophrenia, catatonic type
Axis II	Borderline personality disorder
Axis III	Hypertension
Axis IV	Psychosocial stressor: death of mother Severity: 5 (extreme)
Axis V	Current global assessment of functioning: 30 (behavior influenced by delusions)

TABLE 2–4. **DSM-III-R GLOBAL ASSESSMENT OF FUNCTIONING SCALE (GAF SCALE)**

Consider psychological, social, and occupational functioning on a hypothetical continuum of mental health-illness. Do not include impairment in functioning due to physical (or environmental) limitations.

Note: Use intermediate codes when appropriate, e.g., 45, 68, 72.

Code

90 | 81	**Absent or minimal symptoms** (e.g., mild anxiety before an exam), **good functioning in all areas, interested and involved in a wide range of activities, socially effective, generally satisfied with life, no more than everyday problems or concerns** (e.g., an occasional argument with family members).
80 | 71	**If symptoms are present, they are transient and expectable reactions to psychosocial stressors** (e.g., difficulty concentrating after family argument); **no more than slight impairment in social, occupational, or school functioning** (e.g., temporarily falling behind in school work).
70 | 61	**Some mild symptoms** (e.g., depressed mood and mild insomnia) **OR some difficulty in social, occupational, or school functioning** (e.g., occasional truancy, or theft within the household), **but generally functioning pretty well, has some meaningful interpersonal relationships.**
60 | 51	**Moderate symptoms** (e.g., flat affect and circumstantial speech, occasional panic attacks) **OR moderate difficulty in social, occupational, or school functioning** (e.g., few friends, conflicts with co-workers).
50 | 41	**Serious symptoms** (e.g., suicidal ideation, severe obsessional rituals, frequent shoplifting) **OR any serious impairment in social, occupational, or school functioning** (e.g., no friends, unable to keep a job).
40 | 31	**Some impairment in reality testing or communication** (e.g., speech is at times illogical, obscure, or irrelevant) **OR major impairment in several areas, such as work or school, family relations, judgment, thinking, or mood** (e.g., depressed man avoids friends, neglects family, and is unable to work; child frequently beats up younger children, is defiant at home, and is failing at school).
30 | 21	**Behavior is considerably influenced by delusions or hallucinations OR serious impairment in communication or judgment** (e.g., sometimes incoherent, acts grossly inappropriately, suicidal preoccupation) **OR inability to function in almost all areas** (e.g., stays in bed all day; no job, home, or friends).
20 | 11	**Some danger of hurting self or others** (e.g., suicide attempts without clear expectation of death, frequently violent, manic excitement) **OR occasionally fails to maintain minimal personal hygiene** (e.g., smears feces) **OR gross impairment in communication** (e.g., largely incoherent or mute).
10 | 1	**Persistent danger of severely hurting self or others** (e.g., recurrent violence) **OR persistent inability to maintain minimal personal hygiene OR serious suicidal act with clear expectation of death.**

Used with permission, APA.

After diagnosis, there are four other areas to be covered:

1. **Psychodynamic formulation**—the defense mechanism used to control anxiety, summary of psychologic factors, including precipitating events, that account for illness. See Table 2-5 for defense mechanisms.
2. **Differential diagnosis**—list other mental/physical disorders that have to be ruled out.
3. **Prognosis**—describe the course of the illness and expected outcome based on history, mental status, and good or bad prognostic factors.
4. **Treatment plan**—describe type of treatment, i.e., psychotherapy, drug therapy, behavior modification, hospitalization. Counseling by psychologist, social worker, vocational guidance. Assess patient's cooperativeness, reliability, judgment, insight, and intelligence and its impact on treatment.

VII. Definitions of signs and symptoms found in mental status examination

Abstraction. Ability to separate a quality from an object and to think or to perform symbolically, e.g., boat is concrete, sailing is abstract. Impaired in OMD, schizophrenia.

Affect. Subjective feeling tone that accompanies an idea or mental representation; objective behavioral component described as blunted (severely reduced), flat (absent), restricted (reduced), appropriate (harmonious), inappropriate (out of harmony), and labile (unstable). One of Bleuler's four A's, impaired in schizophrenia.

Aggression. Hostile or angry feelings, thoughts, or actions directed toward an object or person. Seen in impulse control disorders, explosive disorders, mania.

Agitation. Tension state in which anxiety is manifested in psychomotor area with hyperactivity and general perturbation. Seen in depression, schizophrenia, mania.

Ambivalence. Coexistence of opposing attitudes or emotions, e.g., love and hate, toward a given person or thing at the same time. One of Bleuler's four A's, seen in schizophrenia.

Amnesia. Loss of memory manifested by total or partial inability to recall past experiences. Seen in OMD, psychogenic fugue.

    Retrograde (RA). Loss of past/remote/long-term memory. Occurs in dementia.

    Anterograde (AA). Loss of immediate/short-term memory. Occurs after trauma, drug intake, transient ischemic attack.

    Localized. Loss of memory for an isolated event; not a total loss of memory; also referred to as **lacunar amnesia** and **patch amnesia**. Seen in brain lesions, anxiety, fugue.

Anhedonia. Absence of pleasure in acts that normally are pleasurable. Most common symptom in depression.

Anxiety. Feeling of dread, impending doom. Seen in anxiety disorders, schizophrenia.

Apathy. Lack of feeling, emotion, interest, or concern. Common in depression.

Aphasia. Impaired or absent communication by speech, writing, or signs, due to dysfunction of brain centers in the dominant hemisphere.

Apraxia. Disorder of voluntary movement, consisting of partial or complete incapacity to execute purposeful movements; motor and sensory systems intact.

Ataxia. Inability to coordinate muscles in the execution of voluntary movement. Seen in cerebellar lesions, tardive dyskinesia.

Autistic thinking. Form of subjective thinking with total disregard of reality. One of Bleuler's four A's, seen in schizophrenia.

Automatism. Activity is carried out without person's conscious knowledge.

Blocking. Sudden cessation in the train of thought or in the midst of a sentence; also known as **thought deprivation**. Common in schizophrenia.

Catalepsy. Inordinate maintenance of postures or physical attitudes; synonymous with **flexibilitas cerea** or **waxy flexibility**. Seen in catatonic type of schizophrenia.

Cataplexy. Temporary paralysis or immobilization and collapse caused by strong emotions. Part of narcolepsy.

Catatonia. Type of schizophrenia characterized by periods of physical rigidity, negativism, excitement, and stupor.

    Catatonic excitement. Marked agitation, impulsivity, and aggressive behavior.

    Catatonic rigidity. Rigid posturing and stereotypic behavior.

Circumstantiality. Thought and speech associated with unnecessary detail, is usually relevant to a question, and an answer is ultimately given. Seen in schizophrenia, obsessive-compulsive disorder.

Clang association. Association, i.e., relationship, based on similarity of sound, without regard for differences in meaning. Common in mania.

Clouding of consciousness. Impairment of orientation, perception, and attention. Seen in OMD.

Cognition. Quality of knowing, including perceiving, recognizing, judging, sensing, reasoning, and imagining. Impaired in OMD, mental retardation.

Coma. Profoundest degree of stupor in which all consciousness is lost; no voluntary activity of any kind. Has organic basis.

Compulsion. Irresistible impulse to perform an irrational act. Seen in impulse control and obsessive-compulsive disorders.

Concrete thinking. Inability to form the whole from its parts; inability to abstract. Seen in schizophrenia.

Confabulation. Fabrication of stories in response to questions about situations or events that are not recalled.

Conflict. Mental struggle that arises from simultaneous operation of opposing impulses, drives, or external (environmental) or internal demands. Termed intrapsychic when conflict is between forces within the personality; termed extrapsychic when it is between the self and the environment.

Confusional state. Disturbed orientation in respect to time, place, or person.

Consciousness. Awareness of one's own internal thoughts and feelings and ability to recognize external environment. Impaired in OMD, fugue, dissociative states.

Coprolalia. Involuntary utterance of vulgar or obscene words. Seen in Tourette's disorder.

Déjà entendu. Feeling that one is hearing or perceiving what one has heard before. Seen in anxiety disorders, fatigue.

Déjà vu. Feeling that one is seeing or experiencing what one has seen before. Seen in anxiety disorders, fatigue.

Delusion. False belief, i.e., not shared by others, that is firmly maintained, even though contradicted by social reality. Most common in schizophrenia.

> **Grandiose delusion.** Belief that one is possessed of greatness, **megalomania**; such ideas are referred to as **delusions of grandeur**. Seen in schizophrenia, mania, tertiary syphilis.

> **Infidelity delusion.** False belief that a loved one is unfaithful. A variation is that a person of high social status is deeply in love with the individual. Occurs more often in women; is called **erotomania, Clérembault's syndrome, delusional loving, amorous paranoia**.

> **Somatic delusion.** Belief that patient's body or parts of the body are diseased or distorted.

> **Persecutory (paranoid) delusion.** Excessive or irrational suspiciousness and distrustfulness of others, characterized by systematized delusions of persecution. Seen in paranoid schizophrenia.

Depersonalization. Patients feel that they have lost their personal identity and are different, strange, or unreal. Part of dissociative disorder.

Depression. Feeling tone characterized by sadness, apathy, pessimism, and a sense of loneliness. Part of bipolar disorder, major depression.

Derealization. Feeling of changed reality; environment is strange or unreal. Common in anxiety and dissociative disorders.

Dereism. Mental activity not in accordance with reality, logic, or experience.

Disorientation. Loss of awareness of position of self in relation to space, time, or other persons; confusion.

Distractibility. Patient changes from topic to topic in accordance with stimuli from within and from without. Seen in mania.

Dysarthria. Difficulty in speech production due to incoordination of speech apparatus.

Dyskinesia. Any disturbance of movement.

Echolalia. Imitative repetition of speech of another. Seen in schizophrenia.

Echopraxia. Imitative repetition of movements of another. Sometimes seen in catatonic schizophrenia.

Ecstasy. State of elation beyond reason and control; trance state of overwhelming emotion, e.g., religious fervor.

Elation. Affect consisting of feelings of euphoria, triumph, intense self-satisfaction, or optimism.

Euphoria. Exaggerated feeling of physical/emotional well-being, usually of psychologic origin. Seen in OMDs and in toxic and drug-induced states.

Exaltation. Excessively intensified sense of well-being. Seen in mania.

Fear. Unpleasant emotional and physiologic response to recognized sources of danger, to be distinguished from anxiety.

Flight of ideas. Rapid shifting from one topic to another; also called **topical flight**; themes can sometimes be followed. Part of manic episode.

Grandiosity. Feelings of great importance; absurd exaggeration. Seen in mania, schizophrenia.

Hallucination. Sensory perception for which there is no external stimulus. Seen in schizophrenia, toxic psychoses.

   Auditory hallucination. Associated with sound. Most common in schizophrenia.

   Gustatory hallucination. Associated with taste.

   Haptic hallucination. Associated with sensation of touch. Common in DTs, cocainism.

   Hypnagogic hallucination. Hallucination occurring during state between wakefulness and sleep, i.e., just before falling asleep. Normal mental phenomenon.

   Hypnopompic hallucination. Occurs upon awakening.

   Induced hallucination. Hallucination aroused in one person by another; also called **folie à deux.**

   Lilliputian hallucination. Hallucinated object appears reduced in size; also called microptic hallucination. Seen in toxic psychoses.

   Visual hallucination. Associated with sight.

Hypermnesia. Exaggerated memory; ability to recall material not ordinarily available to memory process.

Hypochondriasis. Somatic overconcern with and morbid attention to details of body functioning; exaggeration of any symptom. Part of hypochondriacal neurosis.

Ideas of reference. Incorrect interpretation of casual incidents and external events as directly referring to oneself. May reach sufficient intensity to constitute delusions.

Ideas of unreality. Thoughts that events are artificial, illusory, unpredictable, or do not exist. Seen in schizophrenia, anxiety disorders, dissociative disorders.

Ideé fixe. Fixed idea; describes a compulsive drive, an obsessive idea, or a delusion.

Illusion. Erroneous perception; false response to a sensory stimulus. Seen in schizophrenia, toxic psychoses.

Incoherence. Quality or state of being loose; lacking cohesion.

Insight. Knowledge of objective reality of a situation; person is aware of a mental problem.

Intelligence quotient (I.Q.). Numerical rating determined through psychological testing that indicates approximate relationship of a person's mental age (MA) to chronologic age (CA). Expressed mathematically as $I.Q. = \dfrac{MA}{CA} \times 100$.

Intoxication. OMD due to recent ingestion or presence in the body of a chemical agent, causing maladaptive behavior because of its effects on the central nervous system.

Judgment. Ability to recognize true relation of ideas; capacity to draw correct conclusions from experience. Impaired in schizophrenia, OMD.

La belle indifférence. Literally, "beautiful indifference." Seen in certain patients with conversion disorders who show an inappropriate lack of concern about their disabilities.

Logorrhea. Uncontrollable, excessive talking. Seen in mania, schizophrenia.

Loosening of associations. Various disturbances of associations that render speech (and thought) inexact, vague, diffuse, unfocused. One of Bleuler's four A's. Seen in schizophrenia.

Macropsia. False perception that objects are larger than they really are. Seen in drug intoxication states.

Magical thinking. Conviction that thinking equates with doing. Characterized by lack of realistic relationship between cause and effect. Occurs in dreams, children, primitive peoples, and patients under a variety of conditions. Seen in obsessive-compulsive disorder.

Mannerism. Gesture or other form of expression peculiar to a given person. Seen in schizophrenia.

Memory. Ability, process, or act of remembering or recalling; ability to reproduce what has been learned or experienced.

> **Recent memory.** Refers to events over past few days.
> **Remote memory.** Refers to events in distant past; also called long-term memory.
> **Immediate (short-term) memory.** Refers to immediate retention, i.e., events of the past few moments. Also known as working or buffer memory.

Mood. Feeling tone, particularly as experienced internally by the person.

> **Mood-congruent.** In harmony; mood-appropriate; ideas consistent with mood. Common in bipolar disorder.
> **Mood-incongruent.** Mood-inappropriate; ideas out of harmony with mood. Common in schizophrenia.

Mutism. Inability to speak. Common in catatonic schizophrenia, fugue states.

Negativism. Opposition or resistance, either covert or overt, to outside suggestions or advice. May be seen in schizophrenia.

Neologism. New word created by the patient, which is often a blend of other words. Seen in schizophrenia.

Nihilism. Feelings of nonexistence and hopelessness. Common in depression. May assume delusional proportions.

Obsession. Idea, emotion, or impulse that repetitively and insistently forces itself into consciousness, although it is unwelcome. Part of obsessive-compulsive disorder.

Orientation. Awareness of one's self in relation to time, place, and person. Lost in OMD.

Panic. Sudden, overwhelming anxiety of such intensity that it produces terror and physiologic changes.

Paucity of speech. Limited use of speech. Seen in autistic disorder, catatonic schizophrenia, major depression.

Perseveration. Involuntary, excessive continuation or recurrence of a response or activity, most often verbal. Seen in schizophrenia, e.g., perseverative speech.

Phobia. A morbid fear associated with extreme anxiety. Part of phobic disorder.

Psychomotor retardation. Slowed psychic activity, motor activity, or both. Seen in depression, catatonic schizophrenia. Opposite can also occur, i.e., psychomotor agitation.

Stereotypy. Constant, almost mechanical, repetition of any action. Common in schizophrenia.

Stilted speech. Formal, stiff speech pattern.

Stupor. State in which a person does not react to or is unaware of the surroundings. Due to neurologic or psychiatric disorders. In catatonic stupor, the unawareness is more apparent than real.

Thought broadcasting. Delusion about thoughts being aired to the outside world. Seen in schizophrenia. One of Schneider's first rank symptoms.

Thought disorder. Disturbance of speech, communication, or content of thought, e.g., delusions, ideas of reference, poverty of thought, flight of ideas, perseveration, loosening of associations. Can be caused by a functional emotional disorder or an organic condition. Characteristic of schizophrenia.

Thought insertion. Delusion that thoughts are placed into the mind by outside influences. One of Schneider's first rank symptoms, seen in schizophrenia.

Tic. Sudden involuntary muscle movement. Seen in tic disorders.

Verbigeration. Stereotyped and seemingly meaningless repetition of words or sentences.

Word salad. Mixture of words and phrases that lack comprehensive meaning or logical coherence. Commonly seen in schizophrenic states.

TABLE 2–5. **DEFENSE MECHANISMS.**

Unconscious intrapsychic processes that provide relief from emotional conflict and anxiety. Conscious efforts are frequently made for the same reasons, but true defense mechanisms are unconscious.

Compensation—an attempt to make up for real or imagined inadequacies and deficiencies by overdeveloping other areas.

Conscious control—the awareness of how one's mental functioning affects one's behavior and the ability to use this knowledge accordingly.

Conversion—intrapsychic conflicts that would otherwise give rise to anxiety are, instead, given symbolic external expression. The repressed ideas or impulses, and the psychological defenses against them, are converted into a variety of somatic symptoms involving the nervous system, e.g., paralysis, pain, or loss of sensory function.

Denial—the resolution of emotional conflict and anxiety by disavowing external reality factors that are intolerable (a disregard for a disturbing reality). Common in narcissistic personality.

Displacement—emotions, ideas, or wishes are transferred from their original object, person, or situation to a more acceptable substitute. Common in phobias.

Dissociation—the splitting off of clusters of mental contents from conscious awareness. A defense mechanism central to hysterical conversion and dissociative disorders.

Identification—an individual patterns himself/herself after some other person that he/she admires.

Introjection—loved, hated, or feared external objects are symbolically absorbed within oneself; the converse of projection.

Isolation—the affect attached to an idea is rendered unconscious, leaving the conscious idea emotionally neutral; central to obsessive-compulsive disorder.

Projection—what is emotionally unacceptable in oneself is unconsciously rejected and attributed to others, i.e., one's wishes, desires, and fears are displaced onto another person. Seen in delusional disorders.

Rationalization—an individual attempts to justify feelings, motives, or behavior that otherwise would be unreasonable, illogical, or intolerable.

Reaction formation—an individual adopts the attitudes, behaviors, ideas, and affects that are the opposite of the ones he/she harbors, e.g., excessive moral zeal may be a reaction to strong but repressed asocial impulses.

Regression—partial or symbolic return to more infantile patterns of reacting or thinking.

Repression—banishing from consciousness internal reality factors, e.g., impulses, desires, or affects, that are unacceptable. Although not subject to voluntary recall, repressed material may emerge in disguised form.

Resistance—the opposition displayed toward bringing repressed (or unconscious) material into awareness.

Sublimation—process by which an unacceptable drive or behavior is diverted into a more personally and socially acceptable form of behavior.

Symbolization—process by which some mental representation or object comes to stand for some other representation or object. This mechanism underlies dream formation and such symptoms as conversion reactions, obsessions, and compulsions.

Undoing (or restitution)—something that is unacceptable and already done is symbolically acted out in reverse, e.g., by restitutive gifts or making up, in order to relieve anxiety or guilt. Seen in obsessive-compulsive disorder.

For more detailed discussion of this topic, see Leon RL, Bowden CL, Faber RA: The Psychiatric Interview, History, and Mental Status Examination, Sec. 9.1, pp 449–462; Kaplan HI, Sadock BJ: Psychiatric Report, Sec. 9.2, pp 462–467; Kaplan HI, Sadock BJ: Typical Signs and Symptoms of Psychiatric Illness, Sec. 9.3, pp 468–475; Yager J: Clinical Manifestations of Psychiatric Disorders, Chap. 10, pp 555–558, in *CTP/V*.

3

Organic Mental Syndromes and Disorders

I. General introduction

A. Definition. **Organic** implies brain dysfunction. **Syndrome** is a constellation of signs and symptoms. **Disorder** implies a presumed or known etiology (although DSM-III-R often uses "disorder" instead of "syndrome" when a specific etiology seems probable).

All of these diagnoses require a psychologic or behavioral abnormality associated with transient or permanent brain dysfunction. Often, there is a fine line between functional and organic disease.

B. General approach to the organic patient. Usually, chronic organic mental syndromes are more subtle and slowly progressive in their clinical presentations than are acute organic mental syndromes. Although the etiologic factors are often self-apparent in acute syndromes, this is usually not the case in chronic syndromes.

1. Nonspecific signs of chronic organicity

a. Intellectual, memory, and cognitive impairment (shallow thoughts, lack of intellectual flexibility, perseveration, poor judgment).

b. Change in personality.

c. Disinhibition (inappropriateness or exacerbation of underlying personality traits).

d. Poverty of speech with decreased vocabulary and use of cliches.

e. Prominent visual hallucinations.

f. Affect initially may be depressed, anxious, and labile, but it may progress to be shallow, apathetic, and empty.

C. Clinical evaluation

1. History. May be time-consuming and require information from others. Need information about premorbid condition.

2. Physical. Emphasize neurologic, but do not overlook other systems.

3. Mental status. Carefully evaluate cognition but not to the point of missing other information, especially appearance and general behavior, mood/affect, and thought content and process.

4. Cognitive evaluation. Screening tests by psychiatrists are nonspecific but sensitive to a wide range of impairments (orientation, attention and concentration, memory, general information, intelligence). Develop a routine. Suspicious findings usually warrant an extensive cognitive evaluation.

5. Lab tests

a. **Psychometric assessment** (psychological testing)—more sensitive to organicity; standardized; can utilize probabilities in interpretation; requires patient cooperation. Psychologist needs to be guided about where to focus.

b. Skull x-ray, electroencephalogram (EEG), computed tomography (CT), magnetic resonance imaging (MRI), lumbar puncture, brain scan, and angiography, as indicated.

D. Six general DSM-III-R categories of organic conditions

1. Delirium and dementia—global impairment.
2. Amnestic syndrome and organic hallucinosis—selective areas of impaired cognition.
3. Organic delusional, mood, and anxiety syndromes—similar to functional disorders, but they imply a probable organic etiology.
4. Organic personality syndrome.
5. Intoxication and withdrawal—defined by etiology, but not enough to meet criteria for one of the other syndromes.
6. Organic mental syndrome not otherwise specified (NOS)—residual category.

II. Delirium

A. Definition. An acute organic mental syndrome in which the cognitive impairment is relatively global. Delirium is often reversible, and the course is usually brief.

B. Diagnosis, signs and symptoms

TABLE 3–1.   **DSM-III-R DIAGNOSTIC CRITERIA FOR DELIRIUM**

A. Reduced ability to maintain attention to external stimuli (e.g., questions must be repeated because attention wanders) and to appropriately shift attention to new external stimuli (e.g., perseverates answer to a previous question).

B. Disorganized thinking, as indicated by rambling, irrelevant, or incoherent speech.

C. At least two of the following:

(1) reduced level of consciousness, e.g., difficulty keeping awake during examination
(2) perceptual disturbances: misinterpretations, illusions, or hallucinations
(3) disturbance of sleep-wake cycle with insomnia or daytime sleepiness
(4) increased or decreased psychomotor activity
(5) disorientation to time, place, or person
(6) memory impairment, e.g., inability to learn new material, such as the names of several unrelated objects after 5 minutes, or to remember past events, such as history of current episode of illness

D. Clinical features develop over a short period of time (usually hours to days) and tend to fluctuate over the course of a day.

E. Either (1) or (2):

(1) evidence from the history, physical examination, or laboratory tests of a specific organic factor (or factors) judged to be etiologically related to the disturbance
(2) in the absence of such evidence, an etiologic organic factor can be presumed if the disturbance cannot be accounted for by any nonorganic mental disorder, e.g., manic episode accounting for agitation and sleep disturbance

Used with permission, APA.

C. Epidemiology. Common among hospitalized patients—about 10% in all hospitalized patients, 20% in postburn patients, 30% in intensive care unit (ICU) patients. Very young and elderly more susceptible to delirium. Patients with a previous history of delirium are more likely to have another episode of delirium. Brain-damaged patients also more susceptible.

D. Etiology. There are multiple etiologies, including infection, fever, metabolic imbalance, hepatic or renal disease, endocrine dysfunctions, thiamine deficiency, psychoactive substance intoxication or withdrawal, postoperative states, severe blood loss, cardiac arrhythmias or heart failure, hypertensive encephalopathy, following head trauma, following seizures, side effects of many medications, certain focal brain lesions (right parietal lobe and medial surface of occipital lobe), and sensory deprivation, e.g., blind or deaf patients. Delirium may be thought of as a common pathway for any brain insult.

E. **Lab tests.**   Delirium is a medical emergency that demands identification of the cause as rapidly as possible. If the likely cause is not apparent, then a complete medical workup should be immediate. Even if an apparent cause is identified, there may be multiple causes. The workup should include vital signs, complete blood count (CBC) with differential, erythrocyte sedimentation rate (ESR), complete blood chemistries, liver and renal function tests, urinalysis, urine toxicology, electrocardiogram (EKG), chest x-ray, CT scan of head, and lumbar puncture (if indicated). EEG often shows diffuse slowing throughout.

F. **Differential diagnosis**
   1. Dementia.

TABLE 3–2.   **CLINICAL DIFFERENTIATION OF DELIRIUM AND DEMENTIA**

	Delirium	Dementia
History	Acute disease	Chronic disease
Onset	Rapid	Insidious (usually)
Duration	Days - weeks	Months - years
Course	Fluctuating	Chronically progressive
Level of consciousness	Fluctuating	Normal
Orientation	Impaired, at least periodically	Intact initially
Affect	Anxious, irritable	Labile but not usually anxious
Thinking	Often disordered	Decreased amount
Memory	Recent memory is markedly impaired	Both recent and remote are impaired
Perception	Hallucinations common (especially visual)	Hallucinations less common (except sundowning)
Psychomotor	Retarded, agitated, or mixed	Normal
Sleep	Disrupted sleep/wake cycle	Less disruption of sleep/wake cycle
Attention and awareness	Prominently impaired	Less impaired
Reversibility	Often reversible	Majority not reversible

Note: Demented patients are more susceptible to delirium, and delirium superimposed on dementia is common.

   2. Schizophrenia and mania.   Usually do not have the rapidly fluctuating course of delirium, nor do they show impaired level of consciousness or prominently impaired cognition.

3. **Dissociative disorders.** May show spotty amnesia but lack the global cognitive impairment and abnormal psychomotor and sleep patterns of delirium.
G. **Course and prognosis.** The course is usually rapid. In some cases, the delirium may spontaneously clear. Delirium may also rapidly progress to death or permanent dementia, if untreated. If the underlying cause is treated, there may be a rapid recovery. Some residual deficits, however, may persist.
H. **Treatment.** Identify the cause and reverse it. Correct metabolic abnormalities; ensure proper hydration, electrolyte balances, and nutrition; optimize the sensory environment for the patient, e.g., decreased stimuli for a delirium tremens patient and appropriate increased stimulation for a patient delirious from sensory deprivation. Low doses of a high potency antipsychotic may be used for agitation, e.g., haloperidol (Haldol) 2–5 mg orally or intramuscularly every 4 hours as needed. Benzodiazepines, e.g., lorazepam (Ativan) 1–2 mg orally or intramuscularly every 4 hours as needed, can also be used for agitation or insomnia, especially in a patient who may be at risk for seizures, e.g., alcohol withdrawal or withdrawal from sedative/hypnotics.

III. Dementia

A global impairment of intellect without impaired consciousness. These patients have an enormous socioeconomic impact on the health care system because they require such great amounts of care. Also, as the population ages, the number of demented persons increases geometrically.
A. **Definition.** A loss of cognitive and intellectual functions sufficiently severe to interfere with social or occupational functioning. The essential deficit is a loss of memory, both short- and long-term. Abstract thinking and judgment are also frequently impaired, and there are often other signs of higher cortical involvement. With time, there can be a marked change in personality.
B. **Diagnosis, signs and symptoms.** See Table 3-3.
C. **Epidemiology.** Primarily a syndrome of the elderly, although it may be diagnosed at any age after which the intelligence quotient (I.Q.) is stabilized (3–4 years of age). May be as common as 5% in persons over age 65 and 20% in persons over age 80. Increasing age is the most important risk factor. One-fourth of demented patients have some treatable illness. One-tenth of all dementias are reversible.
D. **Etiology.** Most common cause is Alzheimer's disease followed by multi-infarct dementia (MID) (mixed forms are also common). Acquired immune deficiency syndrome (AIDS) is also a common cause. See Table 3-4 for other causes of dementia.
E. **Lab tests.** The first priority—identify a potentially reversible cause for the dementia. The next priority—identify other treatable medical conditions that may otherwise worsen the dementia (cognitive decline is often precipitated by other medical illness). The workup should include vital signs, CBC with differential, ESR, complete blood chemistries, serum B_{12} and folate levels, liver and renal function tests, thyroid function tests, urinalysis, urine toxicology, EKG, chest x-ray, CT scan or MRI of head, and lumbar puncture.

TABLE 3–3.   **DSM-III-R DIAGNOSTIC CRITERIA FOR DEMENTIA**

A. Demonstrable evidence of impairment in short- and long-term memory. Impairment in short-term memory (inability to learn new information) may be indicated by inability to remember three objects after 5 minutes. Long-term memory impairment (inability to remember information that was known in the past) may be indicated by inability to remember past personal information (e.g., what happened yesterday, birthplace, occupation) or facts of common knowledge (e.g., past Presidents, well-known dates).

B. At least one of the following:
  (1) impairment in abstract thinking, as indicated by inability to find similarities and differences between related words, difficulty in defining words and concepts, and other similar tasks
  (2) impaired judgment, as indicated by inability to make reasonable plans to deal with interpersonal, family, and job-related problems and issues
  (3) other disturbances of higher cortical function, such as aphasia (disorder of language), apraxia (inability to carry out motor activities despite intact comprehension and motor function), agnosia (failure to recognize or identify objects despite intact sensory function), and "constructional difficulty" (e.g., inability to copy three-dimensional figures, assemble blocks, or arrange sticks in specific designs)
  (4) personality change, i.e., alteration or accentuation of premorbid traits

C. The disturbance in A and B significantly interferes with work or usual social activities or relationships with others.

D. Not occurring exclusively during the course of delirium.

E. Either (1) or (2):
  (1) there is evidence from the history, physical examination, or laboratory tests of a specific organic factor (or factors) judged to be etiologically related to the disturbance
  (2) in the absence of such evidence, an etiologic organic factor can be presumed if the disturbance cannot be accounted for by any nonorganic mental disorder, e.g., major depression accounting for cognitive impairment

Used with permission, APA.

F. Differential diagnosis

1. Normal aging. Associated with a decreased ability to learn new material and a slowing of thought processes. In addition, there is a syndrome of benign senescent forgetfulness, which does not show a progressively deteriorating course. However, neither of these includes an impairment in social or occupational functioning, which is part of the definition of dementia.

2. Depression in the elderly may present as symptoms of cognitive impairment, which has led to the term "pseudodementia." The apparently demented patient is really depressed and responds well to antidepressants or electroconvulsive therapy (ECT). Many demented patients also become depressed as they begin to comprehend their progressive cognitive impairment. Often, in patients with both dementia and depression, a treatment trial with antidepressants or ECT is warranted. Table 3-5 differentiates dementia from depression.

3. Delirium is also characterized by global cognitive impairment, and demented patients can often have a superimposed delirium. The course of dementia usually tends to be more chronic and lacks the prominent features of rapid fluctuations, acute onset, impaired attention, changing level of consciousness, psychomotor disturbances, acutely disturbed sleep-wake cycle, and prominent hallucinations or delusions that characterize delirium.

TABLE 3–4.   **DISEASES THAT CAUSE DEMENTIA**[a]

Parenchymatous diseases of the central nervous system
    Alzheimer's disease (primary degenerative dementia)
    Pick's disease (primary degenerative dementia)
    Huntington's disease
    Parkinson's disease[b]
    Multiple sclerosis
Systemic disorders
    Endocrine and metabolic disorders
        Thyroid disease[b]
        Parathyroid disease[b]
        Pituitary-adrenal disorders[b]
        Posthypoglycemic states
    Liver disease
        Chronic progressive hepatic encephalopathy[b]
    Urinary tract disease
        Chronic uremic encephalopathy[b]
        Progressive uremic encephalopathy (dialysis dementia)[b]
    Cardiovascular disease
        Cerebral hypoxia or anoxia[b]
        Multi-infarct dementia[b]
        Cardiac arrhythmias[b]
        Inflammatory diseases of blood vessels[b]
    Pulmonary disease
        Respiratory encephalopathy[b]
Deficiency states
    Cyanocobalamin deficiency[b]
    Folic acid deficiency[b]
Drugs and toxins[b]
Intracranial tumors[b] and brain trauma[b]
Infectious processes
    Creutzfeldt-Jakob disease[b]
    Cryptococcal meningitis[b]
    Neurosyphilis[b]
    Tuberculosis and fungal meningitis[b]
        Viral encephalitis
        Human immunodeficiency virus (HIV)-related disorders
            (e.g., AIDS and AIDS-related complex [ARC])
Miscellaneous disorders
    Hepatolenticular degeneration[b]
    Hydrocephalic dementia[b]
    Sarcoidosis[b]
    Normal pressure hydrocephalus[b]

[a]Adapted from Wells CE: Organic syndromes: dementia. In *Comprehensive Textbook of Psychiatry*, ed 4, HI Kaplan and BJ Sadock, eds, Williams & Wilkins, Baltimore, 1985, p. 855.
[b]Conditions calling for specific therapeutic intervention.

G. Course and prognosis.   Because about 10% of dementias are reversible, e.g., hypothyroidism, central nervous system (CNS) syphilis, subdural hematoma, B_{12} deficiency, uremia, and hypoxia, the course in these cases depends on the speed with which the cause is reversed. If the cause is reversed too late, there may be residual deficits with a subsequently stable course if there has not been extensive brain damage.

    For the cases in which there is no identifiable cause, such as primary degenerative dementia of the Alzheimer type, the course is likely to be a slowly progressively deteriorating one. The patient may become lost in familiar places, later be unable to handle money, even later fail to recognize family members, and eventually become incontinent of stool and urine.

TABLE 3-5. DEMENTIA VERSUS DEPRESSION

Feature	Organic Dementia	Pseudodementia
Age	Usually elderly	Nonspecific
Onset	Vague	Days to weeks
Course	Slow, worse at night	Rapid, even through day
History	Systemic illness or drugs	Mood disorder
Awareness	Unaware, unconcerned	Aware, distressed
Organic signs	Often present	Absent
Cognition[a]	Prominent impairment	Personality changes
Mental status		Variable deficits in different
examination	Consistent, spotty deficits	modalities
	Approximates, confabulates, perseverates	Apathetic, "I don't know"
	Emphasizes trivial accomplishments	Emphasizes failures
	Shallow or labile mood	Depressed
Behavior	Appropriate to degree of cognitive impairment	Incongruent with degree of cognitive impairment
Cooperation	Cooperative but frustrated	Uncooperative with little effort
CT/EEG	Abnormal	Normal

[a]Benzodiazepines and barbiturates worsen cognitive impairments in the demented patient, whereas they help the depressed patient to relax.

H. Treatment. Treatment is generally supportive. Ensure proper treatment of any concurrent medical problems. Maintain proper nutrition, exercise, and activities. Provide an environment that provides frequent cues for orientation to day, date, place, and time. As functioning decreases, nursing home placement may be necessary. Often, cognitive impairment may become worse at night (*sundowning*). Some nursing homes have successfully developed a schedule of nighttime activities to help manage this problem.

Supportive therapy, group therapy, and referral to organizations for families of demented patients can help them to cope and to feel less frustrated and helpless.

Pharmacologic. In general, barbiturates and benzodiazepines should be avoided, since they can worsen cognition. For agitation, low doses of an antipsychotic are effective, e.g., haloperidol 2 mg orally or intramuscularly, or thioridazine (Mellaril) 25–50 mg orally. Some clinicians suggest a short-acting benzodiazepine for sleep, e.g., triazolam (Halcion) 0.25 mg orally, but this may cause futher memory deficits the next day.

IV. Primary degenerative dementia of the Alzhemier type (DAT)
A. Definition. A progressive dementia in which all known reversible causes have been ruled out. Two types—**senile**, with onset at age 65 or greater, and **presenile**, with onset before age 65. The distinction between senile and presenile dementia is a conventional one not based on any real differences other than age of onset.
B. Diagnosis, signs and symptoms

TABLE 3-6. DSM-III-R DIAGNOSTIC CRITERIA FOR PRIMARY DEGENERATIVE DEMENTIA OF THE ALZHEIMER TYPE

A. Dementia
B. Insidious onset with a generally progressive deteriorating course
C. Exclusion of all other specific causes of dementia by history, physical examination, and laboratory tests

Used with permission, APA.

C. **Epidemiology.** Essentially the same as for dementia. DAT may be more common in women, but this may be an artifact of women's longer life expectancy. Relatives of DAT patients are more likely than the general population to develop DAT. There is a high concordance rate among twins. There are some forms of DAT that run in families, and in these families DAT follows a pattern of autosomal dominant transmission. DAT in one family has been linked to an anomaly on chromosome 21.

The relationship between DAT and Down syndrome has lent further support to genetic hypotheses of DAT. All Down syndrome patients who live into the third decade develop the characteristic brain histopathologic abnormalities found in DAT patients.

Rates of DAT are lower in nonindustrialized countries, but this may be an artifact of their lower level of medical care and thus decreased sensitivity in making the diagnosis.

D. **Etiology.** Hypothetical risk factors include maternal age at birth, exposure to aluminum, history of head trauma, deficiencies of brain choline, autoimmunity, and others. A viral theory exists but lacks scientific support (two other dementing diseases—*kuru* and Creutzfeldt-Jakob disease—have been shown to be caused by transmissible viruses). None of these hypotheses has been clearly proven for DAT. The only known risk factor is increasing age.

E. **Pathology.** The characteristic neuropathologic changes first described by Alois Alzheimer are neurofibrillary tangles, senile plaques, and granulovacuolar degenerations. These changes can also appear with normal aging, but they are always present in brains of DAT patients. They are most prominent in the amygdala, hippocampus, cortex, and basal forebrain. A definitive diagnosis of Alzheimer's disease can only be made histopathologically. That these pathologic structures in the brain contain high amounts of aluminum is the basis of the aluminum toxicity theory of etiology. Clinical diagnosis of DAT should only be considered either possible or probable Alzheimer's disease.

Other abnormalities that have been found in DAT patients include diffuse cortical atrophy on CT or MRI, enlarged ventricles, and decreased brain acetylcholine metabolism. The finding of low levels of acetylcholine explains why these patients are highly susceptible to anticholinergic effects of medication and has led to development of choline replacement strategies for treatment.

F. **Course and prognosis.** Same as for dementia.

G. **Treatment.** Same as for dementia.

V. Multi-infarct dementia (MID)

A. **Definition.** Dementia due to cerebrovascular disease. Usually, dementia progresses in a stepwise fashion with each recurrent infarct. Patients will notice one specific moment when their functioning became worse and will improve slightly over subsequent days until their next infarct. Often, neurologic signs will be present. Impaired cognition may be patchy with some areas intact.

B. Diagnosis, signs and symptoms

TABLE 3–7. **DSM-III-R DIAGNOSTIC CRITERIA FOR MULTI-INFARCT DEMENTIA**

A. Dementia

B. Stepwise deteriorating course with "patchy" distribution of deficits (i.e., affecting some functions, but not others) early in the course

C. Focal neurologic signs and symptoms (e.g., exaggeration of deep tendon reflexes, extensor plantar response, pseudobulbar palsy, gait abnormalities, weakness of an extremity)

D. Evidence from history, physical examination, or laboratory tests of significant cerebrovascular disease (recorded on Axis III) that is judged to be etiologically related to the disturbance

Used with permission, APA.

C. **Epidemiology.** Less common than DAT. More common in men than in women. Onset at an earlier age. Risk factors include hypertension, heart disease, and other risk factors for stroke.

D. **Lab tests.** CT scan or MRI will show infarcts.

E. **Differential diagnosis**

1. **DAT.** MID may be difficult to differentiate from DAT. Obtain a good history of the course of the disease, noting whether the onset was abrupt, the course insidious or stepwise, and whether neurologic impairment was present. Identify MID risk factors and obtain brain image. If a patient has features of both MID and DAT, then the diagnosis should be mixed DAT/MID.

2. **Depression.** MID patients may also become depressed, as described above in patients with pseudodementia. Depression is unlikely to produce focal neurologic findings. If present, depression should be diagnosed and treated.

3. **Strokes and transient ischemic attacks (TIAs).** Generally do not lead to a progressively demented patient. The deficits in TIA are, by definition, transient. A completed stroke patient may have some cognitive deficits, but unless there is a massive loss of brain tissue, a single stroke generally will not cause dementia.

F. **Treatment.** The treatment is to identify and reverse the cause of the strokes. Hypertension, diabetes, and cardiac disease must be treated. Nursing home placement may be necessary if impairment is severe. Treatment is supportive and symptomatic. Antidepressants, antipsychotics, and benzodiazepines can be used, but these brain-damaged patients may develop side effects from any psychoactive drug.

VI. Pick's disease

This relatively rare primary degenerative dementia is clinically very similar to DAT. However, there is prominent frontal lobe involvement, and frontal signs of disinhibited behavior may present early. Reactive gliosis present in frontal and temporal lobes. Diagnosis often made at autopsy, although CT or MRI can show prominent frontal lobe involvement.

VII. Creutzfeldt-Jakob disease

This rapidly progressive degenerative dementing disease is caused by a transmissible slow virus. Onset usually occurs in the 40s or 50s. The very first signs of this disease may be vague somatic complaints or unspecified feelings of anxiety. Other signs include ataxia, extrapyramidal signs, choreoathetosis, and dysarthria. Fatal, usually within 2 years of diagnosis. CT scan shows atrophy in cortex and cerebellum. Characteristic EEG in later stages. No known treatment.

VIII. Huntington's disease (Huntington's chorea)

A. **Definition.** A genetic autosomal dominant disease with complete penetrance (chromosome 4) characterized by choreoathetoid movement and dementia. A person with one parent with Huntington's disease has a 50% chance of developing the disease.

B. **Diagnosis.** Onset usually in 30s to 40s (patient may frequently already have children), asymptomatic initially. Choreiform movements usually present first and become progressively more severe. Later, dementia presents often with psychotic features. Dementia may first be described by the patient's family as a personality change. Look for a family history.

C. **Associated psychiatric complications**
   1. 25% personality changes.
   2. 25% schizophreniform.
   3. 50% mood.
   4. 25% begin with rapid-onset dementia.
   5. 90% develop dementia.

D. **Epidemiology.** Incidence is 2–6 cases/100,000 people. Appears in all races. Over 1,000 cases have been traced to two brothers who immigrated to Long Island, New York from England. Equal in men and women.

E. **Pathophysiology.** Atrophy of brain with extensive involvement of the basal ganglia and the caudate nucleus in particular.

F. **Course and prognosis.** The course is progressive and usually leads to death 15–20 years after being diagnosed. Suicide is common.

G. **Treatment.** Institutionalization may be needed as chorea progresses. Symptomatic relief of insomnia, anxiety, and depression can be given with benzodiazepines and antidepressants. Psychotic symptoms can be treated with high potency antipsychotics. Genetic counseling is the most important intervention.

IX. Parkinson's disease

A. **Definition.** An idiopathic movement disorder with onset usually in later life, characterized by bradykinesia, resting tremor, pill-rolling tremor, masklike facies, cogwheel rigidity, and shuffling gait. Intellectual impairment is common, and 40–80% of patients become demented. Depression is extremely common and can be considered an organic mood disorder.

B. **Epidemiology.** Annual prevalence in Western hemisphere is 200 cases/100,000 people.

C. **Etiology.** Unknown (for the majority of patients with idiopathic parkinsonism). There are decreased cells in substantia nigra, decreased dopamine, and degeneration of dopaminergic tracts. Parkinsonism can be caused by repeated head trauma and some designer drugs.

D. Treatment.   L-dopa (levodopa [Larodopa, Dopar]) is a dopamine precursor and is often combined with carbidopa, a dopa decarboxylase inhibitor to increase brain dopamine levels. Amantidine (Symmetrel) has also been used synergistically with L-dopa. Some surgeons have tried implanting adrenal medulla tissue into the brain to produce dopamine with some favorable results. Depression is treatable with antidepressants or ECT.

X. Other dementias

Other dementias include Wilson's disease, supranuclear palsy, normal pressure hydrocephalus (dementia, ataxia, incontinence), and brain tumors.

Systemic causes of dementia—thyroid disease, pituitary disease (Addison's or Cushing's), liver failure, dialysis, nicotinic acid deficiency (pellagra causes dementia, dermatitis, diarrhea), B_{12} deficiency, folate deficiency, infections, heavy metal intoxication, chronic alcohol abuse.

XI. Amnestic syndrome

A. Definition.   Impaired short- and long-term memory attributed to a specific organic etiology. Normal in other areas of cognition.

B. Diagnosis, signs and symptoms

TABLE 3–8.   **DSM-III-R DIAGNOSTIC CRITERIA FOR AMNESTIC SYNDROME**

A. Demonstrable evidence of impairment in both short- and long-term memory; with regard to long-term memory, very remote events are remembered better than more recent events. Impairment in short-term memory (inability to learn new information) may be indicated by inability to remember three objects after 5 minutes. Long-term memory impairment (inability to remember information that was known in the past) may be indicated by inability to remember past personal information (e.g., what happened yesterday, birthplace, occupation) or facts of common knowledge (e.g., past Presidents, well-known dates).

B. Not occurring exclusively during the course of delirium, and does not meet the criteria for dementia (i.e., no impairment in abstract thinking or judgment, no other disturbances of higher cortical function, and no personality change).

C. There is evidence from the history, physical examination, or laboratory tests of a specific organic factor (or factors) judged to be etiologically related to the disturbance.

Used with permission, APA.

C. Etiology.   Most common form is due to thiamine deficiency associated with alcohol dependence. May also result from head trauma, surgery, hypoxia, infarction, and herpes simplex encephalitis. Typically, any process that damages certain diencephalic and medial temporal structures, e.g., mammillary bodies, fornix, hippocampus, can cause this syndrome.

D. Differential diagnosis.   Delirium and dementia also have amnesia, but will also have impairments in many other areas of cognition. Factitious disorders may simulate amnesia, but the amnestic deficits will be inconsistent.

E. Treatment.   Identify the cause and reverse it if possible; otherwise, supportive medical procedures, e.g., fluids, blood pressure maintenance.

XII. Transient global amnesia

A. Usually in late middle age or elderly.

   B. Abrupt episodes of profound amnesia in all modalities.

   C. Fully alert, distant memory intact.

   D. Usually lasts several hours.

   E. Very bewildered and confused after episode and may repeatedly ask others about what happened.

   F. Cause unknown but possibly cerebrovascular.

XIII. Organic delusional, mood, and anxiety syndromes; organic hallucinosis

   A. Similar to functional diagnoses except that prominent symptoms are due to a specific organic factor.

   B. Normal in other areas of cognition.

   C. Etiologies include endocrinopathies, deficiency states, connective tissue diseases, CNS disorders, and toxic effects of medications.

XIV. Other syndromes/disorders

A. Organic personality syndrome

   1. Clear, persistent change in personality.

   2. Several types:

     a. Affective instability, irritability, anxiety.

     b. Inappropriate outbursts or aggression.

     c. Impaired social judgment.

     d. Apathy and indifference.

     e. Suspiciousness or paranoid ideation.

   3. This diagnosis is not made in a child or adolescent if the clinical features are of attention-deficit hyperactivity disorder (ADHD).

   4. Etiologies usually involve structural brain damage.

B. Systemic lupus erythematosus (SLE)

   1. One of the collagen vascular diseases with direct CNS involvement (others include polyarteritis nodosa and temporal arteritis).

   2. Mental symptoms common (60%) and may be early.

   3. No characteristic form or pattern.

   4. Delirium most common mental syndrome.

   5. Psychotic depression more common than schizophreniform-like.

   6. May progress to dementia.

   7. Seizures common (50%), including grand mal and temporal lobe.

   8. A variety of movement disorders.

C. Migraine

   1. Psychiatric symptoms in migraine patients:

     a. Memory change: 10%

     b. Delirium: 6%

     c. Hallucinations: 6%

     d. Body image change: 6%

     e. Depression: 4%

   2. Chronic migraine → disability → depression.

   3. High intelligence, obsessive features.

   4. 20–25% lifetime prevalence for entire population.

5. More common in females.
6. Some family patterns.
7. Usually upon awakening, dull, throbbing.
8. Gradual in onset, lasts hours to days.
9. Aura is common with visual hallucination, somatic hallucinations, paresthesias.
10. Precipitated by certain foods, stress, temperature changes.
11. Associated autonomic instability (nausea, vomiting, paroxysmal atrial tachycardia).
12. Etiology may be vasodilation/vasoconstriction, but autonomic dysfunction is also possible.
13. Treatment with analgesics, opiates, hydroxyzine, ergot alkaloids, antiinflamatory drugs.
14. Propranolol (Inderal) used in prophylaxis.
15. Psychotherapy important—separate etiology from treatment, use a rehabilitation model for impaired functioning and symptom control, deal directly with secondary gain. Biofeedback, hypnosis, relaxation techniques, and behavior modification also helpful.
16. Common differential is tension headaches, which are bilateral, daylong, and without prodrome.

D. Multiple sclerosis
1. More common in Northern hemisphere.
2. Psychiatric changes common (75%).
3. Early in course, depression is common.
4. Later, with frontal lobe involvement, disinhibition, and manic-like symptoms, including euphoria.
5. Intellectual deterioration common (60%), ranging from mild memory loss to dementia.
6. Psychosis reported, but rates unclear.
7. Hysteria common, especially late in disease.
8. Symptoms exacerbated by physical or emotional trauma.
9. Must get MRI as workup.

E. Epilepsy
1. Ictal and postictal confusional syndromes.
2. 7% prevalence of psychosis in epilepsy.
3. Epilepsy 3–7 times more common in psychotic patients.
4. 10% lifetime prevalence of psychosis in epileptics.
5. Seizures versus pseudoseizures (See Table 3-9).
6. **Temporal lobe epilepsy (TLE)**
    a. TLE type most likely to have psychiatric symptoms.
    b. Often have schizophreniform-like psychoses.
    c. Often difficult to distinguish from schizophrenia with aggressiveness.
    d. Varied and complex auras that may masquerade as functional illness, e.g., hallucinations, depersonalization, derealization.
    e. Automatisms, autonomic effects, and visceral sensations, e.g.,

TABLE 3–9. **CLINICAL FEATURES DISTINGUISHING SEIZURES AND PSEUDOSEIZURES**[a]

Feature	Organic Seizure	Pseudoseizure
Aura	Common stereotyped	Rare
Timing	Nocturnal common	Only when awake
Incontinence	Common	Rare
Cyanosis	Common	Rare
Postictal confusion	Yes	No
Body movement	Tonic/clonic	Nonstereotyped and asynchronous
Self-injury	Common	Rare
EEG	May be abnormal	Normal
Affected by suggestion	No	Yes
Secondary gain	No	Yes

[a]Note that some patients with organic seizure disorders may also have pseudoseizures.

epigastric aura, stomach churning, salivation, flushing, tachycardia, dizziness.

 f. Altered perceptual experiences, e.g., distortions, hallucinations, depersonalization, feeling remote, feeling something has a peculiar significance, *déjà vu, jamais vu.*

 g. Hallucinations of taste and smell are common and may be accompanied by lip smacking or pursing, chewing, or tasting and swallowing movements.

 h. Subjective disorders of thinking and memory.

 i. Strong affective experiences, most commonly fear and anxiety.

F. Brain tumors

1. Neurologic signs, headache, nausea/vomiting, seizures, visual loss, papilledema, virtually any psychiatric symptoms possible.
2. Symptoms often due to raised intracranial pressure or mass effects rather than direct effects of tumor.
3. Suicidal ideation present in 10%, usually during headache paroxysms.
4. Although rare in a psychiatric practice, most patients with brain tumors have psychiatric symptoms.
   a. Slow tumors → personality change.
   b. Rapid tumors → cognitive change.
5. Frontal lobe tumors—depression, inappropriate affect, disinhibition, dementia, impaired coordination, psychotic symptoms. Often misdiagnosed as primary degenerative dementia, neurologic signs often absent.
6. Temporal lobe tumors—anxiety, depression, hallucinations (especially gustatory and olfactory), TLE symptoms, schizophreniform-like psychosis.
7. Parietal lobe tumors—fewer psychiatric symptoms (anosognosia, apraxia, aphasia); may be mistaken for hysteria.

G. Head trauma

1. Wide range of acute and chronic clinical pictures.
2. Duration of disorientation is an approximate guide to prognosis.
3. Brain imaging shows classic *contrecoup* lesion, edema acutely.
4. Acute—amnesia (post-traumatic amnesia often resolves abruptly), agi-

tation, withdrawn, psychotic (acute post-traumatic psychosis), delirious, among others.

5. Chronic—amnesia, psychosis, mood disorder, personality change, and (rarely) dementia.

6. Factors affecting course—mental constitution, premorbid personality, epilepsy (very strongly affects work ability), environment, litigation, emotional repercussion of injury, response to intellectual losses, and amount and location of brain damage.

7. Within limits, the patient's coping mechanisms may affect the eventual course much more than the actual amount of brain damage.

H. Heavy metal poisoning

1. **Lead.** Abdominal colic, lead neuropathy, lead encephalopathy. May present acutely as delirium, seizures, elevated blood pressure (BP), impaired memory and concentration, headache, tremor, deafness, transient aphasia, and hemianopsia. Chronic headache, depression, weakness, vertigo, hyperesthesia for visual and auditory stimuli. Treatment with calcium lactate, milk, chelating agents.

2. **Mercury.** Mad Hatter's syndrome (thermometers, photoengravers, ore workers, fingerprinters, chemical workers, repairers of electric meters, felt hat industry)—gastritis, bleeding gums, excessive salivation, coarse tremor with coarse jerky movements. Presents as nervous, timid, and shy, blushes easily; embarrasses in social situations; irritable and quarrelsome; loses temper easily.

3. **Manganese** (ore workers, dry batteries, bleaching, welding). Headache; asthenia; torpor; hypersomnia; impotence; uncontrollable laughter and crying; impulses to run, dance, sing, or talk; may commit stupid crimes. Parkinsonism develops later.

4. **Arsenic** (fur and glass industries, insecticides). Chronic—dermatitis, conjunctivitis, lachrymation, anorexia, headache, vertigo, apathy, drowsiness, intellectual impairment, peripheral neuritis. May eventually present as a Korsakoff's psychosis.

5. **Thallium** (pesticides). Tingling, abdominal pain, vomiting, headache, tachycardia, gastritis, offensive breath, alopecia, ataxia, paresthesias, peripheral neuropathy, retrobulbar neuritis, tremor, chorea, athetosis, myoclonic jerking, impaired consciousness, depression, seizures, delirium.

For more detailed discussion of this topic, see Horvath TB, Siever LJ, Mohs RC, Davis KL: Organic Mental Syndromes and Disorders, Chap. 12, pp 599–641, in *CTP/V*.

4

Psychoactive Substance Use Disorders

I. General introduction. Substance abuse occurs in all segments of all societies. The proper evaluation of any patient requires an assessment of substance use. In recent years, hallucinogen, marijuana, and phencyclidine (PCP) abuse has decreased, relative to cocaine abuse, which has risen dramatically, especially through smoking crack (a purified highly addictive form of cocaine, which is distributed in small, inexpensive quantities). The costs of substance abuse to society have been estimated to be a staggering $136 billion per year and include decreased work and school performance, accidents, intoxication while working, absenteeism, violent crime, and theft. Adolescents are the most vulnerable age group for developing substance abuse problems. Males are more at risk than females.

A. Evaluation. Substance-abusing patients are often difficult to detect and evaluate. Not easily characterized into specific categories, they almost always underestimate the amount of substance used, are prone to use denial, are often manipulative, and often fear the consequences of acknowledging the problem. Because these patients may be unreliable, it is necessary to obtain information from other sources, such as family members.

When dealing with these patients, clinicians must present clear, firm, and consistent limits, which will be tested frequently. Such patients usually require a confrontative approach. Although clinicians may feel angered by being manipulated, they should not act on these feelings.

Substance abuse frequently coexists with other psychiatric conditions, such as depressive or anxiety disorders. These conditions, however, are difficult to properly evaluate in the presence of ongoing substance abuse, which itself causes symptoms. Substance abuse is frequently associated with personality disorders, e.g., antisocial, borderline, narcissistic. Depressed, anxious, or psychotic patients may self-medicate with either prescribed or nonprescribed substances. Substance-induced organic mental disorders should always be considered in the evaluation of depression, anxiety, or psychosis.

1. Toxicology. Urine or blood toxicology is useful in confirming suspected substance use. The two types of toxicology tests are screening and confirmatory. Screening tests are sensitive but not specific (many false positives). Confirm positive toxicology screens with a specific confirmatory tests for an identified drug. Although most drugs are well detected in urine, some are best detected in blood, e.g., barbiturates or alcohol. Absolute blood levels can sometimes be useful, e.g., a high level in the absence of clinical signs of intoxication would imply tolerance. Urine toxicology is usually positive for up to 2 days after taking most drugs.

2. Physical examination

a. Carefully consider whether concomitant medical conditions are substance-related. Look specifically for the following:

   i. **Subcutaneous or intravenous abusers** — acquired immune deficiency syndrome (AIDS), scars from intravenous or subcutaneous injection, abscesses, infections from contaminated injections, bacterial endocarditis, drug-induced or infectious hepatitis, thrombophlebitis, tetanus.

  ii. **Cocaine or heroin snorters** — deviated or perforated nasal septum, nasal bleeding, rhinitis.

 iii. **Marijuana smokers, cocaine freebasers, inhalant abusers, crack smokers** — bronchitis, asthma, chronic respiratory conditions.

   b. Determine the pattern of abuse. Is it continuous or episodic? When, where, and with whom is the substance taken? Is it recreational or only in certain social contexts? Find out how much of the patient's life is associated with obtaining, taking, withdrawing from, and recovering from substances. How much do the substances affect the patient's social and work functioning? How does he/she get and pay for the substances? Always specifically describe the substance and route of administration rather than the category, i.e., use "intravenous heroin withdrawal" rather than "opioid withdrawal." If describing polysubstance abuse, list all substances. Substance abusers typically abuse multiple substances.

B. Treatment.   In general, the management of intoxication involves observation for possible overdose, evaluation for possible polysubstance intoxication and concomitant medical conditions, and supportive treatment, such as protecting the patient from injury. The treatment of abuse/dependence involves

1. Period of abstinence (anything that improves abstinence should be used).

2. Long-term teatment lasting at least 6 months (relapse is common). A variety of methods, including individual therapy, group therapy, self-help groups (such as Alcoholics Anonymous, Narcotics Anonymous), therapeutic communities, family groups (such as Al-anon), and chemical maintenance (methadone, disulfiram [Antabuse], naltrexone [Trexan]), as well as a variety of philosophical approaches, including addictive, medical, and moral (or inspirational) models may all be helpful. Find what works for each patient.

C. Common organic mental syndromes associated with psychoactive substances are presented in Table 4-1.

D. Definitions

1. Intoxication.   Maladaptive behavior associated with recent drug ingestion. The effects of intoxication of any drug can vary widely among persons and depend on such factors as dose, circumstances, and underlying personality.

2. Withdrawal.   Psychoactive substance-specific syndrome following cessation of regular use (implies tolerance and indicates dependence).

3. Abuse.   A maladaptive pattern of substance use lasting at least 1 month (or repeatedly over a longer period) and occurring either (1) in hazardous situations or (2) despite knowledge of problems associated with use.

TABLE 4–1. **ORGANIC MENTAL SYNDROMES ASSOCIATED WITH PSYCHOACTIVE SUBSTANCES**

	Intoxi-cation	With-drawal	Delirium	With-drawal Delirium	Delu-sional Disorder	Mood Disorder	Other Syn-dromes
Alcohol	X	X		X			1
Amphetamine and related substances	X	X	X		X		
Caffeine	X	X					
Cannabis	X				X		
Cocaine	X	X	X		X		
Hallucinogen	X (hal-luci-nosis)				X	X	2
Inhalant	X						
Nicotine		X					
Opioid	X	X					
Phencyclidine (PCP) and related substances	X		X		X	X	3
Sedative, hypnotic, or anxiolytic	X	X		X			4

[1]Alcohol Idiosyncratic Intoxication, Alcohol Hallucinosis, Alcohol Amnestic Disorder, Dementia Associated with Alcoholism
[2]Posthallucinogen Perception Disorder
[3]Phencyclidine (PCP) or Similarly Acting Arylcyclohexylamine Organic Mental Disorder NOS
[4]Sedative, Hypnotic or Anxiolytic Amnestic Disorder
Used with permission, APA.

4. Dependence. Psychologic or physical need to continue taking the substance. Dependence on a drug may be physical, psychologic, or both. **Psychologic dependence,** also referred to as habituation, is characterized by a continuous or intermittent craving for the substance. **Physical dependence** is characterized by a need to take the substance to prevent the occurrence of a withdrawal or abstinence syndrome. **Note:** The presence of withdrawal symptoms upon abstinence usually implies dependence. Other than for acute treatment of withdrawal symptoms, the distinction between abuse and dependence is of limited clinical significance. See Table 4-2.

5. Addiction. A nonscientific lay term which still appears despite its official removal from the medical vernacular. Implies psychologic dependence, drug-seeking behavior, physical dependence and tolerance, and associated deterioration of physical and mental health.

II. Opioids. Lifetime risk of opioid dependence is 0.7% in the United States, which has an estimated 600,000 addicts. Opioids include opium derivatives as well as synthetic drugs: opium, morphine, diacetylmorphine (heroin, smack, horse), methadone, codeine, oxycodone (Percodan, Percocet), hydromorphone (Dilaudid), levorphanol (Levo-Dromoran), pentazocine (Talwin), meperidine (Demerol), propoxyphene (Darvon), among others. Table 4-3 lists the duration of action of opioids.

A. Route of administration depends on the drug. Opium is smoked. Heroin is typically injected (intravenously or subcutaneously) or snorted nasally, and may be combined with stimulants for intravenous injection (speedball). Pharmaceutically available opioids are typically taken orally, but some are

TABLE 4–2. **SIGNS AND SYMPTOMS OF PSYCHOACTIVE SUBSTANCE INTOXIFICATION AND WITHDRAWAL**

Substance	Intoxication	Withdrawal
Opioid	Drowsiness Slurred speech Impaired attention or memory Analgesia Anorexia Decreased sex drive Hypoactivity	Craving for drug Nausea/vomiting Muscle aches Lacrimation/rhinorrhea Pupillary dilation Piloerection Sweating Diarrhea Fever Insomnia Yawning
Amphetamine	Perspiration/chills Tachycardia Pupillary dilation Elevated blood pressure Nausea/vomiting Tremor Arrhythmia Fever Convulsions Anorexia/weight loss Dry mouth Impotence Hallucinations Hyperactivity Irritability Aggressiveness Paranoid ideation	Dysphoria Fatigue Sleep disorder Agitation Craving
Cocaine	Same as amphetamines	Same as amphetamines
Sedative-Hypnotic	Slurred speech Incoordination Unsteady gait Impaired attention or memory	Nausea/vomiting Malaise/weakness Autonomic hyperactivity Anxiety/irritability Increased sensitivity to light and sound Coarse tremor Marked insomnia Seizures

also injectable. Heroin is exclusively a drug of abuse and is most commonly abused by lower socioeconomic status patients who often engage in criminal activities to pay for drugs.

B. **Dose** often is difficult to determine by history for two reasons. First, the abuser has no way of knowing the concentration of the heroin he/she has bought and may underestimate the amount (which can lead to accidental overdose if the person suddenly gets one bag containing 15% heroin when the typical amount is 5%). Second, the abuser may overstate the dose in an attempt to get more methadone.

C. **Intoxication**
   1. **Objective signs and symptoms.** Central nervous system (CNS) depression, decreased gastrointestinal (GI) motility, respiratory depression, analgesia, nausea and vomiting, slurred speech, hypotension, brad-

TABLE 4–3.   **DURATION OF ACTION OF OPIOIDS**

Drug	Duration of Action
Heroin	3–4 hours
Meperidine	2–4 hours
Morphine, hydromorphone	4–5 hours
Methadone	12–24 hours
Propoxyphene	12 hours
Pentazocine	2–3 hours

ycardia, pupillary constriction, seizures (in overdose). Tolerant patients still will have pupillary constriction and constipation.

2. **Subjective signs and symptoms.** Euphoria (with heroin described as a total body orgasm), at times anxious dysphoria, tranquility, decreased attention and memory, drowsiness, and psychomotor retardation.

D. **Overdose** can be a medical emergency and is usually accidental. Can result from incorrect estimation of dose or erratic pattern of use in which person has lost previous tolerance to drug. Often caused by combined use with other CNS depressants, e.g., alcohol or sedative-hypnotics. Clinical signs include pinpoint pupils, respiratory depression, CNS depression.

   1. **Treatment**
      a. Intensive care unit (ICU) admission and support vital functions (e.g., intravenous fluids).
      b. Immediate intravenous naloxone (Narcan, an opiate antagonist)—.8 mg (.01 mg/kg for neonates) intravenously and wait 15 minutes.
      c. If no response, give 1.6 mg intravenously and wait 15 minutes.
      d. If still no response, give 3.2 mg intravenously and suspect another diagnosis.
      e. If successful, continue at .4 mg/hour intravenously.

   2. **Always consider possible polyoverdose.** A patient successfully treated with naloxone may wake up briefly only to succumb to a subsequent overdose from another slower-acting drug, e.g., sedative-hypnotic, taken simultaneously. Remember that naloxone will precipitate rapid withdrawal symptoms. It has a short half-life and must be administered continuously until the opioid has been cleared (up to 3 days for methadone). Babies born to opioid-abusing mothers may experience intoxication, overdose, or withdrawal.

E. **Withdrawal** is seldom a medical emergency. Clinical signs are flu-like and include drug craving, anxiety, lacrimation, rhinorrhea, yawning, sweating, insomnia, hot and cold flashes, muscle aches, abdominal cramping, dilated pupils, piloerection, tremor, restlessness, nausea and vomiting, diarrhea, and increased vital signs. Intensity depends on previous dose and on rate of decrease. Less intense with longer half-life drugs, such as methadone; more intense with shorter half-life drugs, such as meperidine. Patients have severe craving for opioid drugs and will demand as well as manipulate for opioids. Beware of fakers and look for piloerection, dilated pupils, tachycardia, hypertension. If objective signs are absent, do not give opioids for withdrawal. The goal of detoxification is to minimize withdrawal symptoms (in order to prevent the patient from abandoning treatment) while steadily decreasing opioid dose. If untreated, no serious medical sequelae of opioid withdrawal occur in otherwise healthy people.

1. Detoxification.   If objective withdrawal signs are present, give methadone 10 mg. If withdrawal persists after 4–6 hours, give an additional 5–10 mg, which may be repeated every 4–6 hours. Total dose in 24 hours equals the dose for the second day (seldom more than 40 mg). Give in a twice-a-day or every day schedule and decrease dose by 5 mg/day for heroin withdrawal; methadone withdrawal may require a slower detoxification. Pentazocine-dependent patients should be detoxified on pentazocine because of its mixed opiate receptor agonist and antagonist properties. Many nonopioid drugs have been tried for opioid detoxification, but the only promising one is clonidine (Catapres), which is a centrally acting alpha-2 agonist effective in the relief of nausea, vomiting, and diarrhea associated with opioid withdrawal (not effective for most other symptoms). Give .1–.2 mg every 3 hours as needed, not to exceed .8 mg/day. Titrate dose according to symptoms. When dose is stabilized, taper over 2 weeks. Hypotension is a side effect. Clonidine is short acting and not a narcotic.

The general approach in withdrawal is one of support, detoxification, and progression to methadone maintenance or abstinence. Patients dependent on multiple drugs, e.g., an opioid and a sedative-hypnotic, should be maintained on a stable dose of one drug while being detoxified from the other. Naltrexone (a long-acting oral opiate antagonist) can be used with clonidine to expedite detoxification. After detoxification, oral naltrexone has been effective in helping to maintain abstinence for up to 2 months.

2. Methadone maintenance is the main long-term treatment for opiate dependence and represents a slow, extended detoxification. Most patients can be maintained on daily doses of 60 mg or less. Although often criticized, methadone maintenance programs do decrease rates of heroin use. A sufficient methadone dose is necessary; use of blood methadone levels may help to determine appropriate dose.

3. Therapeutic communities.   Residential programs that emphasize abstinence and group therapy in a structured environment, e.g., Phoenix House.

III. Sedative-hypnotics.   The major complication of sedative-hypnotic intoxication is overdose with associated CNS and respiratory depression. Although mild intoxication is not in itself dangerous (unless the patient is driving or operating machinery), the possibility of a covert overdose must always be considered. Sedative-hypnotic intoxication is similar to alcohol intoxication, but idiosyncratic aggressive reactions are uncommon. These drugs are often taken with other CNS depressants, e.g., alcohol, which can produce additive effects. Withdrawal is dangerous and can lead to delirium or seizures.

Sedative-hypnotics are the most commonly prescribed psychoactive drugs. Lifetime prevalence of abuse or dependence is 1.1%. Sedative-hypnotics are taken orally. Usually, at least several months of daily use is necessary to develop dependence, but there are large interindividual differences. Because most of these drugs have legitimate uses, they have become part of the establishment as well as the drug abuse culture. Many middle-aged patients begin taking benzodiazepines for insomnia or anxiety, become dependent, and then seek out multiple physicians to prescribe them. In the drug abuse culture, sedative-hypnotics are used for their euphoriant effects, to augment the effects of such other CNS depressant drugs as opioids or alcohol, or to temper the excitatory and anxiogenic effects of stimulants, e.g., cocaine. Barbiturates have now been replaced largely by benzodiazepines for two reasons: (1) benzodiazepines have a much larger therapeutic index (lethal dose much greater than effective dose), and (2) barbiturates rapidly induce hepatic microsomal enzymes, causing physiologic tolerance, whereas the benzodiazepines do not.

A. Drugs

    1. Benzodiazepines. Diazepam (Valium), chlordiazepoxide (Librium), flurazepam (Dalmane), lorazepam (Ativan), alprazolam (Xanax), triazolam (Halcion), oxazepam (Serax), temazepam (Restoril), and others.

    2. Barbiturates. Secobarbital (Seconal), pentobarbital (Nembutal), and others.

    3. Others. Meprobamate (Equanil, Miltown), methaqualone (Quaalude), glutethimide (Doriden), ethchlorvynol (Placidyl), chloral hydrate (Noctec).

B. Intoxication.   See Table 4-2. Intoxication also can cause disinhibition and amnestic disorder.

C. Withdrawal.   See Table 4-2. A potentially life-threatening condition, which often requires hospitalization. There are large interindividual differences in tolerance, and the daily doses taken by some patients can be very large. All sedative-hypnotics have cross tolerance with each other and alcohol. The degree of sedative-hypnotic tolerance can be measured with the pentobarbital challenge test, which identifies the dose of pentobarbital needed to prevent withdrawal.

    1. Pentobarbital challenge test (other drugs can also be used).

      a. Give pentobarbital 200 mg orally.

      b. Observe for intoxication after 1 hour, e.g., sleepiness, slurred speech, or nystagmus.

      c. If not intoxicated, give another 100 mg of pentobarbital every 2 hours (maximum 500 mg over 6 hours).

      d. Total dose given to produce mild intoxication is equivalent to daily abuse level of barbiturates.

      e. Substitute phenobarbital 30 mg (longer half-life) for each 100 mg of pentobarbital.

      f. Decrease by about 10%/day.

      g. Adjust rate if signs of intoxication or withdrawal are present.

IV. Stimulants (not including cocaine).   Extremely addicting and dangerous. Powerful anorectic effects. Amphetamines are usually taken orally, but also can be injected or snorted. The clinical syndromes associated with amphetamines are similar to those associated with cocaine, although the usual (oral) route of amphetamine administration produces a less rapid euphoria and consequently is less addictive. Commonly abused by students, long-distance truck drivers, and other groups who desire prolonged wakefulness and attentiveness. Intravenous amphetamine abuse is highly addictive but recently has been displaced by cocaine. Amphetamines cause release of dopamine (dopamine model of schizophrenia). May cause hallucinations and delusions, which are symptomatically identical to an acute schizophreniform psychosis.

A. Drugs

1. Amphetamine (Benzedrine).
2. Dextroamphetamine (Dexedrine).
3. Methamphetamine (Methedrine).
4. Phenmetrazine (Preludin).

V. Cocaine (crack, snow, rock, freebase, lady).   The effects of cocaine are pharmacologically similar to other stimulants, but its widespread use warrants a separate discussion.

A natural product of the coca plant, cocaine has been used for its psychoactive effects in many cultures for centuries. Before its high addictiveness was well known, it was widely used as a stimulant and euphoriant. Cocaine is usually snorted, but can be smoked or injected. To be smoked, cocaine hydrochloride must be purified into a freebase form. The availability of a crystallized form of freebase cocaine (crack) in small, inexpensive amounts (about $10 for a 65–100 mg dose) in recent years has led to an epidemic of crack use, which has had devastating effects on society. Lower socioeconomic groups have been particularly susceptible, leading to the further decay of many urban neighborhoods from its use and associated crime. Crack is smoked, has a rapid onset of action, and is highly addictive. The typical addict image previously associated with the heroin abuser now also applies to the crack abuser.

Smoking cocaine produces an onset of action comparable to an intravenous injection and is equally addictive. The euphoria is intense, and there is a risk of dependence after only one dose. Like amphetamines, cocaine can be taken in binges lasting up to several days. This phenomenon is partly the result of greater euphoric effects from subsequent doses (sensitization). During binges, the abuser will take the cocaine repeatedly until exhausted or out of drug. This is followed by a crash of lethargy, hunger, and prolonged sleep, followed by another binge. With repeated use, tolerance develops to the euphoriant, anorectic, hyperthermic, and cardiovascular effects.

Intravenous use is associated with usual risks of intravenous drug abuse, including AIDS, septicemia, and venous thrombis. Chronic snorting can lead to a rebound rhinitis, which is often self-treated with nasal decongestants; it also causes nosebleeds and eventually may lead to a perforated nasal septum.

A. Cocaine intoxication.

See Table 4-2. Can cause restlessness, agitation, anxiety, talkativeness, pressured speech, paranoid ideation, aggressiveness, increased sexual interest, heightened sense of awareness, grandiosity, hyperactivity, and other manic-like symptoms. Physical signs include tachycardia, hypertension, pupillary dilation, chills, anorexia, insomnia, and stereotyped movements. Cocaine has also been associated with sudden death through cardiac complications and delirium. Delusional disorders are typically paranoid. In delirium, may have tactile or olfactory hallucinations. Delirium may lead to seizures and death. Treatment is largely symptomatic. Agitation can be treated with restraints, benzodiazepines, or, if severe (delirium or psychosis), low doses of high potency antipsychotics (only as a last resort because these medications lower the seizure threshold). Somatic symptoms, e.g., tachycardia, hypertension, can be treated with beta blockers. Evaluate for possible medical complications.

B. Withdrawal. The most prominent sign of cocaine withdrawal is craving for cocaine. The tendency to develop dependence is related to the route of administration (lower with snorting, higher with intravenous injection or smoking freebase cocaine). Withdrawal symptoms include fatigue, lethargy, guilt, anxiety, and feelings of helplessness, hopelessness, and worthlessness. Chronic use can lead to depression, which may require antidepressant treatment. Observe for possible suicidal ideation. Withdrawal symptoms usually peak in several days, but the syndrome (especially depressive symptoms) may last up to weeks.

VI. Marijuana. Approximately 60% of Americans under age 25 have tried marijuana. Marijuana and hashish contain delta-9-tetrahydrocannabinol (THC), which is the main active euphoriant (many other active cannabinoids are probably responsible for the other varied effects). Sometimes, purified THC also is abused. Cannabinoids usually are smoked, but also can be eaten (delays onset, but can eat very large doses).

A. Cannabis intoxication. Symptoms include euphoria or dysphoria, anxiety, suspiciousness, inappropriate laughter, time distortion, social withdrawal, impaired judgment, and the following objective signs: conjunctival injection, increased appetite, dry mouth, and tachycardia. It also causes a dose-dependent hypothermia and mild sedation. Often used with alcohol, cocaine, or other drugs. Treatment of intoxication usually is not required. Can cause depersonalization or (rarely) hallucinations. More commonly causes a mild delusional disorder, usually persecutory, which seldom requires medication. In very high doses, can cause a mild delirium with panic symptoms or a prolonged cannabis psychosis (may last up to 6 weeks). Chronic use can lead to anxiety or depressed states and an apathetic amotivational syndrome. Dependence and withdrawal are controversial—there are certainly many psychologically dependent abusers, but forced abstinence even in heavy users does not consistently cause a characteristic withdrawal syndrome. Considered a gateway drug, leading to abuse of harder drugs. Urine THC testing is positive for many days after intoxication.

VII. Hallucinogens. About 20% of surveyed Americans under age 25 have used hallucinogens—1–2% within the previous 30 days.

A. Drugs
1. Lysergic acid diethylamide (LSD)
2. Dimethoxymethylamphetamine (DOM, STP)
3. Dimethyltryptamine (DMT)
4. Trimethoxyamphetamine (TMA)
5. Psilocybin
6. Mescaline (peyote, tops, cactus)
7. Methylenedioxymethamphetamine (MDMA, ecstasy)
8. Phencyclidine (PCP, angel dust, hog)—see section on phencyclidine below

B. General considerations. Hallucinogens usually are eaten, sucked out of paper, or smoked (especially PCP). This category includes many different drugs with different effects. Hallucinogens act as sympathomimetics and cause hypertension, tachycardia, hyperthermia, and dilated pupils. Psychologic effects range from mild perceptual changes to frank hallucinations; most users only experience mild effects. Usually used sporadically because of tolerance. Street hallucinogens often contaminated with anticholinergic drugs.

C. Hallucinogen hallucinosis (intoxication)

1. Diagnosis, signs and symptoms. In a state of full wakefulness and alertness, maladaptive behavioral changes (anxiety, depression, ideas of reference, paranoid ideation); changes in perception (hallucinations, illusions, depersonalization); and pupillary dilation, tachycardia or palpitations, sweating, blurring of vision, tremors, and incoordination.

Panic reactions (bad trips) can occur, even in experienced users. The user typically develops the conviction that the disturbed perceptions are real. In the typical bad trip, the user feels as if he/she is going mad, has damaged his/her brain, and will never recover. Treatment involves reassurance and keeping the patient with trusted, supportive people (friends, nurses). In general, avoid using medications, but if patient is severely anxious, benzodiazepines may be used. If the patient is psychotic and agitated, high potency antipsychotics, such as haloperidol (Haldol), fluphenazine (Prolixin), or thiothixene (Navane) may be used (avoid low potency antipsychotics because of anticholinergic effects). A controlled environment is necessary to prevent possible dangerous actions due to grossly impaired judgment. Physical restraints may be required. Prolonged psychosis resembling schizophreniform disorder may occasionally develop in vulnerable patients. Organic delusional syndromes and organic mood disorders (usually depression) may also develop.

D. Posthallucinogen perception disorder. A distressing reexperience of impaired perception after cessation of hallucinogen use, i.e., a distressing flashback. The patient may require low doses of benzodiazepine (acutely) or antipsychotic (if persistent).

VIII. Phencyclidine (PCP) or similarly acting arylcyclohexylamine. PCP is an hallucinogen with different effects whose common use and clinical impact warrant separate discussion. PCP commonly causes paranoia and unpredictable violence, which often brings abusers to medical attention.

A. Intoxication

1. Diagnosis, signs and symptoms. Belligerence, assaultiveness, agitation, impulsiveness, unpredictability, and the following signs: nystagmus, increased blood pressure or heart rate, numbness or diminished response to pain, ataxia, dysarthria, muscle rigidity, seizures, and hyperacusis.

PCP is commonly abused. Typically, it is smoked with marijuana (a laced joint) or tobacco but can be eaten, injected, or snorted nasally. PCP should be considered in patients who describe unusual experiences with marijuana or LSD.

Effects are dose-related. At low doses, PCP acts as a CNS depressant, producing nystagmus, blurred vision, numbness, and incoordination. At moderate doses, PCP produces hypertension, dysarthria, ataxia, increased muscle tone (especially in face and neck), hyperactive reflexes, and sweating. At higher doses, PCP produces agitation, fever, abnormal movements, rhabdomyolysis, myoglobinuria, and renal failure. Overdose can cause seizures, severe hypertension, diaphoresis, hypersalivation, respiratory depression, stupor (with eyes open), coma, and death. Violent actions are common when intoxicated. Because of the analgesic effects, patients may have no regard for their own bodies and may severely injure themselves while agitated and combative. Psychosis, sometimes persistent (may resemble schizophreniform disorder), may develop. This is especially likely in patients with underlying schizophrenia. Other possible complications include delirium, mood disorder, or delusional disorder.

2. Treatment. Isolate the patient in a nonstimulating environment. Do not try to talk down the PCP-intoxicated patient as you might with an anxiety-disordered patient; wait for the PCP to clear first. Urine acidification may increase drug clearance (ascorbic acid or ammonium chloride). Screen for other drugs. If acutely agitated, use benzodiazepines. If agitated and psychotic, a high potency antipsychotic may be used. If physical restraint is required, immobilize the body completely to avoid self-injury (more likely with limb restraints). Recovery is usually rapid. Protect the patient and staff. Always evaluate for concomitant medical conditions.

IX. Inhalants. A wide variety of glues, solvents, and cleaners are volatile and can be inhaled for psychotropic effects. Most are aromatic hydrocarbons; they include gasoline, kerosene, plastic and rubber cements, airplane and household glues, paints, lacquers, enamels, paint thinners, aerosols, polishes, fingernail polish remover, nitrous oxide, amyl nitrate, butyl nitrate, and cleaning fluids.

Inhalants typically are abused by adolescents in lower socioeconomic groups. Some homosexuals use poppers (amyl nitrate, butyl nitrate) during sex to intensify orgasm from the vasodilation, which produces lightheadedness, giddiness, and euphoria.

Symptoms of mild intoxication are similar to intoxication with alcohol or sedative-hypnotics. The diagnosis requires a high level of suspicion. Psychologic effects include mild euphoria, belligerence, assaultiveness, impaired judgment, and impulsiveness. Physical effects include ataxia, confusion, disorientation, slurred speech, dizziness, depressed reflexes, and nystagmus. These can progress to delirium and seizures. Possible toxic effects include reports of brain damage, liver damage, bone marrow depression, peripheral neuropathies, and immunosuppression. Withdrawal is unknown.

Acute treatment is supportive medical care, e.g., fluids and blood pressure monitoring.

X. Caffeine intoxication/dependence. Caffeine is present in coffee, tea, chocolate, cola and other carbonated beverages, cocoa, cold medications, and over-the-counter stimulants. The average cup of coffee contains 100–150 mg of caffeine, whereas tea and cola are about one-half as strong. Stimulants usually contain 100 mg per pill. Intoxication is characterized by restlessness, nervousness, excitement, insomnia, flushed face, diuresis, gastrointestinal disturbance, muscle twitching, rambling flow of thought and speech, tachycardia or cardiac arrhythmia, periods of inexhaustibility, and psychomotor agitation. High doses can increase symptoms of psychiatric disorders, e.g., anxiety, psychosis. Tolerance develops. Withdrawal is usually characterized by headache and lasts 4–5 days. Inquire about all possible sources of caffeine.

XI. Nicotine dependence. Nicotine is taken through tobacco smoking and chewing.

    A. Dependence. Develops rapidly and is strongly affected by environmental conditioning. Often coexists with dependence on other substances, e.g., alcohol, marijuana. Treatments for dependence include hypnosis, aversive therapy, acupuncture, and nicotine nasal sprays and gums. High relapse rates. Smoking is more habit-forming than chewing. Smoking is associated with chronic obstructive pulmonary disease, cancers, coronary heart disease, and peripheral vascular disease. Tobacco chewing associated with peripheral vascular disease.

    B. Withdrawal. Characterized by nicotine craving, irritability, frustration, anger, anxiety, difficulty concentrating, restlessness, bradycardia, and increased appetite. The withdrawal syndrome may last for up to several weeks and is often superimposed on withdrawal from other substances.

    The major points of this chapter are summarized in Table 4-4.

For more detailed discussion of this topic, see Jaffe JH: Drug Dependence: Opioids, Nonnarcotics, Nicotine (Tobacco), and Caffeine, Sec. 13.1, pp 642–686, in *CTP/V*.

TABLE 4-4. PSYCHOACTIVE DRUGS ASSOCIATED WITH ORGANIC MENTAL DISORDERS

Drug	Behavioral Effects	Physical Effects	Lab Findings	Treatment
Opioids: opium, morphine, heroin, meperidine (Demerol), methadone, pentazocine (Talwin)	Euphoria, drowsiness, anorexia, decreased sex drive, hypoactivity, change in personality	Miosis, pruritus, nausea, bradycardia, constipation, needle tracks in arms, legs, groin	Detected in blood up to 24 hours after last dose	For gradual withdrawal: methadone 5–10 mg every 6 hr for 24 hr, then decrease dose for 10 days. For overdose: naloxone (Narcan) 0.4 mg IM every 20 minutes for 3 doses, keep airway open; give O_2
Amphetamine and other sympathomimetics including cocaine	Alertness, loquaciousness, euphoria, hyperactive, irritability, aggressiveness, agitation, paranoid trends, impotence, visual and tactile hallucinations	Mydriasis, tremor, halitosis, dry mouth, tachycardia, hypertension, weight loss, arrhythmias, fever, convulsions, perforated nasal septum (with cocaine)	Detected in blood and urine	For agitation: diazepam (Valium) IM or PO 5–10 mg every 3 hr; for tachyarrhythmias: propanolol (Inderal) 10–20 mg PO q every 4 hr; vitamin CO .5 gm qid PO may increase urinary excretion by acidifying urine
Central nervous system depressants: barbiturates, methaqualone (illegal to make in U.S.), meprobamate, benzodiazepines, glutethimide (Doriden)	Drowsiness, confusion, inattentiveness	Diaphoresis, ataxia, hypotension, seizures, delirium, miosis	Detected in blood	For barbiturates: Substitute 30 mg liquid phenobarbital for every 100 mg barbiturates abused and give in divided doses every 6 hr and then decrease by 20% every other day; may also substitute diazepam (Valium) for barbiturate abused. Give 10 mg every 2–4 hr for 24 hr and then reduce dose; for benzodiazepines; gradual reduction of Valium every other day over 10-day period
Other inhalants: nitrous oxide	Euphoria, drowsiness, ataxia, confusion	Analgesia, respiratory depression, hypotension	None	Hypoxia is treated with O_2 inhalation
Alcohol	Poor judgment, loquaciousness, mood change, aggression, impaired attention, amnesia	Nystagmus, flushed face, ataxia, slurred speech	Blood level between 100 and 200 mg/dl	For delirium: diazepam (Valium) 5–10 mg IM or PO every 3 hr, IM vitamin B complex, hydration; for hallucinosis: haloperidol (Haldol) 1–4 mg every 6 hr IM or PO

Substance	Clinical features	Laboratory findings	Treatment
Hallucinogens: LSD (D-lysergic acid diethylamide), psilocybin (mushrooms), mescaline (peyote), DET (diethyltriptamine), DMT (dimethyltriptamine), DOM or STP (dimethoxymethylamphetamine), MDA (methylene dioxyamphetamine)	8–12 hour duration with flashback after abstinence, visual hallucinations, paranoid ideation, false sense of achievement and strength, suicidal or homicidal tendencies, depersonalization, derealization	Mydriasis, ataxia, hyperemic conjunctiva, tachycardia, hypertension	None	Emotional support ("talking down"); for mild agitation: diazepam (Valium) 10 mg IM or PO every 2 hr for 4 doses; for severe agitation: haloperidol (Haldol) 1–5 mg IM and repeat every 6 hr prn. May have to continue Haldol 1–2 mg per day PO for weeks to prevent flashback syndrome. Phenothiazines may be used only with LSD. Caution: phenothiazines can produce *fatal* results if used with other hallucinogens (DET, DMT, etc) especially if they are adulterated with strychnine or belladonna alkaloids
Phencyclidine (PCP)	8–12 hour duration, hallucinations, paranoid ideation, labile mood, loose associations (may mimic schizophrenia), catatonia, violent behavior, convulsions	Nystagmus, mydriasis, ataxia, tachycardia, hypertension	Detected in urine up to 5 days after ingestion	Phenothiazines contraindicated for first week after ingestion; for violent delusions: haloperidol (Haldol) 1–4 mg IM or PO every 2–4 hr until patient is calm
Volatile hydrocarbons and petroleum derivatives; glue, benzene, gasoline, varnish thinner, lighter fluid, aerosols	Euphoria, clouded sensorium, slurred speech, ataxia, hallucinations in 50% of cases, psychoses, permanent brain damage if used daily over 6 mo	Odor on breath, tachycardia with possible ventricular fibrillation, possible damage of brain, liver, kidneys, myocardium	Relevant to determine tissue damage (SGOT)	For agitation: haloperidol (Haldol) 1–5 mg every 6 hr until calm; avoid epinephrine because of myocardial sensitization
Belladonna alkaloids (found in over-the-counter medications and morning glory seeds): strammonium, homatropine, atropine, scopolomine, hyoscyamine	Hot skin, erythema, weakness, thirst, blurred vision, confusion, excitement, delirium, stupor, coma (anticholinergic delirium)	Dry mouth and throat, mydriasis, twitching, dysphagia, light sensitivity, pyrexia, hypertension followed by shock, urinary retention	None	Antidote is physostigmine (Antilirium) 2 mg IV every 20 min; IV should be controlled at no more than 1 mg/min; watch for copious salivary secretion because of anticholinesterase activity. Propranolol for tachyarrhythmias

Modified from *Desk Reference on Drug Misuse and Abuse*, New York State Medical Society, New York, 1984.

5

Disorders Associated with Alcoholism

I. General introduction. Alcohol, a central nervous system (CNS) depressant and intoxicant, is the most commonly used psychoactive substance in both the mentally healthy and the mentally ill. More than two-thirds of all Americans consume alcohol, and the distinction between recreational/social drinking and alcohol abuse is often vague and unclear.

Alcoholism is defined as the excessive use of ethanol-containing beverages. Although alcoholism does not describe a specific mental disorder, the disorders associated with alcoholism generally can be divided into two groups: (1) disorders related to the direct effects of alcohol on the brain (including alcohol intoxication, uncomplicated withdrawal, withdrawal delirium, hallucinosis, amnestic disorder, dementia, Wernicke's encephalopathy, and Korsakoff's psychosis) and (2) disorders related to behavior associated with alcohol (alcohol abuse/dependence).

II. Alcohol dependence/abuse

A. Definition

1. Alcohol dependence. The excessive use of alcohol that is harmful to physical and mental health. It has three common forms: (1) continuous use of a large quantity of alcohol, (2) heavy use only on weekends or when job functioning is least likely to be impaired, and (3) binges of heavy drinking (lasting days to weeks) interspersed with long periods of sobriety.

2. Alcohol abuse. The continual use of alcohol that interferes with a person's overall functioning and that usually evolves into dependence. Generally, this category describes a person whose drinking problem is not yet sufficient to warrant a diagnosis of alcohol dependence.

B. Epidemiology

1. 13% lifetime prevalence.
2. More prevalent in men than in women (3–4:1), but rates for women may be increasing.
3. Many men and women over age 50 choose abstinence.
4. In the United States, 10% of the drinking population consumes 50% of all alcohol.

C. Etiology. Alcohol dependence runs in families, and children of alcohol-abusing parents are at high risk of developing alcohol abuse whether or not they are raised by their biologic parents. The familial association is strongest for the male child of an alcohol-dependent father. There are ethnic and cultural differences in susceptibility to alcohol and its effects. For example, many Asians show acute toxic effects, such as intoxication, flushing, dizziness, and headache after consuming only minimal amounts of alcohol. Some cultural groups, such as Jews, conservative Protestants, and Asians, have lower rates of alcohol dependence, whereas others, such as Native Americans, Eskimos, and some groups of Hispanic men, show high rates. These findings have led to a genetic theory about the etiology of alcoholism, but a definitive etiology remains unknown.

1. Comorbidity with other mental disorders. Alcohol's sedative effect and its ready availability make it the most commonly used substance for the relief of anxiety, depression, and insomnia. However, chronic use may cause depression, and withdrawal in a dependent individual may cause anxiety. Proper evaluation of depressed or anxious patients who drink heavily may require observation and reevaluation after a period of sobriety lasting up to several weeks. Many psychotic patients medicate themselves with alcohol when prescribed medications do not sufficiently reduce psychotic symptoms or when prescription medications are not available. In bipolar patients, heavy alcohol use often leads to a manic episode. Among the personality-disordered patients, antisocial personalities are particularly likely to develop long-standing patterns of alcohol dependence. Alcohol abuse is prevalent in persons with other substance abuse disorders, and there is a particularly high correlation between alcohol dependence and nicotine dependence.

D. Diagnosis, signs and symptoms

1. Alcohol dependence. Usually, the alcohol dependent/abusing patient will have some alcohol-related impairment in at least one of the following areas: work or school; health; family relationships; social functioning, such as seeing only drinking friends; or legal problems, such as driving while intoxicated or fighting.

TABLE 5-1. DSM-III-R DIAGNOSTIC CRITERIA FOR ALCOHOL AND OTHER PSYCHOACTIVE SUBSTANCE DEPENDENCE

A. At least three of the following:

(1) substance often taken in larger amounts or over a longer period than the person intended

(2) persistent desire or one or more unsuccessful efforts to cut down or control substance use

(3) a great deal of time spent in activities necessary to get the substance (e.g., theft), taking the substance (e.g., chain smoking), or recovering from its effects

(4) frequent intoxication or withdrawal symptoms when expected to fulfill major role obligations at work, school, or home (e.g., does not go to work because hung over, goes to school or work "high," intoxicated while taking care of his or her children), or when substance use is physically hazardous (e.g., drives when intoxicated)

(5) important social, occupational, or recreational activities given up or reduced because of substance use

(6) continued substance use despite knowledge of having a persistent or recurrent social, psychological, or physical problem that is caused or exacerbated by the use of the substance (e.g., keeps using heroin despite family arguments about it, cocaine-induced depression, or having an ulcer made worse by drinking)

(7) marked tolerance: need for markedly increased amounts of the substance (i.e., at least a 50% increase) in order to achieve intoxication or desired effect, or markedly diminished effect with continued use of the same amount

(8) characteristic withdrawal symptoms

(9) substance often taken to relieve or avoid withdrawal symptoms

B. Some symptoms of the disturbance have persisted for at least 1 month, or have occurred repeatedly over a longer period of time.

Used with permission, APA.

Tolerance is the phenomenon of the drinker needing, over time, greater amounts of alcohol to obtain the same effect. The development of tolerance, especially marked tolerance, usually indicates dependence. Mild tolerance for alcohol is common, but severe tolerance, such as that which is possible with other drugs such as opiates and barbiturates, is uncommon. Tolerance varies widely among persons. Dependence may only become apparent to the tolerant patient when he or she is forced to stop and develops withdrawal symptoms.

2. Alcohol abuse

TABLE 5–2. **DSM-III-R DIAGNOSTIC CRITERIA FOR ALCOHOL AND OTHER PSYCHOACTIVE SUBSTANCE ABUSE**

A. A maladaptive pattern of psychoactive substance use indicated by at least one of the following:

    (1) continued use despite knowledge of having a persistent or recurrent social, occupational, psychological, or physical problem that is caused or exacerbated by use of the psychoactive substance
    (2) recurrent use in situations in which use is physically hazardous (e.g., driving while intoxicated)

B. Some symptoms of the disturbance have persisted for at least 1 month, or have occurred repeatedly over a longer period of time.

C. Never met the criteria for psychoactive substance dependence for this substance.

Used with permission, APA.

3. Evaluation. The proper evaluation of the alcohol user requires some suspiciousness on the part of the evaluator. In general, when questioned about the amount of alcohol they consume, most people minimize the amount. When obtaining a history of degree of alcohol use, it might be helpful to phrase questions in a manner likely to elicit positive responses. For example, you might ask, "How much alcohol do you drink?" rather than, "Do you drink alcohol?" Other questions that may give important clues include how often the patient drinks in the morning, how often he/she has **blackouts** (amnesia while intoxicated), and how often friends or relatives have told the patient to cut down on drinking. Always look for subtle signs of alcohol abuse and always inquire about use of other substances. Does the patient seem to be accident prone (head injury, rib fracture, motor vehicle accidents)? Is he/she often in fights? Often absent from work? Are there social or family problems?

E. Treatment. The goal is the prolonged maintenance of total sobriety. Relapses are common. Initial treatment requires detoxification, inpatient if necessary, and treatment of any withdrawal symptoms that are present (see section on alcohol withdrawal). Coexisting mental disorders should be treated when the patient is sober.

1. Insight. Critically necessary but often difficult to achieve. The patient must acknowledge that he or she has a drinking problem. Severe denial may have to be overcome before the patient will cooperate in seeking treatment. Often, this requires the collaboration of family, friends, employers, and others. The patient many need to be confronted with the potential loss of career, family, and health if he or she continues to drink. Individual psychotherapy has been used, but group therapy may be more effective. Group therapy may also be more acceptable to many patients who perceive alcohol dependence as a social problem rather than a personal psychiatric problem.

   2. **Alcoholics Anonymous (AA) and Al-Anon.** Supportive organizations, such as AA (for patients) and Al-Anon (for families of patients), can be effective in maintaining sobriety and helping the family to cope. AA emphasizes the inability of the member to cope with addiction to alcohol alone and encourages dependence on the group for support; AA also utilizes many techniques of group therapy.

   3. **Psychosocial interventions.** Often necessary and very effective.
   a. **Family therapy** — should focus on describing the effects of alcohol use on other family members. Patients must be forced to relinquish the perception of their right to be able to drink and recognize the detrimental effects on the family.

   4. **Psychopharmacotherapy**
   a. **Disulfiram** (Antabuse) (125–500 mg/day; available in 250 mg and 500 mg tablets)—may be used if the patient desires enforced sobriety. Patients taking disulfiram develop an extremely unpleasant reaction when they ingest even small amounts of alcohol. This reaction, caused by an accumulation of acetaldehyde, includes flushing, headache, throbbing in head and neck, dyspnea, hyperventilation, tachycardia, hypotension, sweating, anxiety, weakness, and confusion. Life-threatening complications, although uncommon, can occur. Disulfiram is useful only temporarily to help establish a long-term pattern of sobriety and to change long-standing alcohol-related coping mechanisms.
   b. **Lithium** — probably ineffective in maintaining abstinence in alcohol abusers or treating depression in alcoholics.

   5. **After recovery.** Most experts recommend that a recovered alcohol-dependent patient maintain lifelong sobriety and discourage attempts by recovered patients to learn to drink normally. One of the dogmas of AA is, "It's the first drink that gets you drunk."

F. **Medical complications.** Alcohol is toxic to numerous organ systems. Complications of chronic alcohol abuse (or associated nutritional deficiencies) include cerebral atrophy, cerebellar degeneration, epilepsy, peripheral neuropathy, cardiomyopathy, myopathy, alcoholic hepatitis, cirrhosis, gastritis, pancreatitis, peptic ulcer, and many other gastrointestinal (GI) tract problems. In addition, nutritional deficiencies (e.g., thiamine, vitamin B_{12}, nicotinic acid, folate) often accompany chronic alcoholism. Alcohol use during pregnancy is toxic to the developing fetus and can cause congential defects as well as fetal alcohol syndrome.

III. Alcohol intoxication
A. **Definition.** Recent ingestion of a sufficient amount of alcohol to produce maladaptive behavioral changes.
B. **Diagnosis, signs and symptoms.** Whereas mild intoxication may produce a relaxed, talkative, euphoric, disinhibited person, severe intoxication often leads to more maladaptive changes, which can include aggressiveness, irritability, labile mood, impaired judgment, and impaired social or work functioning, among others.

Persons exhibit at least one of the following: slurred speech, incoordination, unsteady gait, nystagmus, and flushed face. Severe intoxication can lead to withdrawn behavior, psychomotor retardation, blackouts, and eventually obtundation, coma, and death. Common complications of alcohol intoxication include motor vehicle accidents, head injury, rib fracture, criminal acts, homicide, and suicide.

1. **Evaluation.** Conduct a thorough medical evaluation and consider a possible subdural hematoma or a concurrent infection. Always evaluate for possible intoxication with other substances. Alcohol is frequently used in combination with other CNS depressants, such as benzodiazepines and barbiturates. The CNS depressant effects of such combinations can be synergistic and potentially fatal.

Appropriate examination of mental status and diagnosis of other concurrent mental disorders usually require reevaluation after the patient is no longer intoxicated, because almost any psychiatric symptom may acutely be due to alcohol intoxication. Blood alcohol levels are seldom important in the clinical evaluation (except to determine legal intoxication) because there may be differences in tolerance.

C. **Treatment**
1. Usually only supportive.
2. May give nutrients (especially thiamine, B_{12}, folate).
3. May require observation for complications, e.g., combativeness, coma, head injury, falling.

D. **Blackouts.**   Periods of intoxication for which there is complete anterograde amnesia and during which the patient appears awake and alert. Occasionally can last up to days with the intoxicated person performing complex tasks, such as long-distance travel with no subsequent recollection. Brain-damaged persons may be more susceptible to blackouts.

IV. **Alcohol idiosyncratic intoxication** (pathological intoxication).   Maladaptive behavior (often aggressive or assaultive) after ingesting a small amount of alcohol that would not cause intoxication in most people. Uncommon. This behavior must be atypical for the person when he/she is not drinking. Brain-damaged persons may also be more susceptible to alcohol idiosyncratic intoxication.

V. **Alcohol hallucinosis.**   Vivid, persistent hallucinations (often visual and auditory), without delirium, following (usually within 2 days) a decrease in alcohol consumption in an alcohol-dependent person. May persist and progress to a more chronic form, which is clinically similar to schizophrenia. Rare. The male-to-female ratio is 4:1. This disorder usually requires at least 10 years of alcohol dependence. If agitated, may treat with benzodiazepines (e.g., lorazepam [Ativan] 1–2 mg orally or intramuscularly, diazepam [Valium] 5–10 mg orally) or low doses of a high potency antipsychotic, such as haloperidol (Haldol) 2–5 mg orally or intramuscularly as needed every 4–6 hours.

VI. **Alcohol withdrawal.**   Begins within several hours after cessation of, or reduction in, prolonged (at least days) heavy alcohol consumption. May be mild (uncomplicated) or severe (with delirium).

A. Uncomplicated alcohol withdrawal

1. Coarse tremor.
2. At least one of the following: nausea or vomiting, malaise or weakness, tachycardia, hypertension, sweating, anxiety, depressed mood, irritability, transient hallucinations, illusions, headache, insomnia.
3. Common syndrome.

B. Alcohol withdrawal delirium (delirium tremens or DTs).

Usually only occurs after recent cessation of or reduction in severe, heavy alcohol use in medically compromised patients with a long history of dependence. Less common than uncomplicated alcohol withdrawal.

1. **Diagnosis, signs and symptoms**
   a. Delirium.
   b. Marked autonomic hyperactivity, e.g., tachycardia, sweating.
   c. **Associated features** — vivid hallucinations, which may be visual, tactile, or olfactory; delusions; agitation; tremor; fever; and seizures or "rum fits" (if seizures develop, they always occur before delirium).
   d. **Typical features** — paranoid delusions, visual hallucinations of insects or small animals, and tactile hallucinations.

2. **Medical workup**
   a. Complete history and physical.
   b. **Lab tests**—complete blood count (CBC) with differential, electrolytes, calcium, magnesium, blood chemistry panel, liver function tests, bilirubin, blood urea nitrogen (BUN), creatinine, fasting glucose, prothrombin time, albumin, total protein, Hepatitis B surface antigen, B_{12} levels, folate levels, serum amylase, stool guiac, urinalysis, urine drug screen, electrocardiogram (EKG), and chest x-ray. Other possible tests: electroencephalogram (EEG), lumbar puncture (LP), computed tomography (CT) scan of head, and GI series.

3. **Treatment**
   a. Take vital signs every 6 hours.
   b. Observe constantly.
   c. Decrease stimulation.
   d. Correct electrolyte imbalances and treat other coexisting medical problems, e.g., infection, head trauma.
   e. If dehydrated, hydrate.
   f. Chlordiazepoxide (Librium) 25–100 mg orally every 6 hours (other sedative/hypnotics could be substituted, but this is the convention). Use as needed for agitation, tremor, or increased vital signs (temperature, pulse, blood pressure).
   g. Thiamine 100 mg orally 1–3 times/day.
   h. Folic acid 1 mg orally daily.
   i. One multivitamin daily.
   j. Magnesium sulfate 1 g intramuscularly every 6 hours for 2 days (in patients who have had postwithdrawal seizures).
   k. After stabilized, taper chlordiazepoxide by 20% every 5–7 days.

l. Provide medication for adequate sleep.

m. Treat malnutrition if present.

n. This regimen allows for a very flexible dosage range of chlordiazepoxide. Be sure that if prescribing a sedative on a standing regimen that the medication will be held if the patient is asleep or not easily arousable. The necessary total dose of benzodiazepine will vary greatly among patients owing to inherent individual differences, differing levels of alcohol intake, and concomitant use of other substances. Because many of these patients have liver function impairment, it also may be difficult to accurately estimate the sedative's elimination half-life.

Generally, avoid antipsychotics because this class of medications can precipitate seizures. If the patient is agitated, psychotic, and showing signs of benodiazepine toxicity (ataxia, slurred speech) in spite of being agitated, then you may consider using a high potency antipsychotic, such as haloperidol or fluphenazine (Prolixin, Permitil), which is less likely to precipitate seizures than low-potency antipsychotics.

VII. **Alcoholic encephalopathy** (Wernicke's encephalopathy). An acute syndrome caused by thiamine deficiency. Characterized by nystagmus, abducens and conjugate gaze palsies, ataxia, and global confusion. Other symptoms may include confabulation, lethargy, indifference, mild delirium, anxious insomnia, or fear of the dark. Thiamine deficiency usually due to chronic alcohol dependence. Treat with thiamine until opthalmoplegia resolves. May also require magnesium (a cofactor for thiamine metabolism). With treatment, most symptoms resolve except ataxia, nystagmus, and sometimes peripheral neuropathy. A Korsakoff psychosis develops in 84% of patients.

VIII. **Alcohol amnestic disorder** (Korsakoff's psychosis). A chronic syndrome usually related to alcohol dependence, wherein alcohol represents a large portion of caloric intake for years. Caused by thiamine deficiency. Rare. Characterized by retrograde and anterograde amnesia. The patient also often will show confabulation, disorientation, and polyneuritis. In addition to thiamine replacement, clonidine (Catapres) and propranolol (Inderal) may be of some limited use. Often coexists with alcoholic dementia.

IX. **Dementia associated with alcoholism.** This diagnosis should be made when other etiologies of dementia have been excluded and a history of chronic heavy alcohol abuse is evident. The patient must have been free of alcohol for at least 3 weeks. The dementia is usually mild, although a severe form can (rarely) occur. Management is similar to dementia from other etiologies.

For more detailed discussion of this topic, see Goodwin DW: Alcoholism, Sec. 13.2, pp 686–698, in *CTP/V*.

6
Schizophrenia

A. **Definition.** Schizophrenia is a disorder of unknown etiology, which is characterized by psychotic symptoms that significantly impair functioning and that involve disturbances in feeling, thinking, and behavior. The disorder is chronic and generally has a prodromal phase, an active phase with delusions, hallucinations, or both, and a residual phase in which the disorder may be in remission.

B. **History**

   1852. First formally described by Belgian psychiatrist Benedict Morel, who termed it "démence précoce."

   1896. Emil Kraepelin, German psychiatrist, applied term "dementia praecox" to a group of illnesses that began in adolescence and ended in dementia.

   1911. Swiss psychiatrist Eugen Bleuler introduced term "schizophrenia." There are no pathognomonic signs or symptoms; instead, a cluster of characteristic findings make the diagnosis. The diagnostic criteria in current use are from DSM-III-R (Table 6-1). The criteria formulated by Kraepelin, Bleuler (the four A's), and Kurt Schneider (first rank symptoms) are useful criteria (Tables 6-2, 6-3, 6-4); however, DSM-III-R criteria are the most widely used and accepted.

C. **Signs and symptoms**

   1. **Impaired overall functioning.** Below highest level previously achieved or failure to achieve expected level.

   2. **Abnormal content of thought.** For example, delusions, ideas of reference, poverty of content.

   3. **Illogical form of thought.** For example, derailment, loosening of associations, incoherence, circumstantiality, tangentiality, overinclusiveness, neologisms, blocking, echolalia (all incorporated as a thought disorder).

   4. **Distorted perception.** For example, hallucinations: visual, olfactory, tactile, and most frequently, auditory.

   5. **Changed affect.** For example, flat, blunted, silly, labile, inappropriate.

   6. **Impaired sense of self.** For example, loss of ego boundaries, gender confusion, inability to distinguish internal from external reality.

   7. **Altered volition.** For example, inadequate drive or motivation, marked ambivalence.

   8. **Impaired interpersonal functioning.** For example, social withdrawal and emotional detachment, aggressiveness, sexual inappropriateness.

   9. **Change in psychomotor behavior.** For example, agitation versus withdrawal, grimacing, posturing, rituals, catatonia.

   10. **Sensorium.** For example, intact orientation to time, place, and person, intact memory, concreteness.

D. **Diagnosis.** Schizophrenia is a diagnosis based on observation and description of the patient. It is a phenomenologic diagnosis. See Table 6-1.

TABLE 6–1.   **DSM-III-R DIAGNOSTIC CRITERIA FOR SCHIZOPHRENIA**

A. Presence of characteristic psychotic symptoms in the active phase: either (1), (2), or (3) for at least 1 week (unless the symptoms are successfully treated):

(1) two of the following:
  (a) delusions
  (b) prominent hallucinations (throughout the day for several days or several times a week for several weeks, each hallucinatory experience not being limited to a few brief moments)
  (c) incoherence or marked loosening of associations
  (d) catatonic behavior
  (e) flat or grossly inappropriate affect

(2) bizarre delusions involving a phenomenon that the person's culture would regard as totally implausible (e.g., thought broadcasting, being controlled by a dead person)
(3) prominent hallucinations [as defined in (1)(b) above] of a voice with content having no apparent relation to depression or elation, or a voice keeping up a running commentary on the person's behavior or thoughts, or two or more voices conversing with each other

B. During the course of the disturbance, functioning in such areas as work, social relations, and self-care is markedly below the highest level achieved before onset of the disturbance (or, when the onset is in childhood or adolescence, failure to achieve expected level of social development).

C. Schizoaffective disorder and mood disorder with psychotic features have been ruled out, i.e., if a major depressive or manic syndrome has ever been present during an active phase of the disturbance, the total duration of all episodes of a mood syndrome has been brief relative to the total duration of the active and residual phases of the disturbance.

D. Continuous signs of the disturbance for at least 6 months. The 6-month period must include an active phase (of at least 1 week, or less if symptoms have been successfully treated) during which there were psychotic symptoms characteristic of schizophrenia (symptoms in A), with or without a prodromal or residual phase, as defined below.

Prodromal phase: A clear deterioration in functioning before the active phase of the disturbance that is not due to a disturbance in mood or to a psychoactive substance use disorder and that involves at least two of the symptoms listed below.

Residual phase: Following the active phase of the disturbance, persistence of at least two of the symptoms noted below, these not being due to a disturbance in mood or to a psychoactive substance use disorder.

Prodromal or Residual Symptoms:

(1) marked social isolation or withdrawal
(2) marked impairment in role functioning as wage-earner, student, or homemaker
(3) markedly peculiar behavior (e.g., collecting garbage, talking to self in public, hoarding food)
(4) marked impairment in personal hygiene and grooming
(5) blunted or inappropriate affect
(6) digressive, vague, overelaborate, or circumstantial speech, or poverty of speech, or poverty of content of speech
(7) odd beliefs or magical thinking, influencing behavior and inconsistent with cultural norms (e.g., superstitiousness, belief in clairvoyance, telepathy, "sixth sense," "others can feel my feelings," overvalued ideas, ideas of reference)
(8) unusual perceptual experiences (e.g., recurrent illusions, sensing the presence of a force or person not actually present)
(9) marked lack of initiative, interests, or energy

Examples: Six months of prodromal symptoms with 1 week of symptoms from A; no prodromal symptoms with 6 months of symptoms from A; no prodromal symptoms with 1 week of symptoms from A and 6 months of residual symptoms.

E. It cannot be established that an organic factor initiated and maintained the disturbance.

F. If there is a history of autistic disorder, the additional diagnosis of schizophrenia is made only if prominent delusions or hallucinations are also present.

Classification of course. The course of the disturbance is coded in the fifth digit:

1—Subchronic. The time from the beginning of the disturbance, when the person first began to show signs of the disturbance (including prodromal, active, and residual phases) more or less continuously, is less than 2 years but at least 6 months.

TABLE 6–1.   **DSM-III-R DIAGNOSTIC CRITERIA FOR SCHIZOPHRENIA (Continued)**

2—Chronic. Same as above, but more than 2 years.

3—Subchronic with Acute Exacerbation. Reemergence of prominent psychotic symptoms in a person with a subchronic course who has been in the residual phase of the disturbance.

4—Chronic with Acute Exacerbation. Reemergence of prominent psychotic symptoms in a person with a chronic course who has been in the residual phase of the disturbance.

5—In Remission. When a person with a history of schizophrenia is free of all signs of the disturbance (whether or not on medication), "in remission" should be coded. Differentiating schizophrenia in remission from no mental disorder requires consideration of overall level of functioning, length of time since the last episode of disturbance, total duration of the disturbance, and whether prophylactic treatment is being given.

0—Unspecified.

Specify late onset if the disturbance (including the prodromal phase) develops after age 45.

Used with permission, APA.

TABLE 6–2.   **EMIL KRAEPELIN'S CRITERIA**

- Disturbances of attention and comprehension
- Hallucinations, especially auditory (voices)
- Gedankenlautwerden (audible thoughts)
- Experiences of influenced thought
- Disturbances in the flow of thought, above all a loosening of associations
- Impairment of cognitive function and judgment
- Affective flattening
- Appearance of morbid behavior
    Reduced drive
    Automatic obedience
    Echolalia, echopraxia
    Acting out
    Catatonic frenzy
    Stereotypy
    Negativism
    Autism
    Disturbance of verbal expression

Table from the World Health Organization

TABLE 6–3.   **EUGEN BLEULER'S CRITERIA**

I. **Symptomatological criteria**

   Basic or fundamental disturbances
   - Formal thought disorders*
   - Disturbances of affect*
   - Disturbances of the subjective experience of self
   - Disturbances of volition and behavior
   - Ambivalence*
   - Autism*

   Accessory symptoms
   - Disorders of perception (hallucinations)
   - Delusions
   - Certain memory disturbances
   - Modification of personality
   - Changes in speech and writing
   - Somatic symptoms
   - Catatonic symptoms
   - Acute syndrome (such as melancholic, manic, catatonic, and other states)

*"The four A's": association, affect, ambivalence, and autism.
Table from the World Health Organization.

TABLE 6–4.   **KURT SCHNEIDER'S CRITERIA, FIRST AND SECOND RANK SYMPTOMS**

First rank symptoms
- Audible thoughts
- Voices arguing and/or discussing
- Voices commenting
- Somatic passivity experiences
- Thought withdrawal and other experiences of influenced thought*
- Thought broadcasting
- Delusional perceptions
- All other experiences involving made volition, made affect, and made impulses

Second rank symptoms
- Other disorders of perception
- Sudden delusional ideas
- Perplexity
- Depressive and euphoric mood changes
- Feelings of emotional impoverishment
- ". . . and several others as well."

*The symptom "thought insertion" was originally included under other experiences of influenced thought. Table from the World Health Organization.

E. Types of schizophrenia
1. Catatonic
   a. Stupor or mutism.
   b. Negativism.
   c. Rigidity.
   d. Purposeless excitement.
   e. Posturing.
2. Disorganized
   a. Incoherence, marked loosening of associations, or grossly disorganized behavior.
   b. Flat or grossly inappropriate affect.
   c. Does not meet criteria for catatonic type.
3. Paranoid
   a. Preoccupation with systematized delusions or with frequent auditory hallucinations related to a single theme.
   b. None of the following: incoherence, loosening of associations, flat or grossly inappropriate affect, catatonic behavior, grossly disorganized behavior.
4. Undifferentiated type
   a. Prominent delusions, hallucinations, incoherence, or grossly disorganized behavior.
   b. Does not meet the criteria for paranoid, catatonic, or disorganized type.
5. Residual type
   a. Absence of prominent delusions, hallucinations, incoherence, or grossly disorganized behavior.
   b. Continuing evidence of the disturbance through two or more of the residual symptoms.
6. Type I and Type II.   A more recently suggested system proposes classification of schizophrenic patients into type I and type II. This system is based on the presence of positive or negative symptoms, sometimes referred to, respectively, as productive and deficit symptoms. The deficit symptoms include

affective flattening or blunting, poverty of speech or speech content, blocking, poor grooming, lack of motivation, anhedonia, social withdrawal, cognitive defects, and attentional deficits. Positive symptoms include loose associations, hallucinations, bizarre behavior, and increased speech. Type I patients have mostly positive symptoms, and type II patients have mostly negative symptoms.

F. Epidemiology

1. Incidence and prevalence. Lifetime prevalence is approximately 1%. An estimated 2 million Americans suffer from schizophrenia; worldwide, 2 million new cases appear each year. One in 100 Americans is hospitalized at some time for schizophrenia. Prevalence, morbidity, and severity of presentation are greater in urban than in rural areas. Furthermore, morbidity and severity of presentation are greater in industrialized than in nonindustrialized areas.

2. Sex ratio. Male = female.

3. Socioeconomic status. Increased prevalence in lower socioeconomic groups; equal incidence across socioeconomic classes (reflects downward drift theory, which states that although those with the disorder originally may have been born into any socioeconomic class, they eventually will tend to drift downward into the lower socioeconomic classes owing to their significant impairments).

4. Age of onset. Most common between ages 15–35 (50% below age 25). Rare before age 10 or after age 40.

5. Religion. Jews affected less than Protestants and Catholics.

6. Race. Prevalence reported to be higher among blacks and Hispanics than among whites, but investigators believe this may reflect bias on part of diagnosticians. (May also reflect higher percentage of minority people living in lower socioeconomic groups and in industrialized urban areas.)

7. Seasonality. Higher incidences in both winter and early spring (January–April in United States, July–September in southern hemisphere).

8. Inpatient versus outpatient. From 1965–1975, number of schizophrenic patients in hospitals decreased by 40–50%. Currently, up to 80% of schizophrenic patients are treated as outpatients.

9. Cost. Direct and indirect cost to United States approximately $10–12 billion/year.

G. Etiology. Owing to heterogeneity of symptomatic and prognostic presentations of schizophrenia, no single etiologic factor is considered causative. Model most often used is the stress-diathesis model, which states that the person who develops schizophrenia has a specific biologic vulnerability, or diathesis, that is triggered by stress and leads to schizophrenic symptoms. Stresses may be biologic, genetic, psychosocial, or environmental.

1. Genetic. Both single gene and polygenic theories have been proposed (Table 6–5). Although neither theory has been definitively substantiated, the polygenic theory appears to be more consistent with the presentation of schizophrenia.

a. **Consanguinity** — incidence in families is higher than in the general population (Table 6–6). Monozygotic concordance is greater than dizygotic.

b. **Concordance** — proportion of affected twins whose co-twins are or will be affected (Table 6–6).

TABLE 6-5. **FEATURES CONSISTENT WITH POLYGENIC INHERITANCE**

(Number of affected genes determines individual's risk and symptomatic picture)
1. Transmission of disorder possible with two normal parents
2. Presentation of disorder ranges from very severe to less severe
3. More severely affected individuals have a greater number of ill relatives than mildly affected individuals
4. Risk decreases as the number of shared genes decreases
5. Disorder present in both mother's and father's side of family

TABLE 6-6. **GENETICS OF SCHIZOPHRENIA**

		Risk
General population	=	1%
First-degree relatives	=	10–12%
Second-degree relatives	=	5–6%
Child of two schizophrenic parents	=	40%
Dizygotic twin	=	12–15%
Monozygotic twin	=	45–50%

Mother = Father (schizophrenia is not a sex-linked illness. It does not matter which parent has the disorder in terms of risk.)

    c. **Adoption studies** — risk is secondary to biologic parent, not adoptive parent.
       i. Risk to an adopted child (approximately 10–12%) is the same as if the child had been reared by his/her biologic parents.
      ii. An increased prevalence of schizophrenia exists in biologic parents of schizophrenic adoptees over adoptive parents.
     iii. Monozygotic twins reared apart have same concordance rate as twins reared together.
     iv. Children born to nonaffected parents who are raised by a schizophrenic parent do not have increased rates of schizophrenia.
    d. Nine out of every 10 schizophrenic patients have no first-degree relative with schizophrenia.
  2. Biochemical
    a. **Dopamine hypothesis** — schizophrenic symptoms are in part a result of hyperdopaminergic activity caused by hypersensitive dopamine receptors or increased dopamine activity. Antipsychotic medications bind to D_2 dopamine receptors and cause functional decreases in dopamine activity. The mesocortical and mesolimbic central nervous system (CNS) dopaminergic tracts are those most implicated in schizophrenia. Drugs that increase dopamine worsen or trigger psychosis, e.g., amphetamine, cocaine. Dopamine is important in the symptomatic manifestations of schizophrenia, but in a complex way that has not yet been fully elucidated.
    b. **Norephinephrine hypothesis** — increased activity in schizophrenia, leading to increased sensitization to sensory input.
    c. **γ-Aminobutyric acid (GABA) hypothesis** — decreased GABA activity results in increased dopamine activity.
    d. **Serotonin hypothesis** — abnormal serotonin metabolism apparently occurs in some chronic schizophrenic patients, with both hyper- and hyposerotonemia being reported.

e. **Phenylethylamine (PEA)** — an endogenous amine very similar to amphetamine. In increased amounts may be responsible for a generally increased endogenous vulnerability to psychosis.

f. **Hallucinogens** — has been suggested that some endogenous amines may act as substrates for abnormal methylation, resulting in endogenous hallucinogens. No reliable data exist to support this hypothesis.

g. **Enzymes** — monoamine oxidase (MAO), dopamine-β-hydroxylase (DBH), catechol-O-methyltransferase (COMT), and creatinine phosphokinase (CPK) have all been investigated. Findings have included evidence that (1) decreased platelet MAO levels appear to correlate with severe psychopathology in general, (2) DBH inhibitors increase psychosis in some schizophrenic patients, (3) COMT is not consistently elevated or depressed in schizophrenia, (4) elevated levels of CPK are seen in some schizophrenic and manic patients.

h. **Endorphins and prostaglandins** — no conclusive evidence available.

i. **Gluten** — component of wheat protein to which some schizophrenic patients may be intolerant.

3. Psychosocial

a. **Family factors** — patients whose families have high expressed emotion (EE) have higher relapse rates than those whose families have lower expressed emotion. Expressed emotion has been defined as any overly involved, intrusive behavior, be it hostile and critical or controlling and infantilizing. Relapse rates are better when family behavior is modified to lower expressed emotion. Most observers believe that family dysfunction represents a consequence, rather than a cause, of schizophrenia.

b. **Psychodynamic issues** — see Psychodynamic factors (Section J) and Treatment interview (Section M). Understanding which psychosocial stressors may be specific to individual schizophrenic patients is crucial. Knowing what psychologic and environmental stresses are most likely to trigger psychotic decompensation in a patient helps the clinician supportively address these issues and, in the process, helps the patient to feel and remain more in control.

4. Infectious theory.
Evidence for slow virus etiology includes neuropathologic changes consistent with past infections: gliosis, glial scarring, and presence of antiviral antibodies in the serum and cerebrospinal fluid (CSF) of some schizophrenic patients. Increased frequency of perinatal complications and seasonality of birth data also can support an infectious theory.

H. Lab and psychological tests

1. Brain imaging

a. **Computed tomography (CT) scan** — cortical atrophy in 10-35% of patients; enlargement of the lateral and third ventricle in 10-50% of patients; atrophy of the cerebellar vermis and decreased radiodensity of brain parenchyma. There may be correlation between abnormal CT scan findings and presence of negative symptoms (e.g., flattened affect, social withdrawal, psychomotor retardation, lack of motivation), neuropsychiatric impairment, increased frequency of extrapyramidal symptoms from antipsychotic medications, and poorer premorbid history.

    b. **Positron emission tomography (PET)** — in some, decreased frontal and parietal lobe metabolism, relatively high posterior metabolism, and abnormal laterality.

    c. **Cerebral blood flow (CBF)** — in some, decreased resting levels of frontal blood flow, increased parietal blood flow, and decreased whole brain blood flow. When PET scan and CBF studies are placed together with CT scan findings, dysfunction of the frontal lobe is most clearly implicated. Frontal lobe dysfunction may be secondary, however, to pathology elsewhere in the brain.

2. Electroencephalogram (EEG). Most schizophrenic patients have normal EEGs, but some have decreased alpha and increased theta and delta activity; paroxysmal abnormalities; and increased sensitivity to activation procedures, e.g., sleep deprivation.

3. Evoked potential (EP) studies. Initial hypersensitivity to sensory stimulation, with later compensatory blunting of information processing at higher cortical levels.

4. Immunologic studies. In some, atypical lymphocytes and decreased numbers of natural killer cells.

5. Endocrinologic studies. In some, decreased levels of luteinizing hormone (LH) and follicle-stimulating hormone (FSH); diminished release of prolactin and growth hormone when stimulated by gonadotropin-releasing hormone or thyrotropin-releasing hormone (TRH).

6. Neuropsychologic testing. Thematic Apperception Test (TAT) and Rorschach usually reveal bizarre responses. When compared with parents of normal controls, parents of schizophrenic patients show more deviation from normals in projective tests (may be consequence of living with schizophrenic family member). Halstead-Reitan Battery reveals impaired attention and intelligence, decreased retention time, and disturbed problem-solving ability in approximately 20–35% of patients. Schizophrenic patients have decreased intelligence quotients (I.Q.s) when compared with nonschizophrenic patients, although the range of I.Q. scores is wide. Decline in I.Q. occurs with progression of the illness.

I. Pathophysiology. No consistent structural defects; changes noted include decreased number of neurons, increased gliosis, and disorganization of neuronal architecture. Degeneration in limbic system, especially the amygdala, hippocampus, and cingulate cortex, as well as in the basal ganglia, especially substantia nigra and dorsolateral prefrontal cortex.

    Minor (soft) neurologic findings occur in 50–100% of patients: increased prevalence of primitive reflexes, such as grasp reflex, abnormal stereognosis and two-point discrimination, and dysdiadochokinesia (impairment in ability to perform rapidly alternating movements). Paroxysmal saccadic eye movements (inability to follow object through space with smooth eye movements) observed in 50–80% of schizophrenic patients, as well as in 40–45% of first-degree relatives of schizophrenic patients (compared with an 8–10% prevalence in nonschizophrenic persons). This may be a neurophysiologic marker of a vulnerability for schizophrenia. Resting heart rate levels have been found to be higher in schizophrenic patients than in controls and may reflect a hyperaroused state.

J. Psychodynamic factors. Understanding a patient's dynamics (or psychologic conflicts and issues) is critical for complete understanding of the symbolic meaning of symptoms. A patient's internal experience is usually one of confusion and overwhelming sensory input, and defense mechanisms are the ego's attempt to deal with powerful affects. Three major primitive defenses interfere with reality testing: (1) Psychotic projection—inner sensations of aggression, sexuality, chaos, and confusion are projected as occuring in the outside world as opposed to emanating from within; there is confusion about boundaries between inner and outer experience. Projection is major defense underlying paranoia. (2) Reaction formation—turning a disturbing idea or impulse into its opposite. (3) Psychotic denial—involves transformation of confusing stimuli into delusions and hallucinations.

K. Differential diagnosis
1. **Organic mental disorders.** Present with impaired memory, orientation, and cognition; visual hallucinations; signs of CNS damage. Many neurologic and medical disorders can present with symptoms identical to those of schizophrenia, including substance-induced organic mental disorders (e.g., cocaine, phencyclidine [PCP]), CNS infections (e.g., herpes encephalitis), vascular disorders (e.g, systemic lupus erythematosus), complex partial seizures (e.g., temporal lobe epilepsy), and degenerative disease (e.g., Huntington's chorea).
2. **Schizophreniform disorder.** Symptoms may be identical to schizophrenia, but are of less than 6 months' duration. There is also less deterioration and a better prognosis.
3. **Brief reactive psychosis.** Symptoms are of less than 1 month's duration and are secondary to a clearly identifiable psychosocial stress.
4. **Mood disorders.** Both bipolar disorder (mania) and major depression may present with psychotic symptoms similar to schizophrenia. The differential is particularly important because of the availability of specific and effective treatments for the mood disorders. DSM-III-R states that mood symptoms in schizophrenia must be brief relative to the essential criteria. Also, if hallucinations and delusions are present in a mood disorder, they develop after the mood disturbance and do not persist. Other factors that help differentiate mood disorders from schizophrenia include family history, premorbid history, course (e.g., age of onset), prognosis (e.g., absence of residual deterioration following the psychotic episode), and response to treatment. A postpsychotic depression may occur in schizophrenic patients which can be severe enough to be diagnosed as major depression. True depression in these patients must be differentiated from medication side effects, such as sedation, akinesia, and flattening of affect.
5. **Schizoaffective disorder.** Mood symptoms develop concurrently with symptoms of schizophrenia, but delusions or hallucinations must be present for 2 weeks in the absence of prominent mood symptoms during some phase of the illness. The prognosis of this disorder is better than that expected for schizophrenia and worse than that for mood disorders.
6. **Atypical pyschosis.** A psychosis in which there is a confusing clinical feature, such as persistent auditory hallucinations as the only symptom, or specific culture-bound psychoses.

7. **Delusional disorders.** Nonbizarre, systematized delusions of at least 6 months' duration in the context of an intact, relatively high-functioning personality and in the absence of prominent hallucinations or other schizophrenic symptoms. Onset is in middle to late adult life.

8. **Personality disorders.** Generally without psychotic symptoms and, if present, tend to be transient and not prominent. Most important personality disorders in this differential are schizotypal, schizoid, borderline, and paranoid.

9. **Factitious disorder with psychological symptoms and malingering.** No lab test or biologic marker can objectively confirm the diagnosis of schizophrenia. Schizophrenic symptoms are therefore possible to feign for either clear secondary gain (malingering) or deeper psychologic motivations (factitious disorder).

10. **Pervasive developmental disorder (infantile autism).** This diagnosis is made if onset is between 30 months and 12 years. Although behavior may be quite bizarre and deteriorated, there are no delusions, hallucinations, or clear formal thought disorder, e.g., loosening of associations.

11. **Mental retardation.** May have similar intellectual, behavioral, and mood disturbances, which suggest schizophrenia. Generally, however, there are no overt psychotic symptoms, and there is a constant low level of functioning rather than a deterioration. If pyschotic symptoms are present, a diagnosis of schizophrenia may be made concurrently.

12. **Shared cultural beliefs.** Odd beliefs shared and accepted by a cultural group and thus not considered psychotic.

L. **Course and prognosis**

1. **Course.** Prodromal symptoms of anxiety, perplexity, terror, or depression generally precede the onset of schizophrenia, which may be acute or insidious. Prodromal symptoms may be present for months before definitive diagnosis is made. Onset is generally in the late teens and early 20s. Precipitating events, such as emotional trauma, drugs, and separations, may trigger episodes of illness in those predisposed. Classically, the course of schizophrenia is one of deterioration over time, with acute exacerbations superimposed on a chronic picture. Vulnerability to stress is lifelong. Postpsychotic depressive episodes may occur in the residual phase. Over the course of the illness, the more florid positive psychotic symptoms, such as bizarre delusions and hallucinations, tend to diminish in intensity, while the more residual negative symptoms, such as poor hygiene, flattened emotional response, and various oddities of behavior, may actually increase.

   Relapse rates are approximately 40% in 2 years on medication and 80% in 2 years off medication. Suicide is attempted in 50% of patients; 10% are successful. Violence is not greater than in general population. There is increased risk of sudden death, medical illness, and shortened life expectancy.

2. **Prognosis.** Schizophrenic patients in nonindustrialized, developing countries have better prognoses than do patients in industrialized, western societies.

   a. **Good prognosis** schizophrenia is associated with
      i. Acute onset with obvious precipitating factors.
      ii. Good premorbid social and work history (including later age of onset).

iii. Mood symptoms (especially depression).

iv. Paranoid subtype.

v. Possibly catatonic subtype. Some evidence that catatonic schizophrenia may be associated with mood disorders; these patients respond more often to electroconvulsive therapy (ECT) and lithium, and family histories are higher for mood disorders than other schizophrenic subtypes.

vi. Married.

vii. Family history of mood disorder.

viii. Predominance of positive symptoms.

ix. Confusion.

x. Tension, anxiety, hostility.

b. Poor prognosis schizophrenia is associated with

i. Insidious onset with no precipitating factors.

ii. Poor premorbid social and work history (including earlier age of onset).

iii. Withdrawn, autistic behavior.

iv. Disorganized and undifferentiated subtypes.

v. Not married.

vi. Family history of schizophrenia.

vii. History of difficult delivery.

viii. Presence of neurologic signs and symptoms. These include poor cognitive functioning on formal neuropsychiatric testing and abnormalities on CT and PET scans, as well as on EEG and evoked potential studies.

ix. Predominance of negative symptoms.

x. Absence of mood symptoms or overt hostility.

In terms of overall prognosis, some investigators have described a loose rule of thirds: approximately ⅓ of patients lead somewhat normal lives, ⅓ continue to experience significant symptoms but are able to function within society, and the remaining ⅓ may be markedly impaired and require frequent hospitalizations. Approximately 10% of this final third of patients require chronic institutionalization.

M. Treatment. Clinical management of the schizophrenic patient may include hospitalization and antipsychotic medication, as well as psychosocial treatments, such as behavioral, family, group, individual, and social skills and rehabilitation therapies.

1. Psychopharmacologic

a. Choice of drug — antipsychotic drugs ameliorate and reduce the signs and symptoms of schizophrenia. Consider low potency antipsychotic drugs (chlorpromazine [Thorazine]) if patient is hyperactive or agitated. Consider high potency antipsychotic drugs (trifluoperazine [Stelazine]) if patient is withdrawn or lethargic. Clozapine (Clozaril) is used in resistant cases.

In general, both high and low potency drugs are equally effective, but one may work better than another in an individual case.

b. Dosage — use chlorpromazine as reference for relative potency (Table 6–7). Start with 25 mg orally or intramuscularly and raise to 300–1,800 mg daily for acute attacks. Titrate dose upward until therapeutic effect achieved. Haloperidol (Haldol) may be used for rapid tranquilization (1–10 mg orally or intramuscularly over 30-60 minutes); daily dosage may go as high as 100 mg. Long-acting depot fluphenazine (Prolixin, Permitil) concentrate/decanoate (25 mg intramuscularly) or haloperidol can be effective for 14-21 days and is helpful in increasing compliance.

c. **Maintenance** — after signs and symptoms abate and patient is stablized (usually after 4 weeks), dosage can be reduced to lowest level to maintain patient in symptom-free state. After 6 months in remission, drug can be withdrawn for trial period to see if relapse occurs, at which point therapy is reinstituted. Some patients may be on lifelong maintenance therapy to prevent relapse.

d. **Adverse side effects** — adverse effects of antipsychotics are discussed in Chapter 22, Organic Therapy.

If traditional antipsychotic medication alone is ineffective, several other drugs have been reported to cause varying degrees of improvement. The addition of lithium may be helpful in a significant percentage of patients; propranolol (Inderal), benzodiazepines, and carbamazepine (Tegretol) have been reported to lead to improvement in some cases.

TABLE 6–7. **ANTIPSYCHOTICS**

Drug	Average daily oral dose range, mg	Potency ratio compared with 100 mg chlorpromazine
Phenothiazines:		
Aliphatics:		
Chlorpromazine (Thorazine)	400–800	1:1
Piperazines:		
Fluphenazine (Prolixin)	4–20	1:50
Fluphenazine enanthate or		
decanoate	25–100*	
Perphenazine (Trilafon)	8–32	1:10
Trifluoperazine (Stelazine)	6–20	1:20
Piperidines:		
Thioridazine (Mellaril)	200–600	1:1 (approx)
Butyrophenones:		
Haloperidol (Haldol)	8–32	1:50
Haloperidol decanoate	+	1:50
Thioxanthenes:		
Chlorprothixene (Taractan)	400–800	1:1
Thiothixene (Navane)	15–30	1:25
Oxoindoles:		
Molindone (Moban, Lidone)	40–200	1:10
Dibenzoxazepines:		
Loxapine (Loxitane)	60–100	1:10

*Intramuscular injection, long-acting, every 1-3 weeks
+ Intramuscular injection, long-acting, administered at monthly intervals. Initial dose should not exceed 100 mg, and clinical experience at doses greater than 300 mg/month has been limited.

2. **Electroconvulsive therapy.**   Used effectively in small percentage of schizophrenic patients, particularly those of the catatonic subtype. Patients with an illness duration of less than 1 year are most responsive.

3. **Psychosocial.**   Antipsychotic medication alone is not as effective in treating

schizophrenic patients as when the drugs are coupled with psychosocial interventions.

a. **Behavior therapy**

 i. **Token economy** — desired behaviors are positively reinforced by rewarding targeted behaviors with specific tokens, such as trips or privileges. Intent is for reinforced behavior to generalize to the world outside of hospital ward.

b. **Group therapy** — focus is on support and social skills development (activities of daily living). Groups are especially helpful in decreasing social isolation and increasing reality testing.

c. **Family therapy** — family therapy techniques can significantly decrease relapse rates for the schizophrenic family member. High expressed emotion family interaction can be diminished through family therapy. Multiple family groups (MFGs), in which family members of schizophrenic patients discuss and share issues, have been particularly helpful in this regard.

d. **Supportive psychotherapy** — traditional insight-oriented psychotherapy is not recommended in treating schizophrenic patients, whose egos are too fragile. Supportive therapy, which may include advice, reassurance, education, modeling, limit setting, and reality testing, is generally the therapy of choice. The rule is that as much insight as a patient desires and can tolerate is an acceptable goal.

e. **Interview techniques** — one must first understand as much as possible what schizophrenic patients may be feeling and thinking. Schizophrenic patients are described as having extremely fragile ego structures, which leave them open to an unstable sense of self and others, primitive defenses, and severely impaired ability to modulate external stress.

 The critical task for the interviewer is to establish contact with the patient in a manner that allows for a tolerable balance of autonomy and interaction.

 i. There is both a deep wish for and a terrible fear of interpersonal contact, called the need-fear dilemma.

 ii. The fear of contact may represent the fear of a fundamental intrusion, resulting in delusional fears of personal and world annihilation as well as loss of control, identity, and self.

 iii. The wish for contact may represent fears that, without human interaction, the individual is dead, nonhuman, mechanical, or permanently trapped.

 iv. Schizophrenic patients may project their own negative, bizarre, and frightening self-images onto others, leading the interviewer to feel as uncomfortable, scared, or angry as the patient. Aggressive or hostile impulses are particularly frightening to these patients and may lead them to disorganization in thought and behavior.

 v. Offers of help may be experienced as coercion, attempts to force the individual into helplessness, or being devoured.

f. **Suggestions for the psychiatric and psychotherapeutic interview: "Do's and don'ts"** — there is no one right thing to say to a schizophrenic patient. The most important job of the interviewer is to help to diminish the inner chaos, loneliness, and terror that the schizophrenic patient is feeling. The challenge is to convey empathy without being regarded as being dangerously intrusive.

1. **Don't try to argue** or rationally persuade the patient out of a delusion. Efforts to convince the patient that a delusion is not real will generally lead to more tenacious assertions of delusional ideas.

2. **Do listen.** How patients experience the world, e.g., dangerous, bizarre, overwhelming, invasive, is conveyed through their thought content and process. Listen for the feelings behind the delusional ideas—are they afraid, sad, angry, hopeless? Do they feel as though they have no privacy, no control? What is their image of themselves?

3. **Do acknowledge** these feelings to the patient, simply and clearly. For example, when the patient tells you, "When I walk into a room, people can see inside my head and read my thoughts," you might respond with, "What is that like for you?"

4. **Don't feel you have to say anything.** Careful listening can convey that you believe the person is human with something important to say.

5. **Be flexible** about interview times, both the number of visits and how long each visit lasts. If a patient can only tolerate 10 minutes, tell him/her that you will be back again later. Be clear and reliable about when you will be seeing the patient; it can be an indicator of your trustworthiness.

6. **Be straightforward** with a patient—don't pretend that you believe a delusion is actually true, but convey that you believe the delusion is true for the patient. Represent reality to the patient—the challenge is to be a consistent source of reality-testing without making the patient feel humiliated or rejected. For example, if a patient says, "This song on the radio was written just for me, can't you hear the message?" You might respond, "I can hear that the song is about feeling sad after losing someone, and that you must be feeling like that yourself."

7. **Use yourself** as an instrument—pay attention to how the patient makes you feel, because this often reflects the patient's characteristic style of interaction. Be careful to sort out whether you are feeling something in direct response to the patient as opposed to something else going on in your life, e.g., are you annoyed because you had a fight with a supervisor that morning or because the patient is making subtle, insulting remarks about doctors?

8. **Don't automatically laugh** at a patient when something is said that strikes you as funny. Actively psychotic people will describe delusions that can sound absurd or humorous, but clearly the patient does not experience them as funny. Laughing at a patient can convey disrespect and a lack of understanding of the underlying terror and despair that many patients feel. Keeping this in mind can help to decrease the urge to laugh. Laughter can be appropriate, such as when a patient purposefully tells you a joke. Humor can be an indication of health, unless it is used excessively or inappropriately.

9. **Do respect** a paranoid patient's need for distance and control. Many paranoid patients feel more comfortable with a certain formality and respectful aloofness, as opposed to expressions of warmth and empathy.

10. **Do answer certain personal questions**—try to turn the interview back to the patient. Answering some personal questions may help patients talk more freely

about themselves. For example, if the patient asks "Are you married?" you might respond, "Can you tell me why that's important to you?" *Patient*: "I just want to know; are you married?" *Interviewer*: "I will tell you, but let's talk a bit first about why that information is so important to you."

For more detailed discussion of this topic, see Karno M, Norquist GS: Schizophrenia: Epidemiology, Sec. 14.1, pp 699–705; Berman KF, Weinberger DR: Schizophrenia: Brain Structure and Function, Sec. 14.2, pp 705–717; Wyatt RJ, Kirch DG, DeLisi LE: Schizophrenia: Biochemical, Endocrine, and Immunological Studies, Sec. 14.2b, pp 717–732; Cloninger CR: Schizophrenia: Genetic Etiological Factors, Sec. 14.2c, pp 732–744; McGlashan TH: Schizophrenia: Psychodynamic Theories, Sec. 14.2d, pp 745–756; Grebb JA, Cancro R: Schizophrenia: Clinical Features, Sec. 14.3, pp 757–777; Kane JM: Schizophrenia: Somatic Treatment, Sec. 14.4, pp 777–792; Liberman RP, Mueser KT, Schizophrenia: Psychosocial Treatment, Sec. 14.5, pp 792–806; Schwartz DP: Schizophrenia: Individual Psychotherapy, Sec. 14.6, pp 806–815, in *CTP/V*.

7

Delusional and Other Psychotic Disorders

I. Delusional disorder

A. Definition. Disorder in which the primary, if not the sole, manifestation is a delusion that is fixed and unshakeable; previously known as paranoid disorder.

B. Signs and symptoms. Delusions are of at least 1 month's duration and are well systematized as opposed to bizarre or fragmented. Patient's emotional response to the delusional system is congruent with and appropriate to the content of the delusion. Personality remains intact or deteriorates minimally. Patients often are hypersensitive and hypervigilant, which may lead, despite their high-functioning capacities, to a relatively socially isolated existence. Under nonstressful circumstances, the patient may be judged to be without evidence of mental illness.

C. Diagnosis

TABLE 7–1. **DSM-III-R DIAGNOSTIC CRITERIA FOR DELUSIONAL DISORDER**

A. Nonbizarre delusion(s) (i.e., involving situations that occur in real life, such as being followed, poisoned, infected, loved at a distance, having a disease, being deceived by one's spouse or lover) of at least 1 month's duration.

B. Auditory or visual hallucinations, if present, are not prominent [as defined in schizophrenia, A(1)(b)].

C. Apart from the delusion(s) or its ramifications, behavior is not obviously odd or bizarre.

D. If a major depressive or manic syndrome has been present during the delusional disturbance, the total duration of all episodes of the mood syndrome has been brief relative to the total duration of the delusional disturbance.

Specify type: The following types are based on the predominant delusional theme. If no single delusional theme predominates, specify as unspecified type.

Erotomanic Type
Delusional disorder in which the predominant theme of the delusion(s) is that a person, usually of higher status, is in love with the subject.

Grandiose Type
Delusional disorder in which the predominant theme of the delusion(s) is one of inflated worth, power, knowledge, identity, or special relationship to a deity or famous person.

Jealous Type
Delusional disorder in which the predominant theme of the delusion(s) is that one's sexual partner is unfaithful.

Persecutory Type
Delusional disorder in which the predominant theme of the delusion(s) is that one (or someone to whom one is close) is being malevolently treated in some way. People with this type of delusional disorder may repeatedly take their complaints of being mistreated to legal authorities.

Somatic Type
Delusional disorder in which the predominant theme of the delusion(s) is that the person has some physical defect, disorder, or disease.

Unspecified Type
Delusional disorder that does not fit any of the previous categories, e.g., persecutory and grandiose themes without a predominance of either; delusions of reference without malevolent content.

Used with permission, APA.

D. Epidemiology. Incidence is approximately 1-3 new cases per 100,000. Prevalence reported at 0.03%, but may be higher because many patients do not seek help voluntarily. Women outnumber men by a slight margin. Age of onset from the mid-20s into the 90s, with average age of 40 years.

E. Etiology

  1. Genetic. Genetic studies indicate that delusional disorder is neither a subtype nor an early or prodromal stage of schizophrenia or mood disorder. No increased risk of schizophrenia or mood disorder in first-degree relatives.

  2. Biologic. Patients may have discrete defects in the limbic system and basal ganglia.

  3. Psychosocial. Delusional disorder is primarily psychosocial in origin. Common background characteristics include histories of physical/emotional abuse; cruel, erratic, and unreliable parenting; and overly demanding and perfectionistic upbringings. Basic trust (Erikson) does not develop, with the child believing that the environment is consistently hostile and potentially dangerous. Other psychosocial factors include a history of deafness, blindness, social isolation and loneliness, recent immigration or other abrupt environmental changes, and advanced age.

F. Lab and psychological tests. No lab test can be applied to help make diagnosis. Projective psychological tests reveal a preoccupation with paranoid or grandiose themes and issues of inferiority, inadequacy, and anxiety.

G. Pathophysiology. No known pathophysiology except those cases with discrete anatomic defects of limbic system or basal ganglia.

H. Psychodynamic factors. Defenses used: (1) denial, (2) reaction formation, (3) projection. Major defense is projection—symptoms are a defense against unacceptable ideas and feelings. Patients deny feelings of shame, humiliation, and inferiority; turn any unacceptable feelings into their opposites through reaction formation (inferiority into grandiosity); and project any unacceptable feelings outward onto others.

I. Differential diagnosis

  1. Organic delusional disorder. Organic disorders that may mimic delusional disorder include hypothyroidism and hyperthyroidism, Parkinson's disease, multiple sclerosis, Alzheimer's disease, substance abuse, tumors, and trauma to the basal ganglia.

  2. Paranoid personality disorder. No true delusions are present in the personality disorder, although overvalued ideas that verge on being delusional may be present. Predisposition to delusional disorder exists.

  3. Paranoid schizophrenia. More likely to present with prominent auditory hallucinations, personality deterioration, and more marked disturbance in role functioning. Age of onset tends to be younger in schizophrenia.

  4. Major depression. Depressed patients may have paranoid delusions secondary to mood disturbance, but the mood disturbance is primary and prominent with such associated characteristics as vegetative symptoms, positive family history, and response to antidepressants.

  5. Bipolar disorder. Manic patients may have grandiose or paranoid delusions, which are clearly secondary to the primary and prominent mood disorder; associated with such characteristics as euphoric and labile mood, positive family history, and response to lithium.

J. Course and prognosis. Disorder tends to be chronic and unremitting in 30–50% of patients. Less satisfactory response to pharmacotherapy than patients with delusional symptoms associated with schizophrenia or mood disorder. Psychotherapy difficult because of lack of trust.

K. Treatment. Rarely enter therapy voluntarily; rather, are brought by concerned friends and relatives. Establishing rapport is difficult; patient's hostility is fear-motivated. Successful psychotherapy may enable patient to have better social adaption in spite of persistent delusion.

1. Hospitalization. Hospitalization is necessary if patient is unable to control suicidal or homicidal impulses; if there is extreme impairment, e.g., refusing to eat due to delusion about food poisoning; or if there is a need for a thorough organic workup.

2. Psychopharmacotherapy. Patients tend to refuse medications because of suspiciousness. Severely agitated patient may require intramuscular antipsychotic medication. Otherwise, low dose antipsychotics, e.g., 2 mg haloperidol (Haldol), may be tried. Delusional patients are more likely to react to side effects with delusional ideas; thus, a very gradual increase in dose is recommended to diminish the likelihood of disturbing side effects. Antidepressant may be of use with severe depression.

3. Psychotherapy: "Do's and Don'ts"
  a. Don't argue with or challenge the patient's delusions. A delusion may become even more entrenched if the patient feels it must be defended.
  b. Don't pretend that you believe the delusion is true, since you must represent reality to the patient. However, **do** listen to the patient's concerns about the delusion and try to understand what the delusion may mean specifically in terms of the patient's self-esteem.
  c. Do respond sympathetically to the fact that the delusion is disturbing and intrusive in the patient's life and offer to help the patient develop ways to live more comfortably with the delusion.
  d. Do understand that the delusional system may be a means of grappling with profound feelings of shame and inadequacy and that the patient may be hypersensitive to any imagined slights or condescensions, even when unintended.
  e. Do be very straightforward, honest, and upfront in all your dealings with the patient, since these patients are hypervigilant to being "tricked" or deceived. Explain side effects of medications and why you are giving medications, e.g., to help with anxiety, irritability, insomnia, anorexia; be reliable and on time for appointments; schedule regular appointments.
  f. Do examine what particular life stresses or life experiences triggered the first appearance of the delusion and try to understand what it was about these stresses that led to patient's feelings of shame or inadequacy. Understand that other similar stresses or experiences in the patient's life may exacerbate delusional symptoms. Help the patient develop alternative means of responding to stressful situations.

II. Schizoaffective disorder

A. Definition. A disorder with concurrent features of both schizophrenia and a mood disorder that cannot be diagnosed as either one separately.

B. Diagnosis, signs and symptoms

TABLE 7-2. **DSM-III-R DIAGNOSTIC CRITERIA FOR SCHIZOAFFECTIVE DISORDER**

A. A disturbance during which, at some time, there is either a major depressive or a manic syndrome concurrent with symptoms that meet the A criterion of schizophrenia.

B. During an episode of the disturbance, there have been delusions or hallucinations for at least 2 weeks, but no prominent mood symptoms.

C. Schizophrenia has been ruled out (i.e., the duration of all episodes of a mood syndrome has not been brief relative to the total duration of the psychotic disturbance).

Used with permission, APA.

C. Epidemiology. Lifetime prevalence less than 1%; there is no difference in prevalence between men and women.

D. Etiology. Some patients may be misdiagnosed; they are actually schizophrenic with prominent mood symptoms or have a mood disorder with prominent schizophrenic-like symptoms. There is no increased prevalence of schizophrenia in schizoaffective families, but there is increased prevalence of mood disorders in schizoaffective families. See etiology of schizophrenia and mood disorders for additional data.

E. Differential diagnosis. Any organic condition that causes either schizophrenic-like or mood symptoms must be considered. Any psychiatric condition that presents similarly to schizophrenia or a mood disorder must also be considered.

F. Course and prognosis. Poor prognosis associated with positive family history of schizophrenia, early and insidious onset without precipitating factors, predominance of psychotic symptoms, and poor premorbid history. Schizoaffective patients have a better prognosis than schizophrenic ones and a worse prognosis than mood disorder patients. Schizoaffective patients respond more often to lithium and are less likely to have a deteriorating course than schizophrenic patients.

G. Treatment. Antidepressant or antimanic treatments should always be attempted, and antipsychotic medication should be used to control acute psychotic symptoms.

III. Schizophreniform disorder

A. Definition. Symptom presentation identical to schizophrenia except that symptoms resolve within 6 months and there is a return to normal functioning.

B. Diagnosis, signs and symptoms

TABLE 7-3. **DSM-III-R DIAGNOSTIC CRITERIA FOR SCHIZOPHRENIFORM DISORDER**

A. Meets criteria A and C of schizophrenia

B. An episode of the disturbance (including prodromal, active, and residual phases) lasts less than 6 months. (When the diagnosis must be made without waiting for recovery, it should be qualified as "provisional.")

C. Does not meet the criteria for brief reactive psychosis, and it cannot be established that an organic factor initiated and maintained the disturbance.

Used with permission, APA.

  C. Epidemiology. Data are unavailable; however, the disorder may be less
  than half as common as schizophrenia.
  D. Etiology. Related more to mood disorders than to schizophrenia. In general,
  schizophreniform patients have more mood symptoms and a better prognosis
  than schizophrenic patients. Schizophrenia occurs less often in families of
  schizophreniform patients than in schizophrenic patients, but more frequent
  than in families of mood disorder patients.
  E. Differential diagnosis. Identical to that of schizophrenia.
  F. Course and prognosis. Good prognostic features include absence of blunted
  or flat affect, good premorbid functioning, confusion and disorientation at the
  height of the psychotic episode, shorter duration, acute onset, and onset of
  prominent psychotic symptoms within 4 weeks of any first noticeable change
  in behavior.
  G. Treatment. Antipsychotic medications should be used to treat psychotic
  symptoms, but should be withdrawn after 3-6 months. Recurrent episodes
  warrant a trial with lithium. Psychotherapy is critical in helping patients to
  understand and deal with their psychotic experiences.

IV. Brief reactive psychosis
  A. Definition. Symptoms are of less than 1 month's duration and follow an
  obvious stress in the patient's life.
  B. Signs and symptoms. Similar to those observed in other psychotic disorders, but with an increase in volatility and lability, confusion, disorientation,
  and affective symptoms.
  C. Diagnosis
  D. Epidemiology. No definitive data available. More highly associated in
  persons with preexisting personality disorders and in those who have previously experienced major stressors, such as disasters or dramatic cultural changes.
  E. Etiology. Mood disorders more common in the families of these patients.

TABLE 7–4. **DSM-III-R DIAGNOSTIC CRITERIA FOR BRIEF REACTIVE PSYCHOSIS**

A. Presence of at least one of the following symptoms indicating impaired reality testing (not culturally sanctioned):

(1) incoherence or marked loosening of associations
(2) delusions
(3) hallucinations
(4) catatonic or disorganized behavior

B. Emotional turmoil, i.e., rapid shifts from one intense affect to another, or overwhelming perplexity or confusion

C. Appearance of the symptoms in A and B shortly after, and apparently in response to, one or more events that, singly or together, would be markedly stressful to almost anyone in similar circumstances in the person's culture.

D. Absence of the prodromal symptoms of schizophrenia, and failure to meet the criteria for schizotypal personality disorder before onset of the disturbance.

E. Duration of an episode of the disturbance of from a few hours to 1 month, with eventual full return to premorbid level of functioning. (When the diagnosis must be made without waiting for the expected recovery, it should be qualified as "provisional.")

Used with permission, APA.

Psychosocial stress triggers psychotic episode. Psychosis is understood as defensive response in person with inadequate coping mechanisms.

F. Differential diagnosis. Organic etiologies must be ruled out—in particular, drug intoxication and withdrawal. Seizure disorders must also be considered. Schizophrenia, mood disorders, and transient psychotic episodes associated with borderline and schizotypal personality disorders must be ruled out.

G. Course and prognosis. Good prognostic indicators include a severe precipitating stressor (usually followed within hours by the psychosis), confusion and lability during the episode, good premorbid history, negative family history for schizophrenia, and short duration of symptoms (may last a few hours to days).

H. Treatment. Acute hospitalization may be required; antipsychotic medications may not be necessary, because often the symptoms can resolve very quickly on their own. If medication is required, use as low a dose as possible and discontinue as soon as possible. Psychotherapy is extremely important to address the nature and significance of the specific social stress that triggered the psychotic episode. Patients must build more adaptive and less devastating means of coping with future stress.

V. Induced psychotic disorder

A. Definition. Delusional system shared by two or more persons; previously called shared paranoid disorder and *folie à deux*.

B. Signs and symptoms. Persecutory delusions are most common, and the key presentation is the sharing and blind acceptance of these delusions between two people. Suicide or homicide pacts may be present.

C. Diagnosis

TABLE 7–5.   **DSM-III-R DIAGNOSTIC CRITERIA FOR INDUCED PSYCHOTIC DISORDER**

A. A delusion develops (in a second person) in the context of a close relationship with another person, or persons, with an already established delusion (the primary case).

B. The delusion in the second person is similar in content to that in the primary case.

C. Immediately before the onset of the induced delusion, the second person did not have a psychotic disorder or the prodromal symptoms of schizophrenia.

Used with permission, APA.

D. Epidemiology. The disorder is rare; more common in women and in persons with physical disabilities that make them largely dependent on another person. 95% of cases involve family members, the most common relationship being between two sisters.

E. Etiology. The cause is primarily psychologic; however, there may be genetic input because it most often affects members of the same family. There is a risk of schizophrenia in the families of people with this disorder. Psychologic or psychosocial factors include a socially isolated relationship in which one person is submissive and dependent and the other is dominant with an established psychotic system.

F. **Psychodynamic factors.** The dominant psychotic personality maintains some contact with reality through the submissive partner, while the submissive personality is desperately anxious to be cared for and accepted by the dominant partner. A strongly ambivalent relationship often exists between the two.

G. **Differential diagnosis.** Rule out a personality disorder, malingering, and factitious disorder in the submissive partner. Organic etiologies must always be considered.

H. **Course and prognosis.** Recovery rates vary; some are as low as 10-40%. Traditionally, the submissive partner is separated from the dominant, psychotic partner with ideal outcome of a rapid diminution in the psychotic symptoms. If symptoms do not remit, the submissive individual may meet the criteria for a major psychotic disorder, such as schizophrenia or delusional disorder.

I. **Treatment.** Separate the two individuals and help the more submissive, dependent partner develop other means of support to compensate for the loss of the relationship. Antipsychotic medications are beneficial.

VI. Psychotic disorder not otherwise specified (NOS)

A. **Definition.** Patients whose psychotic presentation does not meet the diagnostic criteria for any established psychotic disorder; also known as atypical psychoses.

B. **Signs and symptoms.** This diagnostic category includes disorders that present with various psychotic features, e.g., delusions, hallucinations, loosening of associations, catatonic behaviors, but that cannot be delineated as any specific disorder. The disorders may include rare or exotic syndromes, such as specific culture-bound syndromes.

C. **Diagnosis**

TABLE 7–6. **DSM-III-R DIAGNOSTIC CRITERIA FOR PSYCHOTIC DISORDER NOT OTHERWISE SPECIFIED (ATYPICAL PSYCHOSIS)**

Disorders in which there are psychotic symptoms (delusions, hallucinations, incoherence, marked loosening of association, catatonic excitement or stupor, or grossly disorganized behavior) that do not meet the criteria for any other nonorganic psychotic disorder. This category should also be used for psychoses about which there is inadequate information to make a specific diagnosis. (This is preferable to "diagnosis deferred," and can be changed if more information becomes available.) This diagnosis is made only when it cannot be established that an organic factor initiated and maintained the disturbance.

Examples:
(1) psychoses with unusual features (e.g., persistent auditory hallucinations as the only disturbance)
(2) postpartum psychoses that do not meet the criteria for an organic mental disorder, psychotic mood disorder, or any other psychotic disorder
(3) psychoses with confusing clinical features that make a more specific diagnosis impossible

Used with permission, APA.

D. **Postpartum psychosis**
1. **Definition.** Syndrome occurring after childbirth characterized by severe depression and delusions.
2. **Diagnosis, signs and symptoms.** Most cases occur 2-3 days postpartum. Initial complaints of insomnia, restlessness, and emotional lability progress to confusion, irrationality, delusions, obsessive concerns about infant. Thoughts of wanting to harm baby or self are characteristic.

3. **Epidemiology.**   Occurs in 1-2 per 1,000 deliveries. Most episodes occur in primiparas.

4. **Etiology.**   Usually secondary to underlying mental illness, such as schizophrenia or bipolar disorder.

   a. Sudden change in hormonal levels after parturition may contribute.

   b. Psychodynamic conflicts about motherhood—unwanted pregnancy, trapped in unhappy marriage, fears of mothering.

5. **Differential diagnosis**

   a. **Postpartum blues** — normal period of emotional lability occurs postpartum in majority of women. Clears spontaneously. No evidence of psychotic thinking.

   b. **Drug-induced depression** — associated with postanesthetic states, such as that after cesarean section or scopolamine-meperidine (Demerol) analgesia (twilight sleep).

   c. **Organic mental syndrome** — rule out infection, hormonal imbalance, e.g., hypothyroidism, encephalopathy associated with toxemia of pregnancy, preeclampsia.

6. **Course and prognosis.**   Risk of infanticide, suicide, or both is high in untreated cases. Supportive family network, good premorbid personality, and appropriate treatment associated with good to excellent prognosis.

7. **Treatment.**   Suicidal precautions in presence of suicidal ideation. Do not leave infant alone with mother if delusions are present or if there are ruminations about infant's health.

   a. **Pharmacologic** — medication for primary symptoms: antidepressants for suicidal ideation and depression; antianxiety agents for agitation, insomnia (e.g., lorazepam [Ativan] 0.5 mg every 4-6 hours); lithium for manic behavior; antipsychotic agents for delusions (e.g., haloperidol [Haldol] 0.5 mg every 6 hours).

   b. **Psychologic** — psychotherapy, both indvidual and marital, to deal with intrapsychic or interpersonal conflicts. Consider discharging mother and infant to home only after arrangements for temporary homemaker are in place to reduce environmental stresses associated with care of newborn.

E. **Autoscopic psychosis.**   Rare hallucinatory psychosis during which patient sees a phantom or spectre of his/her own body. Usually psychogenic in origin, but consider irritable lesion of temporoparietal lobe. Responds to reassurance, antipsychotic medications, or both.

F. **Capgras syndrome.**   Delusion that persons in the environment are not their real selves but are doubles imitating the patient or imposters imitating someone else. May be part of schizophrenic illness. Treat with antipsychotic medication. Psychotherapy is useful in understanding dynamics of the delusional belief, e.g., distrust of certain real persons in the environment.

G. **Cotard's syndrome.**   Delusions of nihilism, e.g., nothing exists, body has disintegrated, world is coming to an end. Usually seen as part of schizophrenia or severe bipolar disorder. May be early sign of Alzheimer's disease. May respond to antipsychotic or antidepressant medication.

For more detailed discussion of this topic, see Manschreck TC: Delusional (Paranoid) Disorders, Chap. 15, pp 816–829; Procci WR: Schizoaffective Disorder, Schizophreniform Disorder, and Brief Reactive Psychosis, Sec. 16.1, pp 830–842; Neppe VM, Tucker GJ: Atypical, Unusual, and Cultural Psychoses, Sec. 16.2, pp 842–852; Inwood DG: Postpartum Psychotic Disorders, Sec. 16.3 pp 852–858, in *CTP/V*.

8

Mood (Affective) Disorders

I. General introduction

Mood is a sustained emotional tone perceived along a normal continuum of sad to happy. Mood disorders are characterized by abnormal feelings of depression or euphoria with associated psychotic features in some severe cases. Mood disorders are divided into bipolar and depressive disorders.

II. Depression
A. Signs and symptoms
1. Data obtained from history
   a. Anhedonia—inability to experience pleasure.
   b. Withdrawal from friends or family.
   c. No motivation, low frustration tolerance.
   d. Vegetative signs:
      1. Loss of libido.
      2. Weight loss and anorexia.
      3. Weight gain and hyperphagia.
      4. Low energy level; fatigability.
      5. Abnormal menses.
      6. Early morning awakening (terminal insomnia); approximately 75% of depressed patients have sleep difficulties, either insomnia or hypersomnia.
      7. Diurnal variation (symptoms worse in morning).
   e. Constipation.
   f. Dry mouth.
   g. Headache.
2. Data obtained from mental status examination (MSE)
   a. **General appearance and behavior** — psychomotor retardation or agitation, poor eye contact, tearful, downcast, inattentive to personal appearance.
   b. **Affect** — constricted, intense.
   c. **Mood** — depressed, irritable, frustrated, sad.
   d. **Speech** — little or no spontaneity, monosyllabic, long pauses, soft, low, monotone.
   e. **Thought content** — 60% of depressed patients have suicidal ideation, and 15% of depressed patients commit suicide; obsessive rumination; pervasive feelings of hopelessness, worthlessness, and guilt; somatic preoccupations; indecisiveness; poverty of content; hallucinations and delusions (mood-congruent themes of guilt, poverty, nihilism, deserved persecution, somatic preoccupation); little spontaneity.
   f. **Sensorium** — distractable, difficulty concentrating, complaints of poor memory, apparent disorientation; abstract thought may be impaired.

g. **Insight/judgment** — impaired due to cognitive distortions of personal worthlessness.

B. Diagnosis

Table 8–1.   **DSM-III-R DIAGNOSTIC CRITERIA FOR MAJOR DEPRESSIVE EPISODE**

Note: A "major depressive syndrome" is defined as criterion A below.

A. At least five of the following symptoms have been present during the same two-week period and represent a change from previous functioning; at least one of the symptoms is either (1) depressed mood, or (2) loss of interest or pleasure. (Do not include symptoms that are clearly due to a physical condition, mood-incongruent delusions or hallucinations, incoherence, or marked loosening of associations.)

(1) depressed mood (or can be irritable mood in children and adolescents) most of the day, nearly every day, as indicated either by subjective account or observation by others

(2) markedly diminished interest or pleasure in all, or almost all, activities most of the day, nearly every day (as indicated either by subjective account or observation by others of apathy most of the time)

(3) significant weight loss or weight gain when not dieting (e.g., more than 5% of body weight in a month), or decrease or increase in appetite nearly every day (in children, consider failure to make expected weight gains)

(4) insomnia or hypersomnia nearly every day

(5) psychomotor agitation or retardation nearly every day (observable by others, not merely subjective feelings of restlessness or being slowed down)

(6) fatigue or loss of energy nearly every day

(7) feelings of worthlessness or excessive or inappropriate guilt (which may be delusional) nearly every day (not merely self-reproach or guilt about being sick)

(8) diminished ability to think or concentrate, or indecisiveness, nearly every day (either by subjective account or as observed by others)

(9) recurrent thoughts of death (not just fear of dying), recurrent suicidal ideation without a specific plan, or a suicide attempt or a specific plan for committing suicide

B. (1) It cannot be established that an organic factor initiated and maintained the disturbance

(2) The disturbance is not a normal reaction to the death of a loved one (uncomplicated bereavement)

Note: Morbid preoccupation with worthlessness, suicidal ideation, marked functional impairment or psychomotor retardation, or prolonged duration suggest bereavement complicated by major depression.

C. At no time during the disturbance have there been delusions or hallucinations for as long as two weeks in the absence of prominent mood symptoms (i.e., before the mood symptoms developed or after they have remitted).

Used with permission, APA.

1. Associated features

a. Somatic complaints may mask depression—in particular, cardiac, gastrointestinal (GI), genitourinary (GU), low back pain, or orthopedic complaints.

b. Content of delusions and hallucinations, when present, tend to be congruent with depressed mood; most common are delusions of guilt, poverty, and deserved persecution, as well as somatic and nihilistic (end of the world) delusions. Mood-incongruent delusions are those with content not apparently related to the predominant mood, such as delusions of thought insertion, broadcasting, and control or persecutory delusions unrelated to depressive themes.

2. Age-specific features.   Depression can present differently at different ages.

a. **Prepubertal** — somatic complaints, agitation, single-voice auditory hallucinations, anxiety disorders, and phobias.

b. **Adolescence** — substance abuse, antisocial behavior, restlessness, truancy, school difficulties, promiscuity, increased sensitivity to rejection, poor hygiene.

  c. **Elderly** — cognitive deficits (memory loss, disorientation, and confusion), pseudodementia or the dementia syndrome of depression, apathy, distractability.

C. Types of depressive disorders

1. Major depression. Severe episodic depressive disorder. Also known as unipolar depression. Symptoms must be present at least 2 weeks and represent a change from previous functioning. More common in women by 2:1. Precipitating event occurs in at least 25% of patients. Diurnal variation with symptoms worse early in morning. Psychomotor retardation or agitation present. Associated with vegetative signs and mood-congruent delusions; hallucinations may be present. Median age of onset—40 years, but can occur at any time. Genetic factor present.

  Melancholic subtype—severe and responsive to biologic intervention.

Table 8–2. **DSM-III-R DIAGNOSITC CRITERIA FOR MELANCHOLIC TYPE (MELANCHOLIA)**

The presence of at least five of the following:

  (1) loss of interest or pleasure in all, or almost all, activities
  (2) lack of reactivity to usually pleasureable stimuli (does not feel much better, even temporarily, when something good happens)
  (3) depression regularly worse in the morning
  (4) early morning awakening (at least 2 hours before usual time of awakening)
  (5) psychomotor retardation or agitation (not merely subjective complaints)
  (6) significant anorexia or weight loss (e.g., more than 5% of body weight in a month)
  (7) no significant personality disturbance before first major depressive episode
  (8) one or more previous major depressive episodes followed by complete, or nearly complete, recovery
  (9) previous good response to specific and adequate somatic antidepressant therapy, e.g., tricyclics, ECT, MAOI, lithium

Used with permission, APA.

  Chronic subtype—present for at least 2 years; more common in elderly men, especially alcohol and substance abusers; and responds poorly to medications. Makes up 10-15% of those with major depression.

2. Dysthymia. Previously known as depressive neurosis. Less severe than major depression, is more common and chronic in women. Insidious onset. Occurs more often in persons with history of chronic stress or acute losses; often coexists with other psychiatric disorders, such as substance abuse, personality disorders, and obsessive-compulsive disorder. Symptoms tend to be worse later in the day. Onset generally in 20s-30s, although there is an early onset type, which begins before age 21. More common among first-degree relatives with major depression. Symptoms should include at least two of the following: poor appetite, overeating, sleep problems, fatigue, low self esteem, poor concentration or difficulty making decisions, and feelings of hopelessness. Secondary type of dysthymia refers to depression secondary to another condition, e.g., anorexia, arthritis.

3. Major depression—seasonal pattern. Depression that comes with shortened daylight in winter and fall and disappears during spring and summer; also known as seasonal affective disorder (SAD). Characterized by hypersomnia, hyperphagia, and psychomotor slowing. Related to abnormal melatonin metabolism. Treated with exposure to bright, artificial light for 3–6 hours/day.

4. **Postpartum depression.** Severe depression beginning shortly after childbirth, usually beginning within 30 days of birth. Most often occurs in women with underlying or preexisting mood or other psychiatric disorder. Symptoms range from marked insomnia, lability, and fatigue to suicide. Homicidal and delusional beliefs can occur about the baby. Can be psychiatric emergency with both mother and baby at risk.

5. **Myxedema madness.** Hypothyroidism associated with fatigability, depression, and suicidal impulses. May mimic schizophrenia with thought disorder, delusions, hallucinations, paranoia, and agitation. More common in women.

6. **Organic mood disorders, depressed type.** Depression secondary to known organic cause, e.g., Cushing's syndrome, propranolol (Inderal) medication (Table 8–3).

TABLE 8–3. **CAUSES OF ORGANIC DEPRESSIONS**

Type	Depression
Pharmacologic	Corticosteroids; contraceptives; Reserpine; α-methyldopa; anticholinesterases; insecticides; amphetamine withdrawal; cimetidine; indomethacin; phenothiazines; thallium; mercury; cycloserine; vincristine; vinblastine
Infectious	General paresis (tertiary syphilis); influenza; acquired immune deficiency syndrome (AIDS); viral pneumonia; viral hepatitis; infectious mononucleosis; tuberculosis
Endocrine	Hypo- and hyperthyroidism; hyperparathyroidism; menses-related; postpartum; Cushing's disease (hyperadrenalism); Addison's disease (adrenal insufficiency)
Collagen	Systemic lupus erythematosus (SLE); rheumatoid arthritis
Neurologic	Multiple sclerosis; Parkinson's disease; head trauma; complex partial seizures (temporal lobe); cerebral tumors; stroke; dementing diseases in early stages; sleep apnea
Nutritional	Vitamin deficiencies (B_{12}, C, folate, niacin, thiamine)
Neoplastic	Cancer of the head of the pancreas; disseminated carcinomatosis

Table adapted from Berkow R, ed: *Merck Manual*, ed 15. Merck Sharp & Dohme Research Laboratories, Rahway, NJ, 1987, p 1515, with permission.

7. **Pseudodementia.** Diagnosed as the dementia syndrome of depression in DSM-III-R. Major depressive disorder presenting as cognitive dysfunction resembling dementia. Occurs in elderly. Occurs more often in patients with previous history of mood disorder. Depression is primary and preeminent, antedating cognitive deficits.

8. **Adjustment disorder with depressed mood.** Moderate depression in response to clearly identifiable stress, which resolves as stress diminishes. Considered a maladaptive response due to either impairment in functioning or excessive and disproportionate intensity of symptoms. Individuals with personality disorders or organic deficits may be more vulnerable.

9. **Grief.** Not a true depressive disorder. Known as uncomplicated bereavement in DSM-III-R. Profound sadness secondary to major loss. May

present very similarly to major depression with anhedonia, withdrawal, and vegetative signs. Remits with time. Differentiated from major depression by absence of suicidal ideation or profound feelings of hopelessness and worthlessness. Usually resolves within a year. May develop into major depressive episode in predisposed individuals.

10. Depression in children. Not uncommon. Same signs and symptoms as adults. Masked depression seen in running away from home, school phobia, substance abuse. Suicide may occur.

11. Double depression. Dysthymic patients who develop superimposed major depression (about 10–15%).

12. Atypical depression. Known as depressive disorder not otherwise specified in DSM-III-R. Depressive features that do not meet criteria for specific mood disorder, such as intermittent dysthymic episodes. Diagnosis is used to describe depression characterized by weight gain and hypersomnia rather than weight loss and insomnia.

III. Mania
A. Signs and symptoms
1. Data obtained from history
a. Erratic and disinhibited behavior:
  1. Excessive spending of money.
  2. Excessive gambling.
  3. Hypersexuality, promiscuity.
b. Overextended in activities and responsibilities.
c. Low frustration tolerance.
d. Vegetative signs:
  1. Increased libido.
  2. Weight loss and anorexia.
  3. Insomnia (expressed as no need to sleep).
  4. Excessive energy.

2. Data obtained from mental status examination (MSE)
a. **General appearance and behavior** — psychomotor agitation, seductive, colorful clothes, excessive makeup, inattention to personal appearance or bizarre combinations of clothes, intrusive, entertaining, threatening, hyperexcited.

b. **Affect** — labile, intense (may have rapid depressive shifts).

c. **Mood** — euphoric, expansive, irritable, demanding, flirtatious.

d. **Speech** — pressured, loud, dramatic, exaggerated, may become incoherent.

e. **Thought content** — highly elevated self-esteem, grandiosity, highly egocentric, delusions and less frequently hallucinations (mood-congruent—themes of inflated self-worth and power; most often grandiose and paranoid).

f. **Thought process** — flight of ideas (if severe, can lead to incoherence), racing thoughts, neologisms, clang associations, circumstantiality, tangentiality.

g. **Sensorium** — highly distractable, difficulty concentrating; memory, if not too distracted, generally intact; abstract thinking generally intact.

h. Insight/judgment — extremely impaired; often total denial of illness and inability to make any organized or rational decisions.

B. Diagnosis

TABLE 8–4. **DSM-III-R DIAGNOSTIC CRITERIA FOR MANIC EPISODE**

Note: A "manic syndrome" is defined as including criteria A, B, and C below. A "hypomanic syndrome" is defined as including criteria A and B, but not C, i.e., no marked impairment.

A. A distinct period of abnormally and persistently elevated, expansive, or irritable mood.

B. During the period of mood disturbance, at least three of the following symptoms have persisted (four if the mood is only irritable) and have been present to a significant degree:

(1) inflated self-esteem or grandiosity
(2) decreased need for sleep, e.g., feels rested after only three hours of sleep
(3) more talkative than usual or pressure to keep talking
(4) flight of ideas or subjective experience that thoughts are racing
(5) distractibility, i.e., attention too easily drawn to unimportant or irrelevant external stimuli
(6) increase in goal-directed activity (either socially, at work or school, or sexually) or psychomotor agitation
(7) excessive involvement in pleasurable activities which have a high potential for painful consequences, e.g., the person engages in unrestrained buying sprees, sexual indiscretions, or foolish business investments

C. Mood disturbance sufficiently severe to cause marked impairment in occupational functioning or in usual social activities or relationships with others, or to necessitate hospitalization to prevent harm to self or others.

D. At no time during the disturbance have there been delusions or hallucinations for as long as 2 weeks in the absence of prominent mood symptoms (i.e., before the mood symptoms developed or after they have remitted).

Used with permission, APA.

C. Types of manic or hypomanic disorders

1. Organic mood disorder, manic type. Symptoms secondary to organic disorder that antedates onset of symptom, e.g., brain tumor, carcinoid syndrome, cocaine (Table 8–5).

TABLE 8–5. **COMMON CAUSES OF ORGANIC MOOD DISORDERS, MANIC TYPE**

Cause	Mania
Pharmacologic	Corticosteroids; levodopa; bromocriptine; cocaine; amphetamines; methylphenidate; most heterocyclic antidepressants; monoamine oxidase inhibitors
Infectious	20% of patients with general paresis (tertiary syphilis); influenza; St. Louis encephalitis; AIDS
Endocrine	Hyperthyroidism (Cushing's); postpartum; menses-related
Collagen	SLE; rheumatic chorea
Neurologic	Multiple sclerosis; Huntington's chorea; Wilson's disease; head trauma; complex partial seizures (temporal lobe); diencephalic and 3rd ventricle tumors; strokes; migraines; neoplasms
Nutritional	Vitamin deficiencies (B_{12}, folate, niacin, thiamine)

Table adapted from Berkow R, ed: *Merck Manual*, ed 15. Merck Sharp & Dohme Research Laboratories, Rahway, NJ, 1987, p 1515, with permission.

2. Mad hatter's syndrome. Chronic mercury poisoning producing manic (sometimes depressive) symptoms.

3. Adolescent mania. Signs of mania masked by substance abuse, alcoholism, antisocial behavior.

4. Rapid cycling bipolar disorder. Alternating manic and depressive episodes separated by intervals of 48-72 hours. Bipolar disorder with mixed or rapid cycling episodes appears to be more chronic than bipolar disorder without alternating episodes.

5. Cyclothymia. Less severe form of bipolar disorder with alternating periods of hypomania and moderate depression. Is chronic and nonpsychotic. Symptoms must be present for at least 2 years. Is equally common in men and women. Onset usually insidious. Substance abuse common. Major depression and bipolar disorder are more common among first-degree relatives than among general population. Onset in late adolescence or early adulthood. Recurrent mood swings may lead to social and professional difficulties. May be responsive to lithium.

6. Bipolar II. Term often used to describe disorder in which individual has had at least one depressive episode and at least one hypomanic episode. In DSM-III-R, this would be officially classified as bipolar disorder not otherwise specified.

IV. Depression and mania
A. Summary of clinical differences

TABLE 8–6. **CLINICAL DIFFERENCES BETWEEN DEPRESSION AND MANIA**

	Depressive Syndrome	Manic Syndrome
Mood	Depressed, irritable, or anxious (the patient may, however, smile or deny subjective mood change and instead complain of pain or other somatic distress)	Elated, irritable, or hostile
	Crying spells (the patient may, however, complain of inability to cry or to experience emotions)	Momentary tearfulness (as part of mixed state)
Associated psychologic manifestations	Lack of self-confidence; low self-esteem; self-reproach	Inflated self-esteem; boasting; grandiosity
	Poor concentration; indecisiveness	Racing thoughts; clang associations (new thoughts triggered by word sounds rather than meaning); distractibility
	Reduction in gratification; loss of interest in usual activities; loss of attachments; social withdrawal	Heightened interest in new activities, people, creative pursuits; increased involvement with people (who are often alienated because of the patient's intrusive and meddlesome behavior); buying sprees; sexual indiscretions; foolish business investments
	Negative expectations; hopelessness; helplessness; increased dependency	
	Recurrent thoughts of death and suicide	
Somatic manifestations	Psychomotor retardation; fatigue Agitation	Psychomotor acceleration; eutonia (increased sense of physical well-being)
	Anorexia and weight loss, or weight gain	Possible weight loss from increased activity and inattention to proper dietary habits
	Insomnia, or hypersomnia	Decreased need for sleep
	Menstrual irregularities; amenorrhea	
	Anhedonia; loss of sexual desire	Increased sexual desire

TABLE 8–6.   **CLINICAL DIFFERENCES BETWEEN DEPRESSION AND MANIA (Continued)**

Psychotic symptoms	Delusions of worthlessness and sinfulness Delusions of reference and persecution Delusions of ill health (nihilistic, somatic, or hypochondriacal) Delusions of poverty Depressive hallucinations in the auditory, visual, and (rarely) olfactory spheres	Grandiose delusions of exceptional talent Delusions of assistance; delusions of reference and persecution Delusions of exceptional mental and physical fitness Delusions of wealth, aristocratic ancestry, or other grandiose identity Fleeting auditory or visual hallucinations

Table from Berkow R, ed: *Merck Manual*, ed 15. Merck Sharp & Dohme Research Laboratories, Rahway, NJ, 1987, p 1518, with permission.

B. Epidemiology

Table 8–7.   **EPIDEMIOLOGY OF DEPRESSIVE AND MANIC DISORDERS**

	Depression	Mania
Incidence (new cases per year)	1/100 men 3/100 women	1.2/100 men 1.8/100 women
Prevalence (existing cases)	2-3/100 men 5-10/100 women	1/100 men and women
Lifetime expectancy	10% men 20% women	1% men and women
Sex	2:1 women/men	Men = women (may be slightly higher in women)
Age	40—mean age men/women 10% occur after age 60 Small peak in adolescence 50% occur before age 40	30—mean age men/women
Race	No difference	No difference
Sociocultural	↑ risk with family history of alcohol/depression/parental loss before age 13 slighty ↑ risk in lower socioeconomic groups	↑ risk with family history of mania/bipolar illness No difference urban/rural Slightly increased in higher socioeconomic groups
Family history (see also Etiology, Genetic)	(Evidence for heritability stronger for bipolar disorder than for depression) Approximately 10-13% risk for first-degree relatives Monozygotic concordance rate higher than dizygotic but ratio not as high as seen in bipolar	20-25% risk for first-degree relatives 50% of bipolar patients have parent with mood disorder Child with one bipolar parent = 25% risk of developing disorder Child with two bipolar parents = 50-75% risk Bipolar monozygotic concordance rate = 40-70% Bipolar dizygotic concordance rate = 20%

C. Etiology
1. Biologic
a. Hormonal — in general, neuroendocrine abnormalities probably reflect disruptions in biogenic amine input to the hypothalamus. Hyperactive

hypothalamic-pituitary-adrenal axis in depression leading to increased cortisol secretion. Also in depression—blunted release of thyroid-stimulating hormone (TSH); decreased growth hormone (GH), decreased follicle-stimulating hormone (FSH), decreased luteinizing hormone (LH), and decreased testosterone. Changes in immune functions (decreased) in both mania and depression.

b. **Chemistries** — decreased biogenic amine (norepinephrine, serotonin, dopamine) activity in depression—increased in mania. Biogenic amine metabolites 5-hydroxyindoleacetic acid (5-HIAA) (from serotonin), homovanillic acid (HVA) (from dopamine), 3-methoxy-4-hydroxyphenylglycol (MHPG) (from norepinephrine)—altered in blood, urine, and cerebrospinal fluid (CSF). Some assaultive, violent, depressed suicidal patients show decreased 5-HIAA in CSF. Dysregulation of adrenergic-cholinergic system with cholinergic dominance.

c. **Sleep** — abnormalities in 60-65% of mood disorder patients. In depression, increased rapid eye movement (REM) density in first half of sleep, increased REM time overall, decreased REM latency (beginning of first REM period after falling asleep), decreased stage 4 sleep. Multiple awakenings common in mania, with overall decrease in sleep time.

d. **Genetic** — both bipolar and major depressive disorders run in families, but evidence for heritability higher for bipolar disorder.

One parent with bipolar disorder   — 25% chance in child.
Two parents with bipolar disorder   — 50-75% chance in child.
One monozygotic twin bipolar   — 40-70% chance in other twin.
    — Dizygotic twins about 20%.
One parent with depressive disorder   — 10-13% chance in child.

Concordance rates in depression variable but monozygotic:dizygotic ratio lower than for bipolar disorder.

Dominant gene on short arm of chromosome 11 associated with catecholamine metabolism dysfunction found in one Amish family with a strong history of bipolar disorder.

2. **Psychosocial**

a. **Psychoanalytic** — symbolic or real loss of loved person (love object) perceived as rejection. Mania and elation viewed as defense against underlying depression. Rigid superego serves to punish person for guilt feelings about unconscious sexual or aggressive impulses. Freud described internalized ambivalence toward love object, which can produce a pathologic form of mourning if the object is lost or perceived as lost. This mourning takes the form of a major depression with feelings of guilt, worthlessness, and suicidal ideation.

b. **Cognitive** — cognitive triad of Aaron Beck: (1) negative self view ("things are bad because I'm bad"); (2) negative interpretation of experience (everything has always been bad); (3) negative view of future (anticipation of failure). Learned helplessness is a theory that describes depression as occurring when a person is helpless to control events. Theory derives from observed behavior of experimental animals given unexpected random shocks from which they could not escape.

D. Tests
1. Lab tests

a. **Dexamethasone suppression test (DST)** — nonsuppression (a positive DST) due to hypersecretion of cortisol secondary to hyperactivity of hypothalamic-pituitary-adrenal axis. Abnormal in 50% of major depressives. Of limited clinical usefulness owing to frequency of false-positives and negatives. **Thyroid-stimulating hormone (THS)**—diminished release in response to thyrotropin-releasing hormone (TRH); reported in both depression and mania. **Prolactin release**—decreased in response to tryptophan. Tests are not definitive.

2. Psychological tests

a. **Zung Self-Rating Scale** — scored by patients; index of depressive intensity; **Hamilton Depression Scale**—scored by examiner; **Rorschach Test**—standardized set of 10 inkblots scored by examiner—few associations, slow response time in depression; **Thematic Apperception Test (TAT)**—series of 30 pictures depicting ambiguous situations and interpersonal events. Patient creates a story about each scene—depressives will create depressed stories, manics more grandiose and dramatic ones.

b. **Psychophysiology** — no gross brain changes. Enlarged cerebral ventricles on computed tomography (CT) scan in some patients with mania or psychotic depression; diminished basal ganglia blood flow in some depressive patients.

c. **Psychodynamics** (see also Etiology, Psychosocial) — in depression, introjection of ambivalently viewed lost object leading to an inner sense of conflict, guilt, rage, pain, and loathing; a pathologic mourning, which becomes depression as ambivalent feelings meant for introject are directed at self. In mania, feelings of inadequancy and worthlessness converted by means of denial, reaction formation, and projection to grandiose delusions.

E. Differential diagnosis

1. Organic mood disorder.
Depression/mania secondary to drugs or medical illness: cocaine, amphetamine, propranolol, steroids, brain tumor, metabolic illness. Cognitive deficits usually present. (See also Tables 8–3 and 8–4.)

2. Schizophrenia.
Acutely, schizophrenia can look exactly like an acute manic episode or an episode of major depression with psychotic features. To differentiate, must rely on such factors as family history, course, premorbid history, and response to medication. Depression or mania with presence of mood-incongruent delusions or hallucinations, such as thought insertion and broadcasting; loose associations or flight of ideas; poor reality testing; inattention to personal hygiene; or bizarre behavior can be mistaken for schizophrenia and may have a poorer prognosis than depression or mania with mood-congruent psychotic features.

3. Dysthymia/cyclothymia.
Chronic, signs of depression or elation not as severe, no hallucinations or delusions; "subaffective" disorders.

4. Grief.
Self-limited, no suicidal ideation, no severe decrease in self-esteem.

5. **Substance abuse.** History of drug use when combined with depression or bipolar disorder called dual diagnosis. Must always rule out when patient presents with depressive or manic symptoms.
6. **Personality disorder.** Lifelong behavioral pattern associated with rigid defensive style; depression may occur more readily after stressful life event due to inflexibility of coping mechanisms. Manic episode may also occur more readily in predisposed people with preexisting personality disorder. Can diagnose both simultaneously with mood disorder on Axis I and personality disorder on Axis II.
7. **Schizoaffective disorder.** Signs and symptoms of schizophrenia accompany prominent mood symptoms. Course and prognosis between that of schizophrenia and mood disorders.
8. **Pseudodementia.** (Dementia syndrome of depression) cognitive impairment in elderly occurs as a result of depression. Not a true dementia associated with brain damage or dysfunction. Responsive to electroconvulsive therapy (ECT) or antidepressant medication.

F. **Course and prognosis.** 15% of depressed patients eventually commit suicide. Untreated, average depressed episode lasts about 10 months. At least 75% of affected patients have second episode of depression—most common in first 6 months after initial episode. Average number of depressive episodes in a lifetime is five. Prognosis generally good: 50% recover, 30% partially recover, 20% have chronic course. About 20-30% of dysthymic or cyclothymic patients develop major depression ("double depression") or mania. 45% of manic episodes recur. Untreated, manic episodes last 3-6 months with high rate of recurrence (average of 10 recurrences). 80-90% of manic patients eventually experience a full depressive episode. Prognosis fair: 15% recover; 50-60% partially recover (multiple relapses with good interepisodic functioning), and one-third have some evidence of chronic symptoms and social deterioration.

G. **Treatment of depression.** Acute major depression is treatable in 70-80% of patients.
1. **Pharmacologic.** Indicated in almost all major depressions and may be used in some cases of dysthymia. See Table 8-8.
   a. Begin with heterocyclic antidepressants at lowest dose and monitor over 2-3 week period. Response usually seen within 4 weeks. About 75% of patients respond positively. If symptoms are still present at 4-6 weeks, serum drug levels should be obtained.
   b. Triiodothyronine (T_3), lithium, or amphetamine may be added to supplement the heterocyclic antidepressant. If symptoms still persist, a second heterocyclic antidepressant from a different class may be tried.
   c. If symptoms still do not improve, try a monoamine oxidase inhibitor (MAOI). MAOI is quite safe with reasonable dietary restrictions of tyramine-containing substances.
   d. Newer serotonergic antidepressants should be considered when anticholinergic side effects need to be avoided.
   e. Maintenance treatment for at least 6 months with antidepressants helps to prevent relapse. Chronic treatment may be indicated in patients with

TABLE 8–8.   **ANTIDEPRESSANT MEDICATIONS USED TO TREAT DEPRESSION**

Antidepressant	Sedation	Anticholinergic	Dosage Range (Mg/day)
III° and II° amine tricyclic antidepressants			
Amitriptyline	+ + +	+ + +	50–300
↓			
Nortriptyline*	+ +	+ +	50–150
Imipramine	+ +	+ +	50–300
↓			
Desipramine*	+	+	50–300
Other tricyclic antidepressants			
Doxepin	+ + +	+ +	50–300
Trimipramine	+ + +	+ +	50–400
Clomipramine	+ +	+ +	50–300
Protriptyline	±	+ + +	10–60
Newer antidepressants			
Amoxapine	+ +	+	150–600
Maprotiline	+ +	+	50–300
Trazodone	+ + +	0	150–600
Fluoxetine	±	0	20–80
Bupropion	±	±	200–450

*Arrows indicate biotransformed secondary amine tricyclic; such transformation is usually complete with imipramine and variable with amitriptyline.
Table adapted from Berkow R, ed: *Merck Manual*, ed 15. Merck Sharp & Dohme Research Laboratories, Rahway, NJ, 1987, p 1523, with permission.

recurrent major depressions. Lithium appears to be effective as an adjunct in treating recurrent major depression.

   f. ECT useful in refractory major depressions; also indicated when rapid therapeutic response is desired or when side effects of antidepressant medications must be avoided. (ECT is underused as first-line antidepressant treatment.)

   g. If there is family history of positive response to particular drug, that drug should be tried first.

   h. Lithium should be first-line antidepressant in treatment of the depression of bipolar disorder. A heterocyclic antidepressant, T_3, or MAOI may be added as necessary.

2. **Psychologic.** Psychotherapy in conjunction with antidepressants has been shown to be more effective than either treatment alone in treatment of major depression.

   a. **Cognitive therapy** — based on correcting chronic distortions in thinking, which lead to depression, in particular the cognitive triad; feelings of helplessness and hopelessness about oneself, one's future, and one's past. Short-term treatment with interactive therapist and assigned homework aimed at testing and correcting negative cognitions and the unconscious assumptions that underlie them.

   b. **Behavior therapy** — based on premises of learning theory (classical and operant conditioning)—generally short-term and highly structured; aimed at specific, circumscribed undesired behaviors. The operant conditioning technique of positive reinforcement may be an effective adjunct in the treatment of depression.

  c. Interpersonal therapy (IPT) — developed as specific short-term treatment for nonbipolar, nonpsychotic, outpatient depression. Emphasis on ongoing, current interpersonal issues as opposed to unconscious, intrapsychic dynamics.

  d. Psychoanalytically oriented psychotherapy — insight-oriented therapy of indeterminate length aimed at achieving understanding of unconscious conflicts and motivations that may be fueling and sustaining depression.

  e. Supportive psychotherapy — therapy of indeterminate length with primary aim to provide emotional support. Indicated particularly in acute crisis, such as grief, or in period of time when patient is beginning to recover from a major depression but is not yet able to engage in more demanding, interactive therapy.

  f. Group therapy — not indicated for acutely suicidal patients. Other depressed patients may benefit from support, ventilation, and positive reinforcement of groups, as well as from interpersonal interaction and immediate correction of cognitive and transference distortions by other group members.

  g. Family therapy — particularly indicated when patient's depression is disrupting family stability, when depression is related to family events, or when depression is supported or maintained by family patterns.

H. Treatment of bipolar disorder
1. Pharmacologic

  a. Lithium is treatment of choice; effective in 80% of patients. With acute manic symptoms, lithium plus an antipsychotic (generally haloperidol [Haldol]) is necessary because the clinical response to lithium generally takes 7-10 days. A complete lithium trial should last at least 4 weeks before deciding to discontinue.

  b. A lithium blood level of 0.8-1.2 mEq/L is generally necessary for control of acute symptoms. A lower blood level, e.g., 0.4-0.8 mEq/L, is often sufficient nonacutely as a maintenance level. For most adult patients, reasonable starting dose is 300 mg three times/day. Eventual dose usually ranges between 900-2,100 mg/day. Toxicity can occur quickly at blood levels close to therapeutic levels, e.g., 2.0 mEq/L and above.

  c. The need for maintenance lithium is determined by the patient's history of previous severe manic episodes. Maintenance dose should be the lowest possible amount that controls symptoms and produces minimal side effects. If manic symptoms occur while patient is on lithium, an antipsychotic may be added or dose of lithium increased.

  d. Lithium is treatment of choice for the depressed phase of bipolar disorder, both acutely and prophylactically. If episodes of major depression occur while a patient is on lithium, an antidepressant may be added or dose of lithium increased.

  e. Pretreatment workup for lithium includes a serum creatinine level, electrolyte screen, thyroid function tests, complete blood count (CBC), electrocardiogram (EKG), and a pregnancy test as indicated. Lithium toxicity is potentially fatal and may consist of vomiting, severe diarrhea, severe tremor, ataxia, seizures, mental confusion, focal neurologic signs, hyperreflexia, dysarthria and coma. Generally, less serious adverse effects include gastric distress, weight gain, tremor, fatigue, and mild cognitive deficits. Other adverse effects involve the kidneys, thryoid, heart, and skin. Lithium is teratogenic and has been associated with birth defects affecting the heart.

f. After 4 weeks, if lithium is ineffective by itself in controlling manic symptoms, other drugs may be tried, in particular, carbamazepine (Tegretol), either alone or in conjunction with lithium. Other drugs used in treatment of mania include valproic acid (Depakene), verapamil (Isoptin, Calan), clonidine (Catapres), and clonazepam (Klonopin).

g. The usual initial dose of carbamazepine is 200 mg 2 times/day, increased by 200 mg/day each week until plasma level of 6-8 mg/L is achieved. Usual daily dose range is 1,200 to 2,000 mg. Pretreatment workup includes CBC with differential and liver function tests. Most serious adverse effects are hepatotoxicity, aplastic anemia, and agranulocytosis; less serious effects include nausea, sedation, dizziness, and blurred vision.

2. Psychologic. Psychotherapy in conjunction with antimanic drugs, e.g., lithium, is more effective than either treatment alone. Psychotherapy is not indicated when a patient is acutely and floridly manic. In this situation, the safety of the patient and others must be paramount, and steps must be taken, pharmacologically and physically, to protect and calm the patient.

a. **Cognitive therapy** — has been studied in relation to increasing compliance with lithium among bipolar patients.

b. **Behavior therapy** — can be most effective during inpatient treatment of manic patients in helping to set limits on impulsive or inappropriate behavior through such techniques as positive and negative reinforcement and token economies.

c. **Psychoanalytically oriented psychotherapy** — can be beneficial in the recovery and stabilization of manic patients, if patient is capable of and desires insight into underlying conflicts that may trigger and fuel manic episodes. Can also help patients understand resistances to medication and thus increase compliance.

d. **Supportive psychotherapy** — indicated particularly during more acute phases and in early recompensation. Some patients may only be able to tolerate supportive therapy, whereas others as they recover may be able to tolerate greater degrees of insight-oriented therapy. Supportive therapy more often indicated with chronic bipolar patients who may have significant interepisodic residual symptoms and social deterioration.

e. **Group therapy** — can be very helpful in challenging denial and defensive grandiosity of manic patients. Useful in addressing such common issues among manic people as loneliness, shame, inadequacy, fear of mental illness, and loss of control. Helpful in reintegrating patients socially.

f. **Family therapy** — particularly important with bipolar patients, because their disorder is strongly familial (20-25% of first-degree relatives) and because acute manic episodes are so disruptive to patients' interpersonal and job relationships. During manic episodes, patient may spend huge amounts of family money or act sexually inappropriate; residual feelings of anger, guilt, and shame among family members must be addressed. Ways to help with compliance and recognizing triggering events can be explored.

For more detailed discussion of this topic, see Mollica RF: Mood Disorders: Epidemiology, Sec. 17.1, pp 859–867; Schildkraut JJ, Green AI, Mooney JJ: Mood Disorders: Biochemical Aspects, Sec. 17.2a, pp 868–879; Gershon ES, Berrettini WH, Goldin LR: Mood Disorders: Genetic Aspects, Sec. 17.26, pp 879–888; Silber A: Mood Disorders: Psychodynamic Etiology, Sec. 17.2c, pp 888–892; Hamilton M: Mood Disorders: Clinical Features, Sec. 17.3, pp 892–913; Post RM: Mood Disorders: Somatic Treatment, Sec. 17.4, pp 913–933; Hirschfeld RMA, Shea MT: Mood Disorders: Psychosocial Treatments, Sec. 17.5, pp 933–944; Docherty JP: Group Psychotherapy of Depression, Sec. 17.6, pp 944–951, in *CTP/V*.

9
Anxiety Disorders

A. Definition

A pathologic state characterized by a feeling of dread accompanied by somatic signs indicative of a hyperactive autonomic nervous system. Differentiated from fear, which is a response to a known cause.

B. Signs and symptoms

TABLE 9–1. SIGNS AND SYMPTOMS OF ANXIETY DISORDERS

Physical Signs	Psychologic Symptoms
Trembling, twitching, feeling shaky	Feeling of dread
Backache, headache	Difficulty concentrating
Muscle tension	Hypervigilance
Shortness of breath, hyperventilation	Insomnia
Fatigability	Decreased libido
Startle response	"Lump in the throat"
Autonomic hyperactivity	"Butterflies in the stomach"
Flushing and pallor	
Tachycardia, palpitations	
Sweating	
Cold hands	
Diarrhea	
Dry mouth (xerostomia)	
Urinary frequency	
Paresthesia	
Difficulty swallowing	

C. Diagnosis, types of anxiety disorders.

The five types of anxiety disorders are (1) panic disorder—massive anxiety, sudden onset, no precipitating factor; (2) generalized anxiety disorder—chronic free-floating anxiety; (3) phobic disorder—anxiety about specific situation or object; (4) obsessive-compulsive disorder—persistent need to repeat thoughts or behaviors, and (5) post-traumatic stress disorder—anxiety following major life stressor. Each disorder is discussed below.

1. Panic disorder. Characterized by spontaneous panic attacks and may be associated with agoraphobia (fear of being in open spaces, outside the home alone, or in a crowd).

Agoraphobia can occur alone, although usually patients have associated panic attacks. Anticipatory anxiety is characterized by the feeling that panic and helplessness or humiliation will occur at some future time. Agoraphobics may become housebound and never leave the home or only go outside with a companion. See Tables 9-2 and 9-3.

2. Generalized anxiety disorder. Characterized by chronic, generalized anxiety for at least 1 month's duration. See Table 9-4.

3. Phobic disorder. Marked by irrational fear of object or situation and the need to avoid it. Divided into **social phobia** (fear of public situation, e.g., public speaking) or **simple phobia** (fear of object, e.g., horses, or isolated situations, e.g., heights).

TABLE 9–2. **DSM-III-R DIAGNOSTIC CRITERIA FOR PANIC DISORDER**

A. At some time during the disturbance, one or more panic attacks (discrete periods of intense fear or discomfort) have occurred that were (1) unexpected, i.e., did not occur immediately before or on exposure to a situation that almost always caused anxiety, and (2) not triggered by situations in which the person was the focus of others' attention.

B. At least four of the following symptoms developed during at least one of the attacks:

(1) shortness of breath (dyspnea) or smothering sensations
(2) dizziness, unsteady feelings, or faintness
(3) palpitations or accelerated heart rate (tachycardia)
(4) trembling or shaking
(5) sweating
(6) choking
(7) nausea or abdominal distress
(8) depersonalization or derealization
(9) numbness or tingling sensations (paresthesias)
(10) flushes (hot flashes) or chills
(11) chest pain or discomfort
(12) fear of dying
(13) fear of going crazy or of doing something uncontrolled

Used with permission, APA.

TABLE 9–3. **DSM-III-R DIAGNOSTIC CRITERIA FOR PANIC DISORDER WITH AGORAPHOBIA**

A. Meets the criteria for panic disorder.

B. Agoraphobia: Fear of being in places or situations from which escape might be difficult (or embarrassing) or in which help might not be available in the event of a panic attack. (Include cases in which persistent avoidance behavior originated during an active phase of panic disorder, even if the person does not attribute the avoidance behavior to fear of having a panic attack.) As a result of this fear, the person either restricts travel or needs a companion when away from home, or else endures agoraphobic situations despite intense anxiety. Common agoraphobic situations include being outside the home alone, being in a crowd or standing in a line, being on a bridge, and traveling in a bus, train, or car.

Used with permission, APA.

TABLE 9–4. **DSM-III-R DIAGNOSTIC CRITERIA FOR GENERALIZED ANXIETY DISORDER**

A. Unrealistic or excessive anxiety and worry (apprehensive expectation) about two or more life circumstances (e.g., worry about possible misfortune to one's child who is in no danger and worry about finances for no good reason, for a period of 6 months or longer, during which the person has been bothered more days than not by these concerns. In children and adolescents, this may take the form of anxiety and worry about academic, athletic, and social performance.)

B. At least six of the following 18 symptoms are often present when anxious (do not include symptoms present only during panic attacks):

Motor tension

(1) trembling, twitching, or feeling shaky
(2) muscle tension, aches, or soreness
(3) restlessness
(4) easy fatigability

Autonomic hyperactivity

(5) shortness of breath or smothering sensations
(6) palpitations or accelerated heart rate (tachycardia)
(7) sweating, or cold clammy hands
(8) dry mouth
(9) dizziness or lightheadedness
(10) nausea, diarrhea, or other abdominal distress
(11) flushes (hot flashes) or chills
(12) frequent urination
(13) trouble swallowing or "lump in throat"

TABLE 9–4.   DSM-III-R DIAGNOSTIC CRITERIA FOR GENERALIZED ANXIETY DISORDER (Continued)

Vigilance and scanning

(14) feeling keyed up or on edge
(15) exaggerated startle response
(16) difficulty concentrating or "mind going blank" because of anxiety
(17) trouble falling or staying asleep
(18) irritability

Used with permission, APA.

4. Obsessive-compulsive disorder.   Recurrent intrusive ideas, impulses, thoughts (obsessions), or patterns of behavior (compulsions) that are ego-alien and produce anxiety if resisted.

TABLE 9–5.   DSM-III-R DIAGNOSTIC CRITERIA FOR SOCIAL PHOBIA

A. A persistent fear of one or more situations (the social phobic situations) in which the person is exposed to possible scrutiny by others and fears that he or she may do something or act in a way that will be humiliating or embarrassing. Examples include being unable to continue talking while speaking in public, choking on food when eating in front of others, being unable to urinate in a public lavatory, hand-trembling when writing in the presence of others, and saying foolish things or not being able to answer questions in social situations.

B. During some phase of the disturbance, exposure to the specific phobic stimulus (or stimuli) almost invariably provokes an immediate anxiety response.

C. The phobic situation(s) is avoided, or is endured with intense anxiety.

D. The avoidant behavior interferes with occupational functioning or with usual social activities or relationships with others, or there is marked distress about having the fear.

E. The person recognizes that his or her fear is excessive or unreasonable.

Used with permission, APA.

TABLE 9–6   DSM-III-R DIAGNOSTIC CRITERIA FOR SIMPLE PHOBIA

A. A persistent fear of a circumscribed stimulus (object or situation) other than fear of having a panic attack (as in panic disorder) or of humiliation or embarrassment in certain social situations (as in social phobia).

B. During some phase of the disturbance, exposure to the specific phobic stimulus (or stimuli) almost invariably provokes an immediate anxiety response.

C. The object or situation is avoided, or endured with intense anxiety.

D. The fear or the avoidant behavior significantly interferes with the person's normal routine or with usual social activities or relationships with others, or there is marked distress about having the fear.

E. The person recognizes that his or her fear is excessive or unreasonable.

Used with permission, APA.

TABLE 9–7.   DSM-III-R DIAGNOSTIC CRITERIA FOR OBSESSIVE-COMPULSIVE DISORDER

A. Either obsessions or compulsions:

Obsessions: (1), (2), and (3):

(1) Recurrent and persistent ideas, thoughts, impulses, or images that are experienced, at least initially, as intrusive and senseless (e.g., a parent's having repeated impulses to kill a loved child, a religious person's having recurrent blasphemous thoughts).

(2) The person attempts to ignore or suppress such thoughts or impulses or to neutralize them with some other thought or action.

(3) The person recognizes that the obsessions are the product of his or her own mind, not imposed from without (as in thought insertion).

TABLE 9–7. **DSM-III-R DIAGNOSTIC CRITERIA FOR OBSESSIVE-COMPULSIVE DISORDER (Continued)**

Compulsions: (1), (2), and (3):

(1) Repetitive, purposeful, and intentional behaviors that are performed in response to an obsession, or according to certain rules or in a stereotyped fashion

(2) The behavior is designed to neutralize or to prevent discomfort or some dreaded event or situation; however, either the activity is not connected in a realistic way with what it is designed to neutralize or prevent, or it is clearly excessive.

(3) The person recognizes that his or her behavior is excessive or unreasonable (this may not be true for young children; it may no longer be true for people whose obsessions have evolved into overvalued ideas).

B. The obsessions or compulsions cause marked distress, are time-consuming (take more than an hour a day), or significantly interefere with the person's normal routine, occupational functioning, or usual social activities or relationships with others.

Used with permission, APA.

5. Post-traumatic stress disorder. Anxiety produced by extraordinary major life stress. Event is relived in dreams and waking thoughts. (Table 9-8).

Table 9–8. **DSM-III-R DIAGNOSTIC CRITERIA FOR POST-TRAUMATIC STRESS DISORDER**

A. The person has experienced an event that is outside the range of usual human experience and that would be markedly distressing to almost anyone (e.g., serious threat to one's life or physical integrity; serious threat or harm to one's children, spouse, or other close relatives and friends; sudden destruction of one's home or community; or seeing another person who has recently been, or is being, seriously injured or killed as the result of an accident or physical violence).

B. The traumatic event is persistently reexperienced in at least one of the following ways:

(1) Recurrent and intrusive distressing recollections of the event (in young children, repetitive play in which themes or aspects of the trauma are expressed)

(2) Recurrent distressing dreams of the event

(3) Sudden acting or feeling as if the traumatic event were recurring (includes a sense of reliving the experience, illusions, hallucinations, and dissociative [flashback] episodes, even those that occur upon awakening or when intoxicated)

(4) Intense psychological distress at exposure to events that symbolize or resemble an aspect of the traumatic event, including anniversaries of the trauma

C. Persistent avoidance of stimuli associated with the trauma or numbing of general responsiveness (not present before the trauma), as indicated by at least three of the following:

(1) Efforts to avoid thoughts or feelings associated with the trauma.

(2) Efforts to avoid activities or situations that arouse recollections of the trauma

(3) Inability to recall an important aspect of the trauma (psychogenic amnesia)

(4) Markedly diminished interest in significant activities (in young children, loss of recently acquired developmental skills such as toilet training or language skills)

(5) Feeling of detachment or estrangement from others

(6) Restricted range of affect (e.g., unable to have loving feelings)

(7) Sense of a foreshortened future (e.g., does not expect to have a career, marriage, children, or a long life)

D. Persistent symptoms of increased arousal (not present before the trauma), as indicated by at least two of the following:

(1) Difficulty falling or staying asleep

(2) Irritability or outbursts of anger

(3) Difficulty concentrating

(4) Hypervigilance

(5) Exaggerated startle response

(6) Physiologic reactivity upon exposure to events that symbolize or resemble an aspect of the traumatic event (e.g., a woman who was raped in an elevator breaks out in a sweat when entering any elevator)

E. Duration of the disturbance (symptoms in B, C, and D) of at least 1 month.

Used with permission, APA.

D. Epidemiology

Table 9–9. **EPIDEMIOLOGY OF ANXIETY DISORDERS**

	Panic Disorder	Phobia	Obsessive-Compulsive Disorder	Generalized Anxiety Disorder	Post-Traumatic Stress Disorder
Prevalence	2-4% of population	Most common anxiety disorder: 3-5% of population	0.05% of population	2-4% of population	0.75% of population
Male:Female	1:1 (without agoraphobia) 1:2 (with agoraphobia)	More common in females 1:2	Males to females 1:1	Males to females 1:2	Males to females 1:2
Age at Onset	Late 20s	Late childhood	Adolescence/early adulthood	Variable; early adulthood	Any age, including childhood
Family History	20% of first-degree (1°) relatives of agoraphobic patients have agoraphobia	May run in families	3-7% in 1° relatives	15-17% of 1° relatives affected	
Twin Studies	20% of 1° relatives have agoraphobia	—	—	80-90% concordance in monozygotic twins; 10-15% in dizygotic twins	—

E. Etiology
1. Biologic
    a. Excessive autonomic reaction with increased sympathetic tone.
    b. Increased release of catecholamines.
    c. Increased norepinephrine metabolites, e.g., 3-methoxy-4-hydroxyphenylglycol (MHPG). Experimental lactate infusion increases norepinephrine, producing anxiety.
    d. Decreased rapid eye movement (REM) latency and stage 4 (similar to depression).
    e. Decreased γ-aminobutyric acid (GABA) causes central nervous system (CNS) hyperactivity (GABA inhibits CNS ability).
    f. Serotonin increase causes anxiety; increased dopaminergic activity associated with anxiety.
    g. Hyperactive center in temporal cerebral cortex.
    h. Locus ceruleus, center of noradrenergic neurons, hyperactive in anxiety states.

2. Psychoanalytic
    a. Unconscious impulses, e.g., sex, aggression, threaten to burst into consciousness and produce anxiety.
    b. Defense mechanisms are used to ward off anxiety.

c. Displacement produces phobias.
d. Reaction formation, undoing, and displacement produce obsessive-compulsive disorder.
e. Breakdown of repression produces panic or generalized anxiety disorder.
f. Agoraphobia related to
  i. Hostile-dependent relationship with companion.
  ii. Fear of aggressive/sexual impulses from self to others or vice versa.

3. Learning theory
a. Anxiety is produced by frustration or stress. Once experienced, it becomes a conditioned response to other, less severe, frustrating or stressful situations.
b. May be learned through identification and imitation of anxiety patterns in parents (social learning theory).
c. Anxiety associated with naturally frightening stimulus, e.g., accident, transferred to another stimulus through conditioning, producing phobia.

F. Psychological tests
1. Rorschach
a. Anxiety responses, e.g., animal movements, unstructured forms, heightened color.
b. Phobic responses, e.g., anatomy forms, bodily harm.
c. Obsessive-compulsive responses, e.g., overattention to detail.

2. Thematic Apperception Test (TAT)
a. Increased fantasy productions.
b. Themes of aggression, sexuality.
c. Feelings of tension.

3. Bender-Gestalt
a. No organic changes.
b. Use of small area in obsessive-compulsive disorder.
c. Spread out on page in anxiety states.

4. Draw-A-Person
a. Attention to head and general detailing in obsessive-compulsive disorder.
b. Body image distortions in phobia.
c. Rapid drawing in anxiety disorders.

5. Minnesota Multiphasic Personality Inventory (MMPI)
a. High hypochondriasis, psychasthenia, hysteria scales in anxiety.

G. Lab tests
1. No specific test for anxiety.
2. See Chapter 24, Laboratory Tests.
3. Nonspecific electroencephalogram (EEG) changes, nonsuppression of dexamethasone suppression test (DST) in some obsessive-compulsive patients.
4. Echocardiogram shows mitral valve prolapse (present in 50% of patients with panic attacks).

H. Pathophysiology
1. No pathognomonic changes noted.
2. In obsessive-compulsive disorder, decreased metabolism on positron emission tomography (PET) in orbital gyrus, caudate nuclei, cingulate gyrus.

3. Increased PET blood flow in right parahippocampus in panic, frontal lobe in anxiety.
4. Mitral valve prolapse in 50% of patients with panic disorder.

I. Psychodynamics

Table 9–10. **PSYCHODYNAMICS OF ANXIETY DISORDERS**

Disorders	Defense	Comment
Phobia	Displacement Symbolization	Anxiety detached from idea or situation and displaced on some other symbolic object or situation.
Agoraphobia	Projection Displacement	Repressed hostility, rage, or sexuality projected on environment, which is seen as dangerous.
Obsessive-compulsive disorder	Undoing Isolation Reaction formation	Severe superego acts against impulses about which patient feels guilty; anxiety controlled by repetitious act or thought.
Anxiety	Regression	Repression of forbidden sexual, agressive, or dependency strivings breaks down.
Panic	Regression	Anxiety overwhelms personality and is discharged in panic state. Total breakdown of repressive defense and regression occurs.
Post-traumatic stress disorder	Regression Repression Denial Undoing	Trauma reactivates unconscious conflicts; ego relives anxiety and tries to master it.

J. Differential diagnosis. Psychologic, medical, neurologic disorders have anxiety as a major component.

1. Depression. 50-70% of depressed patients have anxiety or obsessive brooding; 20-30% of primarily anxious patients also experience depression.

2. Schizophrenia. May be anxious and have severe obsessions in addition to hallucinations or delusions.

3. Mania. Characterized by massive anxiety during manic excitement.

4. Atypical psychoses. Massive anxiety in addition to psychotic features.

5. Adjustment disorder with anxious mood. History of psychosocial stressor within 3 months of onset.

6. Organic anxiety syndrome. Caused by specific organic factor (See Tables 9–11 and 9–12); cognitive impairment present.

7. Substance abuse. Panic/anxiety associated with intoxication (especially caffeine, amphetamine) and withdrawal states.

K. Course and prognosis

1. Panic disorder
   a. Tends to recur daily 2-3 times/week.
   b. Chronic course with remissions and exacerbations.
   c. Prognosis excellent with therapy.

2. Phobic disorder
   a. Chronic course.

Table 9–11.   **MEDICAL AND NEUROLOGIC CAUSES OF ANXIETY**

Neurologic disorders
  Cerebral neoplasms
  Cerebral trauma and postconcussive
    syndromes
  Cerebrovascular disease
  Subarachnoid hemorrhage
  Migraine
  Encephalitis
  Cerebral syphilis
  Multiple sclerosis
  Wilson's disease
  Huntingon's disease
  Epilepsy

Systemic conditions
  Hypoxia
    Cardiovascular disease
    Pulmonary insufficiency
    Anemia

Endocrine disturbances
  Pituitary dysfunction
  Thyroid dysfunction
  Parathyroid dysfunction
  Adrenal dysfunction
  Pheochromocytoma
  Virilization disorders of females

Inflammatory disorders
  Lupus erythematosus
  Rheumatoid arthritis
  Polyarteritis nodosa
  Temporal arteritis

Deficiency states
  Vitamin B_{12} deficiency
  Pellagra

Miscellaneous conditions
  Hypoglycemia
  Carcinoid syndrome
  Systemic malignancies
  Premenstrual syndrome
  Febrile illnesses and chronic infections
  Porphyria
  Infectious mononucleosis
  Posthepatitis syndrome
  Uremia

Toxic conditions
  Alcohol and drug withdrawal
  Amphetamines
  Sympathomimetic agents
  Vasopressor agents
  Caffeine and caffeine withdrawal
  Penicillin
  Sulfonamides
  Cannabis
  Mercury
  Arsenic
  Phosphorus
  Organophosphates
  Carbon disulfide
  Benzene
  Aspirin intolerance

Table from Cummings J: *Clinical Neuropsychiatry*. Grune & Stratton, Orlando, 1985, p 214, with permission.

  b. Phobias may spread if untreated.
  c. Good to excellent prognosis with therapy.
  d. Agoraphobia most resistant of all phobias.
3. Obsessive-compulsive disorder
  a. Chronic course with waxing and waning of symptoms.
  b. Fair prognosis with therapy but some cases intractable.
4. Generalized anxiety disorder
  a. Chronic course; symptoms may diminish as patient gets older.
  b. Over time, patient may develop secondary depression—not uncommon if left untreated.
5. Post-traumatic stress disorder
  a. Chronic course.
  b. Trauma periodically reexperienced over several years.
  c. Worse prognosis with preexisting psychopathologic state.
L. Treatment
1. Pharmacologic
a. Diazepam (Valium)
  i. Supplied—2, 5, 10 mg tablets and 5 mg/mL.
  ii. Dosage—2-10 mg orally 2-4 times/day; 2-10 mg intramuscularly or intravenously for acute agitation.

Table 9–12. **DIFFERENTIAL DIAGNOSIS OF COMMON MEDICAL CONDITIONS MIMICKING ANXIETY**

Angina Pectoris/ Myocardial Infarction (MI)	Electrocardiogram (EKG) with ST depression in angina; cardiac enzymes in MI. Crushing chest pain usually associated with angina/MI. Anxiety pains usually sharp and more superficial.
Hyperventilation Syndrome	History of rapid, deep respirations; circumoral pallor; carpopedal spasm; responds to rebreathing in paper bag.
Hypoglycemia	Fasting blood sugar usually under 50 mg/dL; signs of diabetes mellitus—polyuria, polydypsia, polyphagia
Hyperthyroidism	Elevated triiodothyronine (T_3), thyroxine (T_4); exophthalmos in severe cases.
Carcinoid Syndrome	Hypertension accompanies anxiety; elevated urinary catecholamines (5-hydroxyindoleacetic acid [5-HIAA]).

   iii. Indication—generalized anxiety disorder, post-traumatic stress disorder.

   iv. Side effects—drowsiness, fatigue, hypotension, paradoxical excitement.

   v. Cautions—long-term use can cause physical dependence, i.e., withdrawal symptoms upon abrupt discontinuation; most often in patients with history of alcoholism or drug abuse.

b. Alprazolam (Xanax)

   i. Supplied—0.25, 0.5, 1 mg tablets.

   ii. Dosage—0.25-0.5 mg orally 3 times/day; may be increased to 6-8 mg everyday.

   iii. Indications—rapidly acting, good short-term treatment for panic disorder and agoraphobia.

   iv. Common side effects—drowsiness, cognitive impairment, hypotension.

c. Imipramine (Tofranil)

   i. Supplied—10, 25, 50 mg tablets.

   ii. Dosage—75 mg/day orally to start; increase to 150-300 mg.

   iii. Indications—primarily for mood disorder but useful in panic disorder, social phobia.

Note: In elderly or adolescent patients, start with 25-50 mg/day and increase to 75-100 mg/day. See Chapter 22, Organic Therapy, for other heterocyclic compounds useful in anxiety.

   iv. Common side effects—drowsiness, confusion, anticholinergic effect (dry mouth, tachycardia, arrhythmias), constipation, delayed micturition.

Note: Obtain electrocardiogram (EKG) in patients over age 40 to test cardiac function. Do not prescribe monoamine oxidase inhibitors (MAOIs) until 14 days after imipramine stopped.

d. Tranylcypromine (Parnate)

   i. Supplied—10 mg.

   ii. Dosage—10 mg orally in morning and 10 mg in afternoon; increase to 30-50 mg/day in divided doses.

   iii. Indications—primarily for depression but useful in panic disorder. See Chapter 22 for other MAOIs useful in anxiety.

Note: Do not use in elderly. Do not use with narcotics (especially meperidine [Demerol]), may be fatal.

  iv. Major adverse effect—hypertensive crisis—foods with tryptophan/ tyramine and sympathomimetic agents, other MAOIs, tricyclics, narcotics may produce fatal intracranial bleeding secondary to acute hypertensive episode.

  e. **Buspirone (Buspar)**
   i. Supplied—5 mg tablets.
   ii. Dosage—5 mg twice daily and increase to 15-60 mg/day in divided doses.
   iii. Indications—generalized anxiety disorder.
   iv. Common adverse effects—headache, dizziness.
   Note: Not cross-tolerant to benzodiazepines.

  f. **Propranolol (Inderal)**
   i. Supplied—10 mg tablets.
   ii. Dosage—10 mg orally twice daily and increase to 80-160 mg/day in divided doses; 20-40 mg dose 30 minutes before phobic situation, e.g., public speaking.
   iii. Indications—social phobia.
   iv. Adverse effects—bradycardia, hypotension, drowsiness.
   Note: Do not use with history of asthma. Not useful in chronic anxiety unless caused by hypersensitive beta-adrenergic state.

  g. **Clonazepam (Klonopin)**
   i. Supplied—0.5, 1.0, 2 mg tablets.
   ii. Dosage—0.5 mg twice daily; increase to 2-10 mg/day.
   iii. Indications—generalized anxiety disorder, panic disorder, post-traumatic stress disorder.
   iv. Side effects—drowsiness, ataxia.
   Note: Food and Drug Administration (FDA) approved use is for petit mal, myoclonic, and akinetic seizures, but anxiety disorder is medically approved use.

  h. **Other drugs**
   i. **Clomipramine (Anafranil)**
    (a) Indicated in obsessive-compulsive disorder.
    (b) 150-300 mg/day.
   ii. **Fluoxetine (Prozac)**
    (a) Used primarily in depression, literature reports of use in obsessive-compulsive disorder.
    (b) 20-80 mg/day.

2. **Psychologic.** Some of the anxiety disorders, such as post-traumatic stress disorder, are treated primarily with psychotherapy; others, such as phobias, generalized anxiety, panic disorder, and obsessive-compulsive disorder, are treated with a combination of modalities. The following brief summary of indicated psychologic treatments can be viewed as an introduction to the topic discussed in greater detail in Chapter 21.

  a. **Insight-oriented psychotherapy** — goal is to increase the patient's development of insight into psychologic conflicts, which if unresolved can manifest as symptomatic behavior, such as anxiety, phobias, obsessions and compulsions, and post-traumatic stress. Particularly indicated if (1) anxiety symptoms are clearly secondary to underlying neurotic conflict, (2) anxiety continues to be manifest after behavioral or pharmacologic treatments are instituted, (3) new anxiety symptoms develop after the original symptoms resolve (symptom substitution), and (4) the anxieties are more generalized, less specific, and circumscribed.

b. Behavior therapy — basic assumption is that change can occur without developing psychologic insight into underlying causes. Techniques include positive and negative reinforcement, punishment, systematic desensitization, flooding, implosion, graded exposure, and self-monitoring.

   i. Indicated for clearly delineated, circumscribed, maladaptive behaviors, such as phobias, compulsions, and obsessions. (Compulsive behavior generally more responsive than obsessional thinking.)

   ii. Most current strategies for treatment of anxiety disorders include a combination of pharmacologic and behavioral interventions.

   iii. Current thinking generally maintains that although drugs can reduce anxiety early, treatment with drugs alone leads to equally early relapse. Patients treated with cognitive and behavioral therapies appear to do significantly and consistently better than those receiving drugs alone.

c. Cognitive therapy — based on the premise that maladaptive behavior is secondary to distortions in how people perceive themselves and in how others perceive them. Treatment is short-term and very interactive, with assigned homework and tasks to be performed between sessions, which focus on correcting distorted assumptions and cognitions. Increased emphasis on confronting and examining situations that elicit interpersonal anxiety and associated mild depression.

d. Group therapy — groups range from those that solely provide support and an increase in social skills, to those focusing on relief of specific symptoms, to those that are primarily insight-oriented. Groups may be heterogeneous or homogeneous in terms of diagnosis, with homegeneous groups being most commonly used in the treatment of such diagnoses as post-traumatic stress disorder, in which therapy is aimed at education about and exposure to social skills, with practice provided in a group setting.

For more detailed discussion of this topic, see Uhde TW, Nemiah JC: Panic and Generalized Anxiety Disorder, Sec. 18.1, pp 952–972; Nemiah JC, Uhde TW: Phobic Disorders, Sec. 18.2, pp 972–984; Nemiah JC, Uhde TW: Obsessive-Compulsive Disorder, Sec. 18.3, pp 984–1000; Kinzie JD: Post-Traumatic Stress Disorder, Sec. 18.4, pp 1000–1008, in *CTP/V*.

10

Somatoform Disorders, Factitious Disorders, and Malingering

I. **Somatoform disorders**
   A. **General introduction.** There are six types of somatoform disorders: (1) body dysmorphic disorder, (2) conversion disorder, (3) hypochondriasis, (4) somatization disorder, (5) somatoform pain disorder, and (6) undifferentiated somatoform disorder.

   The essential features of these disorders are the presence of a physical or somatic complaint without any demonstrable organic findings to account for the complaint or without any known physiologic mechanisms to explain the findings. There is also the presumption of associated psychologic factors or unconscious conflicts to account for the presenting syndrome.

   B. **Body dysmorphic disorder (dysmorphophobia)**
   1. **Definition.** Imagined belief (not of delusional proportions) that there is a defect in appearance of all or a part of the body.
   2. **Diagnosis, signs and symptoms.** Patient complains of defect, e.g., wrinkles, hair loss, too small breasts/penis, age spots, stature. Complaint is out of proportion to any minor objective physical abnormality. History of visits to doctors about complaint.

      If a slight physical anomaly is present, the person's concern is grossly excessive; however, the belief is not of delusional intensity, as in delusional disorder, somatic type (i.e., the person can acknowledge the possibility that he or she may be exaggerating the extent of the defect or that there may be no defect at all).
   3. **Epidemiology.** Onset from adolescence through early adulthood. Men are equal to women.
   4. **Etiology.** Unknown. Look for unconscious conflict relating to a distorted body part.
   5. **Lab and psychological tests.** Draw-A-Person test shows exaggeration/dimunition/absence of affected body part.
   6. **Pathophysiology.** No known pathologic abnormalities. Minor body deficits may actually exist upon which imagined belief develops.
   7. **Psychodynamics.** Defense mechanisms include repression (of unconscious conflict), distortion and symbolization (of body part), and projection (believe other persons also see imagined deformity).
   8. **Differential diagnosis.** Distorted body image occurs in schizophrenia, mood disorders, organic mental syndrome, anorexia nervosa, bulimia nervosa, obsessive-compulsive disorder; these must be ruled out.
   9. **Course and prognosis.** Chronic course with repeated visits to plastic surgeons or dermatologists. Secondary depression may occur. In some cases, imagined body distortion progresses to delusional belief.

10. Treatment

a. **Pharmacologic** — antianxiety agents, e.g., benzodiazepines, of limited use. Serotonergic drugs may diminish obsessive ruminations and depression.

b. **Psychologic** — psychotherapy most useful approach; uncovers conflicts relating to symptoms, feelings of inadequacy.

C. Conversion disorder (hysterical neurosis, conversion type)

1. Definition.
Characterized by involuntary alteration or limitation of physical function as a result of psychologic conflict or need, not physical disorder.

2. Diagnosis, signs and symptoms

a. Motor abnormalities—paralysis, ataxia, dysphagia, vomiting, aphonia.

b. Disturbances of consciousness—pseudoseizures, unconsciousness.

c. Sensory disturbances or alterations—blindness, deafness, anosmia, anesthesia, analgesia, diplopia; glove and stocking anesthesia (does not follow known sensory pathways).

d. Close temporal relationship between symptom and stress or intense emotion.

e. Left-sided symptoms more common than right-sided symptoms.

f. The person is not conscious of intentionally producing the symptom.

g. The symptom is not a culturally sanctioned response pattern and cannot, after appropriate investigation, be explained by a known physical disorder.

3. Epidemiology

a. Incidence and prevalence—10% of hospital inpatients; 0.15% of all psychiatric outpatients.

b. Age—early adulthood, but can occur in middle/old age.

c. The male-to-female ratio is 1:2.

d. Family history—higher in family members.

e. More common in low socioeconomic groups and less well-educated persons.

4. Etiology

a. **Biologic**

1. Symptom depends on activation of inhibitory brain mechanisms.
2. Excessive cortical arousal triggers inhibitory central nervous system (CNS) mechanisms at synapses, brain stem, reticular activating system.
3. Increased susceptibility in patients with frontal lobe trauma or other neurologic deficits.

b. **Psychologic**

1. Expression of unconscious psychological conflict, which is repressed.
2. Premorbid personality disorder—avoidant, histrionic.
3. Impulse, e.g., sex or agression, is unacceptable to ego and is disguised through symptom.
4. Identification with family member with same symptoms from real disease.

5. **Lab and psychological tests**
   a. Evoked potential shows disturbed somatosensory perception; diminished or absent on side of defect.
   b. Mild cognitive impairment, attentional deficits, and visuoperceptive changes on Halstead-Reitan Battery.
   c. Minnesota Multiphasic Personality Inventory (MMPI), Rorschach Test show increased instinctual drives, sexual repression, inhibited aggression.
6. **Pathophysiology.** No changes.
7. **Psychodynamics**
   a. *La belle indifférence* is lack of concern that patient has about illness.
   b. Primary gain refers to reduction of anxiety by repression of unacceptable impulse. Symbolization of impulse onto symptom, e.g., paralyzed arm prevents expression of aggressive impulse.
   c. Other defense mechanisms—reaction formation, denial, displacement.
   d. Secondary gain refers to benefits of illness, e.g, compensation from lawsuit (compensation neurosis), avoiding work, being dependent on family. Patient usually lacks insight about this dynamic.
8. **Differential diagnosis.** Major task is to distinguish from organically based disorder. Up to 30% of patients diagnosed have associated physical illness.
   a. **Paralysis** — in conversion, paralysis is inconsistent; it does not follow motor pathways. There are no pathologic reflexes, e.g., Babinski. Spastic paralysis, clonus, cogwheel rigidity absent in conversion disorder.
   b. **Ataxia** — bizarre character in conversion disorder—leg may be dragged and not circumducted as in organic lesion. Astasia-abasia is unsteady gait in which conversion-disordered patient does not fall or injure self.
   c. **Blindness** — no pupillary response seen in most neurologic blindness (*exception*: occipital lobe lesions produce cortical blindness with intact pupillary response). Tracking movements are absent in true blindness. Monocular dyplopia, trilopia, and tunnel vision can be conversion complaint. Tests with distorting prisms and colored lenses used by ophthalmologists to detect hysterical blindness.
   d. **Deafness** — loud noise will awaken sleeping conversion patient but not organic deaf patient. On audiometric tests, variability of response in conversion.
   e. **Sensory loss** — conversion sensory loss does not follow dermatomes; hemisensory loss, which stops at midline, or glove and stocking anesthesia seen in conversion disorder.
   f. **Hysterical pain** — most often relates to head and face, back and abdomen. Look for organic findings—muscular spasm, osteoarthritis.
   g. **Pseudoseizures** — usually no incontinence, loss of motor control, tongue biting in pseudoseizures; presence of aura usual in organic epilepsy. Look for abnormal electroencephalogram (EEG). (Note that 10-15% of normal adult population have abnormal EEG.) Babinski occurs in organic seizure and postictal state but not in conversion seizures.

h. Differentiate conversion from:

1. Schizophrenia—thought disorder.
2. Mood disorder—depression or mania.
3. Malingering and factitious disorder with physical symptoms—difficult to distinguish but malingerers are aware they are faking symptoms and have insight into what they are doing; factitious patients also aware they are faking, but do so because they want to be patients and be in a hospital.

i. Differential diagnosis with amytal interview — intravenous amytal (100 - 500 mg) in slow infusion will often cause conversion symptoms to abate. Example: Patient with hysterical aphonia will begin to talk. Test can be used to aid in diagnosis but is not always reliable.

9. Course and prognosis.   Tends to be recurrent, separated by asymptomatic periods. Major concern is to not miss early neurologic symptom, which then progresses into full-blown syndrome, e.g., multiple sclerosis may begin with spontaneously remitting diplopia or hemiparesis.

10. Treatment

a. Pharmacologic — benzodiazepines for anxiety and muscular tension; antidepressants or serotonergic agents for obsessive rumination about symptoms.

b. Psychologic

i. Insight-oriented therapy is useful in understanding dynamic principles and conflicts behind symptoms. Patient learns to accept sexual/aggressive impulses and not to use conversion disorder as defense.

ii. Behavior therapy used to induce relaxation and to reduce or eliminate need for symptom reduction.

iii. Hypnosis and reeducation of use in uncomplicated situations.

iv. Do not accuse patient of trying to get attention or of not wanting to get better.

v. Narcoanalysis sometimes removes symptoms.

D. Hypochondriasis (hypochondriacal neurosis)

1. Definition.   Morbid fear or belief that one has a serious disease even though none exists.

2. Diagnosis, signs and symptoms

a. Any organ or functional system can be affected. Gastrointestinal (GI) and cardiovascular (CV) most common.

b. Patient believes disease or malfunction is present.

c. Negative physical examination or lab test reassures patient but only for short time, then symptoms return (in somatic delusion, patient cannot be reassured).

d. Duration of the disturbance is at least 6 months.

e. The belief is not of delusional intensity.

3. Epidemiology

a. Incidence/prevalence—10% of all medical patients.

b. Men equal to women.

c. Occurs at all ages; peaks in 30s for men and 40s for women.

    d. Seen in identical twins and in first-degree relatives.

4. Etiology

    a. Psychogenic in origin but patient may have congenital hypersensitivity to bodily functions and sensations and low threshold for pain/physical discomfort.

    b. Aggression toward others turned against self through particular body part.

    c. Organ affected may have important symbolic meaning.

5. Lab and psychological tests

    a. Repeated physical examinations to rule out medical illness are negative.

    b. MMPI shows elevated hysterical scale.

    c. Many color responses on Rorschach test.

6. Psychodynamics. Repression of anger toward others; displacement of anger toward physical complaints; pain and suffering as punishment for unacceptable guilty impulses; undoing.

7. Differential diagnosis. Diagnosis is made by inclusion, *not* by exclusion. Physical disorders must be ruled out; however, 15-30% of patients with hypochondriacal disorder have physical problems. Workup for organic disease may aggravate condition by placing too much emphasis on physical complaint.

    a. Depression — may have a somatic complaint or part of depressive syndrome. Look for signs of depression, e.g., apathy, anhedonia, feelings of worthlessness.

    b. Anxiety disorder — manifested by marked anxiety or obsessive-compulsive signs or symptoms; *la belle indifférence* not present.

    c. Somatization disorder — multiple organ systems involved; vague complaints.

    d. Psychogenic pain disorder — pain is major and usually sole complaint.

    e. Malingering and factitious disorders — history is associated with frequent hospitalizations, marked secondary gain; symptoms lack symbolic value and are under conscious control. *La belle indifférence* not present.

    f. Sexual dysfunction — if sex is complaint, diagnose as sexual disorder.

8. Course and prognosis. Chronic course with remissions. Exacerbations usually associated with identifiable life stress. Good prognosis associated with minimal premorbid personality; poor prognosis with antecedent or superimposed physical disorder.

9. Treatment

    a. Pharmacologic — pharmacologic targeting of symptoms: antianxiety drugs and antidepressant drugs for anxiety and/or depression. Serotonergic drugs useful for depression and obsessive-compulsive disorder. Amytal interview can induce catharsis and potential removal of symptoms; however, usually only temporary.

    b. Psychologic

        i. Insight-oriented dynamic psychotherapy uncovers symbolic meaning of symptom and is useful. Do not confront patient with such statements as, "It's all in your head." Long-term relationship with physician or psychiatrist of value with reassurance that no physical disease is present.

        ii. Hypnosis and behavioral therapy are useful to induce relaxation. Prolonged conversion disorder can produce physical deterioration, e.g., muscle atrophy or contractures, osteoporosis, so attention to these issues is necessary.

E. Somatization disorder
   1. Definition. Somatic complaints not limited to one organ system and not caused by known medical disorder.
   2. History. Previously known as Briquet's syndrome.
   3. Diagnosis, signs and symptoms. Multiple somatic complaints. Patients usually take medication, have many psychologic stresses. Most common complaints are nausea, vomiting, shortness of breath, menstrual. To count a symptom as significant, the following criteria must be met:
   (1) no organic pathology or pathophysiologic mechanism (e.g., a physical disorder or the effects of injury, medication, drugs, or alcohol) to account for the symptom or, when there is related organic pathology, the complaint or resulting social or occupational impairment is grossly in excess of what would be expected for the physical findings
   (2) has not occurred only during a panic attack
   (3) has caused the person to take medicine (other than over-the-counter pain medication), see a doctor, or alter life-style

Symptom list (From DSM-III-R, used with permission, APA)

Note: The seven items in boldface may be used to screen for the disorder. The presence of two or more of these items suggests a high likelihood of the disorder.

Gastrointestinal symptoms:
   (1) **vomiting (other than during pregnancy)**
   (2) abdominal pain (other than when menstruating)
   (3) nausea (other than motion sickness)
   (4) bloating (gassy)
   (5) diarrhea
   (6) intolerance of (gets sick from) several different foods

Pain symptoms:
   (7) **pain in extremities**
   (8) back pain
   (9) joint pain
   (10) pain during urination
   (11) other pain (excluding headaches)

Cardiopulmonary symptoms:
   (12) **shortness of breath when not exerting oneself**
   (13) palpitations
   (14) chest pain
   (15) dizziness

Conversion or pseudoneurologic symptoms:
   (16) **amnesia**
   (17) **difficulty swallowing**

(18) loss of voice
(19) deafness
(20) double vision
(21) blurred vision
(22) blindness
(23) fainting or loss of consciousness
(24) seizure or convulsion
(25) trouble walking
(26) paralysis or muscle weakness
(27) urinary retention or difficulty urinating

Sexual symptoms for the major part of the person's life after opportunities for sexual activity:
(28) **burning sensation in sexual organs or rectum (other than during intercourse)**
(29) sexual indifference
(30) pain during intercourse
(31) impotence

Female reproductive symptoms judged by the person to occur more frequently or severely than in most women:
(32) **painful menstruation**
(33) irregular menstrual periods
(34) excessive menstrual bleeding
(35) vomiting throughout pregnancy

4. Epidemiology
  a. Females greater than males.
  b. 1-2% of all women.
  c. More common in less educated, lower socioeconomic groups.
  d. Usual onset in adolescence and young adulthood.

5. Etiology.
  a. Psychosocial — suppression or repression of anger toward others, with turning of anger toward self, can account for symptoms. Punitive personality organization with strong superego. Low self-esteem common. Identification with parent who models sick role. Some dynamics similar to depression.
  b. Genetic positive family history; present in 10-20% of mothers and/or sisters of affected patients; twins—concordance rate of 29% in monozygotes and 10% in dizygotes.

6. Lab and psychological tests.
Minor neuropsychologic abnormality in some patients, e.g., faulty assessment of somatosensory input.

7. Pathophysiology.
None. Prolonged use of medications may cause adverse side effects unrelated to somatization complaint.

8. Psychodynamics.
Repression of wish or impulse expressed through body complaints. Superego conflicts, partially expressed by symptom. Anxiety converted into specific symptom.

9. Differential diagnosis
  a. Rule out organic cause for somatic symptom.

   b. Multiple sclerosis for weakness.
   c. Epstein-Barr virus for chronic fatigue syndrome.
   d. Porphyria for abdominal pain.
   e. Somatic delusion occurs in schizophrenia.
   f. Panic attacks have cardiovascular symptoms that are intermittent, episodic.
   g. Conversion disorder has fewer symptoms with clearer symbolic meaning.
   h. Factitious disorder—conscious faking of symptoms to achieve patient role; usually eager to be in hospital.
   i. Somatoform pain disorder—pain is usually only complaint.
10. Course and prognosis
   a. Chronic course with few remissions; however, severity of complaints can fluctuate. Complications include unnecessary surgery, repeated medical workups, drug dependence and/or side effects of unnecessary prescribed drugs.
   b. Depression is frequent.
11. Treatment
   a. **Pharmacologic** — avoid psychotropics, except under period of acute anxiety/depression, because patients have tendency to become psychologically dependent. Antidepressants useful in secondary depressions.
   b. **Psychologic** — insight or supportive psychotherapy required on long-term basis to provide understanding of dynamics and/or support through distressing life events; also to follow patient to prevent substance abuse, doctor-shopping, unnecessary procedures or diagnostic tests.
F. Somatoform pain disorder. This disorder is discussed in Chapter 15, Psychosomatic Disorders.
G. Undifferentiated somatoform disorder. This is a category used to describe a partial picture of somatoform disorder (see above). The patient may have multiple somatic complaints but not of sufficient severity or so vague as to not warrant a diagnosis of full somatoform disorder. General fatigue is the most common syndrome.

II. Factitious disorder
A. Definition. Symptoms are deliberately and consciously simulated by patient. May be psychologic (e.g., hallucinations) or physical (e.g., pain).
B. Diagnosis, signs and symptoms
   1. With physical symptoms (also known as Munchausen's syndrome). Intentional production of physical symptoms—nausea, vomiting, pain, seizures. Patients may intentionally put blood in feces or urine, artificially raise body temperature, take insulin to lower blood sugar. "Gridiron abdomen" sign is result of scars from multiple surgical operations.
   2. With psychological symptoms. Intentional production of psychiatric symptoms—hallucinations, delusions, depression, bizarre behavior. Patients may make up story that they suffered major life stress to account for symptoms. *Pseudologia fantastica* consists of making up exaggerated lies that the patient believes. Substance abuse, especially opioids, common in both types.

C. Epidemiology. Unknown. More common in men than in women. Usually adult onset. 5-10% of all hospital admissions are for factitious illness, especially feigned fevers. More common in health care workers.

D. Etiology. Early real illness coupled with parental abuse or rejection is typical. Patient recreates illness as adult in attempt to gain loving attention from doctors. Masochistic gratification for some patients who want surgical procedures. Others identify with important past figure who had psychologic/physical illness.

E. Psychodynamics. Repression, identification with the aggressor, regression, symbolization.

F. Differential diagnosis

   1. Physical illness. Physical examination and laboratory work-up should be done; will be negative. Careful observation by nursing staff to uncover deliberate elevation of temperature, alteration of body fluids.

   2. Somatoform disorder. Symptoms are voluntary in factitious disorder and not caused by unconscious or symbolic factors. *La belle indifférence* not present in factitious disorder. Hypochondriacs do not want to undergo extensive tests or have surgery.

   3. Malingering. Most difficult differential. Malingerers have specific goals, e.g., insurance payments, avoidance of jail term.

   4. Ganser's syndrome. Found in prisoners who give approximate answers to questions and talk past the point. Classified as an atypical dissociative disorder.

G. Course and prognosis. Usually chronic course, which begins in adulthood but may have earlier onset. Frequent consultations with doctors and history of hospitalizations as patient seeks repeated care. High risk of substance abuse over time. Prognosis improves if there is associated depression or anxiety that responds to pharmacotherapy. Risk of death if patient undergoes multiple life-threatening surgical procedures.

H. Treatment

   1. Avoid unnecessary laboratory tests or medical procedures. Confront patient with diagnosis of factitious disorder and feigned symptomatology. Patients rarely enter psychotherapy because of poor motivation; however, working alliance with doctor is possible over time, and patient may gain insights into behavior. Good management, however, more likely than cure. Data bank of patients with repeated hospitalizations for factitious illness available in some areas of country.

   2. Psychopharmacologic therapy is useful with associated anxiety/depression. Substance abuse should be treated if present.

III. Malingering

   A. Definition. Voluntary production of physical or psychologic symptoms in order to accomplish specific goal, e.g., insurance payments, avoid jail term or punishment.

   B. Diagnosis, signs and symptoms. Patient has many vague or poorly localized complaints which are presented in great detail, are easily irritated if doctor is skeptical of history. Psychosocial history reveals a need to avoid some situation, to obtain money, presence of legal problems. Look for defined goal (secondary gain).

C. Epidemiology.   Unknown.

D. Etiology.   Unknown. May be associated with antisocial personality disorder.

E. Differential diagnosis

   1. Factitious disorders.   No obvious secondary gain.

   2. Somatoform disorder.   Symbolic or unconscious component to symptom. Symptoms are not voluntarily and willfully produced.

F. Course and prognosis.   Chronic course with poor prognosis as proved by repeated attempts to manipulate others through feigned illness.

G. Treatment.   Often negative physical and laboratory work-ups. Patient should be monitored as if there were real disease but no treatment offered. At some time, identify areas of secondary gain and encourage patient to ventilate and help provide ways of managing stress. Patient may then be willing to voluntarily give up symptoms.

For more detailed discussion of this topic, see Barsky AJ: Somatoform Disorders, Chap. 19, pp 1009–1027; Sussman N: Factitious Disorders, Chap. 23, pp 1136–1140; Meyerson AT: Malingering, Sec. 28.1, pp 1396–1399, in *CTP/V*.

11

Dissociative Disorders

I. General introduction
   A. Definition. Previously known as hysterical neuroses of the dissociative type, dissociative disorders are now classified into five major types: (1) psychogenic amnesia, (2) psychogenic fugue, (3) multiple personality disorder, (4) depersonalization disorder, and (5) dissociative disorder not otherwise specified (NOS). The common diagnostic feature is a psychologically induced loss of memory, consciousness, or identity. There is also an absence of underlying brain disease.

II. Psychogenic amnesia
   A. Definition. Abrupt loss of important personal memory with the capacity to learn new material preserved. No evidence of organic etiology.
   B. Diagnosis, signs and symptoms. Sudden loss of memory usually precipitated by emotional trauma. Patient is alert and aware of loss. Most common type of loss is localized amnesia in which the events of a short period of time are lost to memory. Apparent indifference to memory loss may be seen; mild clouding of consciousness may occur in some; memory loss may occur in context of a post-traumatic stress disorder.
   C. Epidemiology. See Table 11-1.
   D. Etiology. See Table 11-1.
   E. Lab and psychological tests. Must rule out organic pathology as indicated. Amytal interview can be helpful in distinguishing between organic and psychogenic amnesia; organically amnestic patients tend to worsen under amytal, and psychogenically amnestic patients may have a return of memory.
   F. Psychodynamics. Memory loss believed to be secondary to painful psychologic conflict, which patient has limited emotional resources to confront. Defenses utilized include repression (unconscious blocking of disturbing impulses from awareness), denial (external reality disavowed), and dissociation (separation and independent functioning of one group of mental processes from others). Similar defenses are used in all the dissociative disorders.
   G. Differential diagnosis
      1. Organic mental disorders. Not related to stress, more common in elderly, full return of memory rare and very gradual, clear organic factor in history.
      2. Malingering. Conscious attempt to fake loss of memory for secondary gain.
   H. Course and prognosis. See Table 11-1.
   I. Treatment. Hypnosis, short-acting barbiturates (amytal), psychotherapy (individual, group, supportive and insight-oriented).

Table 11–1. SUMMARY OF DISSOCIATIVE DISORDERS

	Psychogenic Amnesia	Psychogenic Fugue	Multiple Personality Disorder	Depersonalization Disorder
Signs and symptoms	Abrupt onset of loss of memory Patient aware of loss Alert before and after loss	Purposeful wandering, often long distances Amnesia for past life Unaware of loss of memory Assumes new identity Normal behavior during fugue	More than one distinct personality within one person, each of which dominates person's behavior and thinking when it is present Sudden transition from one personality to another Generally, amnesia for other personalities	Persistent sense of unreality about one's body and self Intact reality testing Ego-dystonic
Epidemiology	Most common dissociative disorder More common following disasters or during war F>M Adolescence—young adulthood	Rare More common following disasters or during war Variable sex ratio and age of onset	Not nearly as rare as once thought Adolescence—young adulthood (although may begin much earlier) F>M Increased in first-degree relatives	Although pure disorder is rare, intermittant episodes of depersonalization are common Rare over age 40 May be more common in women
Etiology	Precipitating emotional trauma Rule out organic causes	Heavy alcohol abuse predisposes Borderline, histrionic, schizoid personality disorders predispose Precipitating emotional trauma Rule out organic causes	Severe sexual and psychologic abuse in childhood Seizure disorder reported in 25% of patients Rule out organic causes	Severe stress, anxiety, depression predispose Rule out organic causes
Course and prognosis	Abrupt termination Few recurrences	Usually brief, hours Can last months and involve extensive travel Recovery generally spontaneous and rapid Few recurrences	Most severe and chronic of dissociative disorders Incomplete recovery	Onset usually sudden Tends to be chronic

III. Psychogenic fugue

A. **Definition.** Sudden, severe loss of memory associated with travel, often far from home, and assumption of a new identity.

B. **Diagnosis, signs and symptoms.** Sudden loss of memory associated with purposeful, unconfused travel, often for extended periods of time. Complete loss of memory for past life without awareness of the loss. Assumption of apparently normal, nonbizarre new identity. Perplexity and disorientation, however, may occur.

C. **Epidemiology.** See Table 11–1.

D. **Etiology.** See Table 11–1.

E. **Lab and psychological tests.** Hypnosis and amytal interviews help in clarifying diagnosis.

F. **Differential diagnosis**

   1. **Organic mental disorder.** Wandering is not as purposeful or complex.

   2. **Temporal lobe epilepsy.** Generally no new identity.

   3. **Psychogenic amnesia.** No purposeful travel or new identity.

   4. **Malingering.**

G. **Course and prognosis.** See Table 11–1.

H. **Treatment.** Hypnosis, amytal interviews, psychotherapy (recovery generally spontaneous without treatment).

IV. Multiple personality disorder (MPD)

A. **Definition.** Distinct and separate personalities within the same person, each of which when present dominates the person's attitudes, behavior, and self-view, as though no other personality exists.

B. **Diagnosis, signs and symptoms.** Original personality is generally amnestic for and unaware of other personalities. Transition from one personality to another tends to be abrupt. Some personalities may be aware of aspects of other personalities; each personality may have its own set of memories and associations, and each generally has its own name or description. Different personalities may have different physiologic characteristics, e.g., different eyeglass prescriptions, and different responses to psychometric testing, e.g., different intelligence quotient (I.Q.) scores. Personalities may be of different sexes, ages, or races. One or more of the personalities may exhibit signs of a coexisting psychiatric disorder, such as mood disorder or personality disorder.

C. **Epidemiology.** See Table 11–1.

D. **Etiology.** See Table 11–1.

E. **Lab and psychological tests.** Amytal interviews and hypnosis can help clarify diagnosis. In some studies, positron emission tomography (PET) scans and cerebral blood flow have revealed metabolic differences among different personalities in the same person.

F. **Psychodynamics.** Severe psychologic and physical abuse (most often sexual) in childhood leads to a profound need to distance self from horror and pain. The need to distance leads to an unconscious splitting off of different aspects of the original personality, each personality expressing some necessary emotion or state, e.g., rage, sexuality, flamboyance, competence, which the original personality does not dare express. As the abuse occurs, the child attempts to protect self from trauma by dissociating from the terrifying acts, becoming in essence another person or persons to whom abuse is not occurring and could not occur. These dissociated selves then become a chronic, ingrained method of self-protection from perceived emotional threats.

G. **Differential diagnosis**

1. **Schizophrenic** patients may be delusional in believing they have different identities or are being controlled by others, but the formal thought disorder and social deterioration distinguish schizophrenia from multiple personality disorder.

2. **Malingering** is most difficult differential, and clear secondary gain must raise suspicion.

3. **Borderline personality disorder.** Many patients with coexistent borderline personality disorder may be diagnosed as only having the personality disorder, because the different personalities are mistaken for the characteristic mood, behavior, and interpersonal instability of the borderline patient.

H. **Course and prognosis.** See Table 11–1.

I. **Treatment.** Intensive insight-oriented psychotherapy. Pharmacotherapy has not been very useful. Goals of therapy include reconciliation of disparate, split-off affects by helping patient to understand that the original reasons for the dissociation (overwhelming rage, fear, confusion secondary to abuse) no longer exist and that the affects can be expressed by one whole personality without destroying the self.

V. **Depersonalization disorder**

A. **Definition.** Persistent, recurrent episodes of feeling detached from one's self and body, to extent of feeling mechanical or being in a dream.

B. **Diagnosis, signs and symptoms.** Persistent, recurrent sense of strangeness and unreality about self. Patient aware and disturbed by sense of estrangement from reality. Intact reality testing. Distortion in sense of time and space. Extremities may be experienced as too large or too small. Derealization (sense of strangeness about external world rather than of self) frequently present. Other persons may seem robot-like. Dizziness, depressive and obsessive ruminations, anxiety, and somatic preoccupations commonly occur.

C. **Epidemiology.** See Table 11–1.

D. **Etiology.** See Table 11–1.

E. **Differential diagnosis.** Depersonalization as a symptom can occur in many syndromes, both psychiatric and medical. These primary disorders, e.g., mood disorders, schizophrenia, substance abuse, brain tumors, seizure disorders, must be ruled out. Depersonalization disorder describes the condition in which depersonalization is predominant.

F. **Course and prognosis.** See Table 11–1.

G. **Treatment.** Anxiety responds to anxiolytics and to both supportive and insight-oriented therapy. Usefulness of somatic treatments at this time has not been sufficiently tested.

VI. **Dissociative disorder not otherwise specified (NOS)**

A. **Definition.** Dissociative symptoms present and prominent, but clinical picture does not fully meet specific criteria for dissociative disorder. Disorders in which the predominant feature is a dissociative symptom, i.e., a disturbance or alteration in the normally integrative functions of identity, memory, or consciousness, that does not meet the criteria for a specific dissociative disorder.

Examples:

(1) Ganser's syndrome: the giving of "approximate answers" to questions or "talking past the point," e.g., if asked to add 2 + 2, answering 5; commonly associated with other symptoms, such as amnesia, disorientation, perceptual disturbances, fugue, and conversion symptoms.

(2) Cases in which there is more than one personality state capable of assuming executive control of the individual, but not more than one personality state is sufficiently distinct to meet the full criteria of multiple personality disorder, or cases in which a second personality never assumes complete executive control.

(3) Trance states, i.e., altered states of consciousness with markedly diminished or selectively focused responsiveness to environmental stimuli. In children, this may occur following physical abuse or trauma.

(4) Derealization unaccompanied by depersonalization.

(5) Dissociated states that can occur in persons who have been subjected to periods of prolonged and intense coercive persuasion, e.g., brainwashing, thought reform, or indoctrination while the captive of terrorists or cultists.

(6) Cases in which sudden, unexpected travel and organized, purposeful behavior with inability to recall one's past are not accompanied by the assumption of a new identity, partial or complete.

For more detailed discussion of this topic, see Nemiah JC: Dissociative Disorders (Hysterical Neuroses, Dissociative Type), Chap. 20, pp 1028–1044, in *CTP/V*.

12

Sexual Disorders

I. Sexual dysfunctions

A. **Definition.** Sexual dysfunctions can be symptomatic of biologic problems (biogenic), intrapsychic or interpersonal problems (psychogenic), or a combination of these factors. Sexual function can be adversely affected by stress of any kind, by emotional disorders, or by ignorance of sexual function and physiology. Regardless of etiology, the dysfunction is accompanied by and perpetuates anxiety regarding sexual performance. The dysfunctions can be lifelong (primary) or develop after a period of normal functioning (secondary). The dysfunctions can be generalized or situational, that is, limited to a certain partner or a specific situation, and it can be total or partial. The 10 recognized syndromes of sexual dysfunctions in DSM-III-R are categorized as Axis I disorders. Those attributable entirely to organic factors are coded on Axis III. See Tables 12-1 and 12-2.

TABLE 12-1. **CLASSIFICATION OF SEXUAL DYSFUNCTIONS**

Sexual Response Phase	Phase-Related Dysfunction
I. **Appetitive.** This phase is distinct from any identified solely through physiology and reflects the patient's motivations, drives, and personality. It is characterized by sexual fantasies and the desire to have sex.	1. Hypoactive sexual desire disorder 2. Sexual aversion disorder
II. **Excitement.** This phase consists of an objective sense of pleasure and accompanying physiologic changes; importantly, penile erection in the male and vaginal lubrication in the female.	3. Female sexual arousal disorder 4. Male erectile disorder
III. **Orgasm.** This phase consists of a peaking of sensual pleasure with release of sexual tension, and rhythmic contraction of the perineal muscles and pelvic reproductive organs.	5. Inhibited female orgasm (anorgasmia) 6. Inhibited male orgasm (retarded ejaculation) 7. Premature ejaculation (male)
IV. **Resolution.** This phase entails a sense of general relaxation and muscle relaxation. During it, men are refractory to orgasm for a period of time that increases with age, whereas women are capable of having multiple orgasms without a refractory period.	No dysfunctions

B. **Sexual desire disorders.** In sex therapy clinic populations, lack of desire is one of the most common complaints among married couples, with women more affected than men.

Patients with desire problems may use inhibition of desire defensively to protect against unconscious fears about sex. Lack of desire can also accompany chronic anxiety or depression or the use of drugs that depress the central nervous system (CNS). Desire commonly decreases after major illness or

TABLE 12–2. **SEXUAL DYSFUNCTIONS NOT CORRELATED WITH THE SEXUAL RESPONSE CYCLE**

Category	Dysfunctions
Sexual pain disorders	8. Vaginismus (female) 9. Dyspareunia (female and male)
Other	10. Sexual dysfunctions not otherwise specified Examples: A. No erotic sensation despite normal physiologic response to stimulation, e.g., orgasmic anhedonia B. Female analog of premature ejaculation C. Genital pain occurring during masturbation

surgery. Among married couples, marital discord is the reason most frequently given for the cessation of sexual activity. See Tables 12–3 and 12–4.

TABLE 12–3. **DSM-III-R DIAGNOSTIC CRITERIA FOR HYPOACTIVE SEXUAL DESIRE DISORDER**

Persistently or recurrently deficient or absent sexual fantasies and desire for sexual activity. The judgment of deficiency or absence is made by the clinician, taking into account factors that affect sexual functioning, such as age, sex, and the context of the person's life.

Used with permission, APA.

TABLE 12–4. **DSM-III-R DIAGNOSTIC CRITERIA FOR SEXUAL AVERSION DISORDER**

Persistent or recurrent extreme aversion to, and avoidance of, all or almost all genital sexual contact with a sexual partner.

Used with permission, APA.

C. Sexual arousal disorders. These disorders include male erectile disorder and female arousal disorder. The diagnoses take into account the focus, intensity, and duration of the sexual activity in which the patient engages. If sexual stimulation is inadequate in focus, intensity, or duration, the diagnosis should not be made.

1. Women. The prevalence of female desire disorder is generally underestimated. In one study of subjectively happily married couples, 33% of women described arousal problems.

Difficulty maintaining excitement can reflect psychologic conflicts (discussed under orgasmic inhibition) or physiologic changes. Alterations in testosterone, estrogen, prolactin, and thyroxin levels have been implicated in arousal disorders, as have antihistaminic medications. See Table 12–5.

TABLE 12–5. **DSM-III-R DIAGNOSTIC CRITERIA FOR FEMALE SEXUAL AROUSAL DISORDER**

Either (1) or (2):

(1) persistent or recurrent partial or complete failure to attain or maintain the lubrication-swelling response of sexual excitement until completion of the sexual activity
(2) persistent or recurrent lack of a subjective sense of sexual excitement and pleasure in a female during sexual activity

Used with permission, APA.

2. Men. In erectile disorder, the man has difficulty obtaining or maintaining an erection sufficient for vaginal insertion and thrusting. The incidence of impotence in young men is estimated at 8%. However, this disorder may first appear later in life. Statistics indicate that 20–50% of men have an organic basis for their problem of erectile dysfunction. See Tables 12–6, 12–7, and 12–8.

Medical illness and the use of drugs (prescribed and recreational) are the major causes of organic erectile dysfunction (Tables 12–7 and 12–8).

TABLE 12–6. **DSM-III-R DIAGNOSTIC CRITERIA FOR MALE ERECTILE DISORDER**

Either (1) or (2):

(1) persistent or recurrent partial or complete failure in a male to attain or maintain erection until completion of the sexual activity
(2) persistent or recurrent lack of a subjective sense of sexual excitement and pleasure in a male during sexual activity

Used with permission, APA.

TABLE 12–7. **DISEASES IMPLICATED IN ERECTILE DYSFUNCTION**

Infectious and parasitic diseases
   Elephantiasis
   Mumps

Cardiovascular diseases
   Atherosclerotic disease
   Aortic aneurysm
   Leriche syndrome
   Cardiac failure

Renal and urologic disorders
   Peyronie's disease
   Chronic renal failure
   Hydrocele or varicocele

Hepatic disorders
   Cirrhosis (usually associated with alcoholism)

Pulmonary disorders
   Respiratory failure

Genetics
   Klinefelter's syndrome
   Congenital penile vascular or structural abnormalities

Nutritional disorders
   Malnutrition
   Vitamin deficiencies

Endocrine disorders
   Diabetes mellitus
   Dysfunction of the pituitary-adrenal-testis axis
   Acromegaly
   Addison's disease
   Chromophobe adenoma
   Adrenal neoplasias
   Myxedema
   Hyperthyroidism

Neurologic disorders
   Multiple sclerosis
   Transverse myelitis
   Parkinson's disease
   Temporal lobe epilepsy
   Traumatic or neoplastic spinal cord disease
   CNS tumors
   Amyotropic lateral sclerosis

TABLE 12–7. **DISEASES IMPLICATED IN ERECTILE DYSFUNCTION (Continued)**

Peripheral neuropathies
    General paresis
    Tabes dorsalis

Pharmacologic contributants (Table 12–8)
    Alcohol and other addictive drugs (heroin, methadone, morphine, cocaine, amphetamines, and barbiturates)
    Prescribed drugs (psychotropic drugs, antihypertensive drugs, estrogens, and antiandrogens)

Poisoning
    Lead (plumbism)
    Herbicides

Surgical procedures
    Perineal prostatectomy
    Abdominal-perineal colon resection
    Sympathectomy (frequently interferes with ejaculation)
    Aortoiliac surgery
    Radical cystectomy
    Retroperitoneal lymphadenectomy

Miscellaneous
    Radiation therapy
    Pelvic fracture
    Any severe systemic disease or debilitating condition

TABLE 12–8. **PHARMACOLOGIC AGENTS IMPLICATED IN MALE SEXUAL DYSFUNCTION***

Drug	Impairs Erection	Impairs Ejaculation
Psychiatric drugs		
Tricyclic antidepressants[‡]		
Imipramine (Tofranil)	+	+
Protriptyline (Vivactil)	+	+
Desipramine (Pertofrane, Norpramin)	+	+
Clomipramine (Anafranil)	+	+
Amitriptyline (Elavil)	+	+
Nortriptyline (Aventyl)		
Monoamine oxidase inhibitors		
Tranylcypromine (Parnate)	+	
Mebanazine (Actomal)	+	+
Phenelzine (Nardil)	+	+
Pargyline (Eutonyl)	—	+
Isocarboxazid (Marplan)	—	+
Other mood-active drugs		
Lithium	+	
Amphetamines	+	+
Major tranquilizers[‡]		
Fluphenazine (Prolixin)	+	
Thioridazine (Mellaril)	+	+
Chlorprothixene (Taractan)	—	+
Mesoridazine (Serentil)	—	+
Perphenazine (Trilafon)	—	+
Trifluoperazine (Stelazine)	—	+
Butaperazine (Repoise)	—	+
Reserpine	+	+
Haloperidol (Haldol)	—	+
Minor tranquilizers[§]		
Chlordiazepoxide (Librium)	—	+

TABLE 12–8. **PHARMACOLOGIC AGENTS IMPLICATED IN MALE SEXUAL DYSFUNCTION (Continued)**

Drug	Impairs Erection	Impairs Ejaculation
Antihypertensive drugs		
Clonidine (Catapres)	+	
Methyldopa (Aldomet)	+	+
Spironolactone (Aldactone)	+	—
Hydrochlorothiazide (Apresoline)	+	—
Guanethidine (Ismelin)	+	+
Commonly abused drugs		
Alcohol	+	+
Barbiturates	+	+
Cannibus	+	—
Cocaine	+	+
Heroin	+	+
Methadone	+	—
Morphine	+	+
Miscellaneous drugs		
Antiparkinsonian agents	+	+
Clofibrate (Atromid-S)	+	—
Digoxin (Lanoxin)	+	—
Glutethimide (Doriden)	+	+
Indomethacin (Indocin)	+	—
Phentolamine (Regitine)	—	+
Propranolol (Inderal)	+	—

*Both increase and decrease in libido have been reported with psychoactive agents. It is difficult to separate those effects from the underlying condition or from improvement of the condition. Sexual dysfunction associated with the use of a drug disappears when the drug is discontinued.
†The incidence of erectile dysfunction associated with the use of tricyclic antidepressants is low.
‡Impairment of sexual function is not a common complication of the use of major tranquilizers. Priapism has occasionally occurred in association with the use of thioridazine and trazodone.
§Benzodiazepines have been reported to decrease libido, but in some patients the diminution of anxiety caused by those drugs enhances sexual function.

A number of procedures, from benign to invasive, are used to differentiate organically caused impotence from functional impotence. The most commonly used procedure is the monitoring of nocturnal penile tumescence (erections that occur during sleep), normally associated with rapid eye movement (REM).

A good history is invaluable in determining the etiology. A history of spontaneous erections, morning erections, or good erections with masturbation or with partners other than the usual one is indicative of functional impotence.

Psychologic causes of impotence include unresolved oedipal or preoedipal conflicts, which result in a punitive superego, an inability to trust, or feelings of inadequacy. In an ongoing relationship, erectile dysfunction may reflect difficulties between the partners.

D. Orgasm disorders
  1. Inhibited female orgasm (anorgasmia). Only 5% of married women over age 35 are estimated never to have achieved orgasm. That incidence is higher in unmarried women and younger women. Overall prevalence of inhibited female orgasm is 30%.

Both organic and psychologic factors are implicated in inhibited orgasm. Psychologic factors associated with inhibited orgasm include fears of impregnation or rejection by the sex partner, hostility toward men, feelings of guilt about sexual impulses, or marital conflicts. See Tables 12–9 and 12–10.

TABLE 12–9. **DSM-III-R DIAGNOSTIC CRITERIA FOR INHIBITED FEMALE ORGASM**

Persistent or recurrent delay in, or absence of, orgasm in a female following a normal sexual excitement phase during sexual activity that the clinician judges to be adequate in focus, intensity, and duration. Some females are able to experience orgasm during noncoital clitoral stimulation, but are unable to experience it during coitus in the absence of manual clitoral stimulation. In most of these females, this represents a normal variation of the female sexual response and does not justify the diagnosis of inhibited female orgasm. However, in some of these females, this does represent a psychologic inhibition that justifies the diagnosis. This difficult judgment is assisted by a thorough sexual evaluation, which may even require a trial of treatment.

Used with permission, APA.

TABLE 12–10. **PSYCHIATRIC DRUGS IMPLICATED IN INHIBITED FEMALE ORGASM***

Antidepressant
  Amoxapine (Asendin)[†]
  Fluoxetine (Prozac)

Tricyclic antidepressants
  Imipramine (Tofranil)
  Clomipramine (Anafranil)[‡]
  Nortriptyline (Aventyl)[§]

Monoamine oxidase inhibitors**
  Tranylcypromine (Parnate)
  Phenelzine (Nardil)
  Isocarboxazid (Marplan)

Major tranquilizers
  Thioridazine (Mellaril)
  Trifluoperazine (Stelazine)

*The interrelationship between female sexual dysfunction and pharmacologic agents has been less extensively evaluated than have male reactions. Oral contraceptives are reported to decrease libido in some women and some drugs with anticholinergic side effects may impair arousal as well as orgasm. Benzodiazepines have been reported to decrease libido, but in some patients the diminution of anxiety caused by those drugs enhances sexual function.

Both increase and decrease in libido have been reported with psychoactive agents. It is difficult to separate those effects from the underlying condition or from improvement of the condition. Sexual dysfunction associated with the use of a drug disappears when the drug is discontinued.

[†]Bethanechol (Urecholine) can reverse the effects of amoxapine-induced anorgasmia.
[‡]Clomipramine also is reported to increase arousal and orgasmic potential.
[§]Cyproheptadine reverses nortriptyline-induced anorgasmia.
**MAO-induced anorgasmia dysfunction may be a temporary reaction to the medication, which disappears even though administration of the drug is continued.

2. Inhibited male orgasm. Inhibited male orgasm, also called retarded ejaculation, may have physiologic causes and can follow surgery of the genitourinary tract (prostatectomy), may be associated with neurologic disorders (Parkinson's disease, lumbar or sacral neurologic damage), and is associated with the use of some antihypertensives or phenothiazines.

Primary inhibited male orgasm is usually indicative of more severe psychopathology. In an ongoing relationship, secondary ejaculatory inhibition frequently reflects interpersonal difficulties. See Table 12–11.

TABLE 12–11. **DSM-III-R DIAGNOSTIC CRITERIA FOR INHIBITED MALE ORGASM**

Persistent or recurrent delay in, or absence of, orgasm in a male following a normal sexual excitement phase during sexual activity that the clinician, taking into account the person's age, judges to be adequate in focus, intensity, and duration. This failure to achieve orgasm is usually restricted to an inability to reach orgasm in the vagina, with orgasm possible with other types of stimulation, such as masturbation.

Used with permission, APA.

3. Premature ejaculation.   It is estimated that 30% of the male population have this dysfunction. Premature ejaculation is more prevalent among young men, with a new partner, and among college-educated men than among men with less education; it is thought to be related to concern for partner satisfaction.

Premature ejaculation may be associated with unconscious fears about the vagina. It may also be the result of conditioning if the male's early sexual experiences occurred in situations in which discovery would be embarrassing. A stressful marriage exacerbates the disorder.

This dysfunction is the one most amenable to cure when behavioral techniques are used in treatment. See Table 12–12.

TABLE 12–12. **DSM-III-R DIAGNOSTIC CRITERIA FOR PREMATURE EJACULATION**

Persistent or recurrent ejaculation with minimal sexual stimulation or before, upon, or shortly after penetration and before the person wishes it. The clinician must take into account factors that affect duration of the excitement phase, such as age, novelty of the sexual partner or situation, and frequency of sexual activity.

Used with permission, APA.

E. Sexual pain disorders
  1. Vaginismus.   This dysfunction most frequently afflicts women in higher socioeconomic groups. A sexual trauma, such as rape or childhood sexual abuse, can be the cause. Women with psychosexual conflicts may perceive the penis as a weapon. A strict religious upbringing that associates sex with sin or problems in the dyadic relationship are also noted in these cases. See Table 12–14.

TABLE 12–13. **DSM-III-R DIAGNOSTIC CRITERIA FOR VAGINISMUS**

Recurrent or persistent involuntary spasm of the musculature of the outer third of the vagina that interferes with coitus.

Used with permission, APA.

  2. Dyspareunia.   Organic etiologies (endometriosis, vaginitis, cervicitis, and other pelvic disorders) must be ruled out with this complaint. 30–40% of women with this complaint who are seen in sex therapy clinics have pelvic pathology. An estimated 30% of surgical procedures on the female pelvic or genital area also result in temporary dyspareunia. In the majority of cases, however, dynamic factors are considered causative.

Dyspareunia can occur in men, but it is uncommon and is usually associated with an organic condition, such as Peyronie's disease. See Table 12–14.

TABLE 12–14. **DSM-III-R DIAGNOSTIC CRITERIA FOR DYSPAREUNIA**

A. Recurrent or persistent genital pain in either a male or a female before, during, or after sexual intercourse.

B. The disturbance is not caused exclusively by lack of lubrication or by vaginismus.

Used with permission, APA.

F. Other sexual disorders. See Table 12–15.

TABLE 12–15. **DSM-III-R DIAGNOSTIC CRITERIA FOR SEXUAL DYSFUNCTION NOT OTHERWISE SPECIFIED**

Sexual dysfunctions that do not meet the criteria for any of the specific sexual dysfunctions.

Examples:

  (1) no erotic sensation, or even complete anesthesia, despite normal physiologic component of orgasm
  (2) the female analogue of premature ejaculation
  (3) genital pain occurring during masturbation

Used with permission, APA.

II. Treatment.

Methods that have proved effective singly or in combination include (1) training in behavioral-sexual skills, (2) systematic desensitization, (3) directive marital therapy, (4) psychodynamic approaches, (5) group therapy, (6) pharmacotherapy, and (7) surgery. Evaluation and treatment must address the possibility of accompanying personality disorders and/or physical conditions.

1. **Analytically oriented sex therapy.** One of the most effective treatment modalities is the use of sex therapy (training in behavioral-sexual skills) integrated with psychodynamic and psychoanalytically oriented psychotherapy. The addition of psychodynamic conceptualizations to the behavioral techniques used to treat sexual dysfunctions allows for the treatment of patients with sexual disorders associated with other psychopathology.

2. **Behavioral techniques.** The aim of these techniques is to establish or reestablish verbal and sexual communication between partners. Specific exercises are prescribed to help the couple (or person) with their particular problem.

   Beginning exercises focus on verbal interchange and then on heightening sensory awareness to sight, touch, and smell. Initially, intercourse is prohibited and partners caress each other, excluding stimulation of the genitalia. Performance anxiety is reduced because responses of genital excitement and orgasm are unnecessary for the completion of the initial exercises.

   During these **sensate focus** exercises, patients receive encouragement and reinforcement to reduce their anxiety. They are urged to use fantasies to distract them from obsessive concerns about performance (spectatoring). The expression of mutual needs is encouraged. Resistances, such as claims of fatigue or not enough time to complete the exercises, are common and must be dealt with by the therapist. Genital stimulation is eventually added to general body stimulation. Finally, intromission and intercourse are permitted. Therapy sessions follow each new exercise period, and problems and satisfactions, both sexual and in other areas of the patients' lives, are discussed.

.a. **Specific techniques and exercises**—different techniques are used for specific dysfunctions.

  i. In **vaginismus**, the woman is advised to dilate her vaginal opening with fingers or dilators.

  ii. In **premature ejaculation**, the squeeze technique is used to raise the threshold of penile excitability. The patient or his partner forcibly squeezes the coronal ridge of the glans at the first sensation of impending ejaculation. The erection is diminished and ejaculation is inhibited. A variation is the **stop-start** technique. Stimulation is stopped as excitement increases, but no squeeze is used.

  iii. In **male inhibited desire** or **excitement**, the male is sometimes told to masturbate to demonstrate that full erection and ejaculation are possible.

  iv. In **primary anorgasmia**, the woman is instructed to masturbate, sometimes with the use of a vibrator. The use of fantasy is encouraged.

  v. **Retarded ejaculation** is managed by extravaginal ejaculation initially and gradual vaginal entry after stimulation to the point of near ejaculation.

  b. **Treatment of dysfunctions with behavioral techniques**—has been reported to be successful 40–85% of the time. 10% of refractory cases are estimated to need intensive individual psychotherapy. Approximately one-third of dysfunctional couples refractory to behavioral techniques alone require some combination of marital and sex therapy.

  c. **Organic treatment methods**—include pharmacotherapy: yohimbine, papaverine, psychotropics; and surgery: penile implants, revascularization.

3. **Biological treatment methods**—include pharmacotherapy: yohimbine, papaverine, psychotropics; and surgery: penile implants, revascularization.

III. **Paraphilias.**   These are disorders characterized by sexual impulses, fantasies, or practices that are unusual, deviant, or bizarre. More common in men than in women. Etiology unknown. There may be a biologic predisposition (abnormal electroencephalogram [EEG], hormone levels), which is made manifest by psychologic factors, such as childhood abuse. Psychoanalytic theory holds that paraphilia results from fixation at one of the psychosexual phases of development or is an effort to ward off castration anxiety. Learning theory holds that the act was associated with sexual arousal during childhood and conditioned learning occurred.

Paraphilic activity often has a compulsive quality. Patients repeatedly engage in deviant behavior and are unable to control the impulse. When stressed, anxious, or depressed, there is an increase in deviant behavior. The patient may make numerous resolutions to stop the behavior but is generally unable to abstain for long, and acting out is followed by strong feelings of guilt. Treatment techniques result in only moderate success rates and include insight-oriented psychotherapy, behavior therapy, and pharmacotherapy alone or in combination. Table 12–16 lists the common paraphilias.

For more detailed discussion of this topic, see Sadock VA: Normal Human Sexuality and Sexual Dysfunctions, Sec. 21.1, pp 1045–1061; Levine SL: Gender Identity Disorders of Childhood, Adolescence, and Adulthood, Sec. 21.2, pp 1061–1069; Abel GG: Paraphilias, Sec. 21.3, pp 1069–1085; Gadpaille WJ: Homosexuality, Sec. 21.4a, pp 1086–1096; Sadock VA: Rape, Spouse Abuse, and Incest, Sec. 21.4b, pp 1096–1104, in *CTP/V*.

TABLE 12–16. **PARAPHILIAS**

Disorder	Definition	General Considerations	Treatment
Excretory paraphilias	Defecating (coprophilia) or urinating (urophilia) on a partner or vice versa	Fixation at anal stage of development; klismaphilia (enemas)	Insight-oriented psychotherapy
Exhibitionism	Exposing genitals in public; rare in females	Person wants to shock female—her reaction is affirmation to patient that penis is intact	Insight-oriented psychotherapy, aversive conditioning. Female should try to ignore exhibitionistic male, who is offensive but not dangerous, or call police
Fetishism	Sexual arousal with inanimate objects, e.g., shoes, hair, clothing	Almost always in men. Behavior often followed by guilt	Insight-oriented psychotherapy; aversive conditioning; implosion, i.e., patient masturbates with fetish until it loses its arousal effect (masturbatory satiation)
Frotteurism	Rubbing genitals against female to achieve arousal and orgasm	Occurs in crowded places, such as subways, usually by passive, nonassertive men	Insight-oriented psychotherapy; aversive conditioning; group therapy; antiandrogenic medication
Pedophilia	Sexual activity with children under age 13; most common paraphilia	95% heterosexual, 5% homosexual. High risk of repeat behavior. Fear of adult sexuality in patient; low self-esteem. 10–20% of children have been molested by age 18	Place patient in treatment unit; group therapy; insight-oriented psychotherapy; antiandrogen medication to diminish sexual urge
Sexual masochism	Sexual pleasure derived from being abused physically or mentally or from being humiliated (moral masochism)	Defense against guilt feelings related to sex—punishment turned inwards	Insight-oriented psychotherapy; group therapy
Sexual sadism	Sexual arousal resulting from causing mental or physical suffering to another person	Mostly seen in men. Named after Marquis de Sade. Can progress to rape in some cases	Insight-oriented psychotherapy; aversive conditioning
Transvestic fetishism (Transvestism)	Cross-dressing	Most often used in heterosexual arousal. Most common is male-to-female cross-dressing. Do not confuse with transsexualism—wanting to be of opposite sex	Insight-oriented psychotherapy
Voyeurism (Scoptophilia)	Sexual arousal by watching sexual acts, e.g., coitus or naked person. Can occur in women but more common in men. Variant is listening to erotic conversations, e.g., telephone sex	Masturbation usually occurs during voyeuristic activity. Usually arrested for loitering or Peeping-Tomism	Insight-oriented psychotherapy; aversive conditioning
Zoophilia	Sex with animals	More common in rural areas; may be opportunistic	Behavior modification, insight-oriented psychotherapy

13

Sleep Disorders

I. General introduction

Sleep disturbances are common in the general population and among patients with mental disorders. Insomnia is the most prevalent disorder. Up to 30% of the population suffer from insomnia and seek help for it. Other conditions include excessive daytime sleepiness, difficulty sleeping during desired sleep time, and unusual nocturnal events, such as nightmares or sleepwalking.

Sleep disorders are classified by the Association of Sleep Disorders Centers (ASDC) as four major groupings with considerable overlap: (1) disorders of initiating and/or maintaining sleep (insomnia), (2) disorders of excessive somnolence (hypersomnia), (3) disorders of the sleep-wake schedule (normal sleep but at the wrong time), and (4) disorders associated with sleep stages (parasomnia).

In DSM-III-R, the sleep disorders are divided into two categories: the dyssomnias and the parasomnias. The dyssomnias include insomnia, hypersomnia, and sleep-wake schedule disorder (Table 13–1).

TABLE 13-1. **CLASSIFICATION OF SLEEP DISORDERS**

ASDC classification	DSM-III-R classification
Insomnia	Dyssomnia
Hypersomnia	(insomnia, hypersomnia, sleep-wake schedule
Sleep-wake schedule disorder	disorder)
Parasomnia	Parasomnia

A. **Sleep stages.** Sleep is measured with a polysomnograph, which simultaneously measures brain activity—electroencephalogram (EEG), eye movement—electro-oculogram (EOG), and muscle tone—electromyogram (EMG). Other physiologic tests can be applied during sleep and measured along with the above. EEG findings are used to describe sleep stages (Table 13-2).

TABLE 13-2. **SLEEP STAGES**

Awake	Low voltage, random, very fast
Drowsiness	Alpha waves random and fast (8-12 cycles per second [CPS])
Stage I	Slight slowing, 3-7 CPS, theta waves
Stage II	Further slowing, K complex (triphasic complexes), 12-14 CPS (sleep spindles); this stage marks the onset of true sleep
Stage III	High amplitude, slow waves (delta waves) at 0.5-2.5 CPS
Stage IV	At least 50% delta waves on EEG (stages 3 and 4 constitute delta sleep)
REM sleep	Sawtooth waves, similar to drowsy sleep on EEG

It takes the average person 15–20 minutes to fall asleep. Over the next 45 minutes, one descends to stages 3, 4 (deepest, largest stimulus needed to arouse). Approximately 45 minutes after stage 4, one gets to the first rapid eye movement (REM) period (average REM latency is 90 minutes). As the night progresses, each REM period gets longer and stages 3, 4 disappear. Further into the night, persons sleep more lightly and dream (REM).

B. **Characteristics of REM sleep**
   1. Tonic inhibition of skeletal muscle tone.
   2. Reduced hypercapnic respiratory drive.
   3. Relative poikilothermia (cold bloodedness).
   4. Penile tumescence.

C. **Sleep and aging**
   1. Subjective reports of elderly
      a. Time in bed increases.
      b. Number of nocturnal awakenings increases.
      c. Total sleep time at night decreases.
      d. Time to fall asleep increases.
      e. Dissatisfaction with their sleep.
      f. Tired and sleepy in the daytime.
      g. More frequent napping.
   2. Objective evidence of age-related changes in sleep cycle
      a. Reduced total REM.
      b. Reduced stages 3 and 4.
      c. Frequent awakenings.
      d. Reduced duration of nocturnal sleep.
      e. Need for daytime naps.
      f. Propensity for phase advance.
   3. Sleep disorders that are more common in the elderly
      a. Nocturnal myoclonus.
      b. Restless legs syndrome.
      c. REM sleep behavior disturbance.
      d. Sleep apnea.
      e. Sundowning.
   4. Medications and medical disorders also contribute to the problem.

II. **Classification of sleep disorders**
A. **Disorders of initiating and maintaining sleep (DIMS)**
   1. Also known as the insomnias.
   2. Must have objective daytime sleepiness or subjective sense of feeling unrested in order to be true insomniac. Otherwise, may merely reflect short sleep need.
   3. Insomnia is most prevalent in the elderly. Over 90% of persons over age 60 report unsatisfactory sleep.
   4. Most persons who complain of insomnia are found to have normal sleep when evaluated in the sleep lab. They do not have a psychiatric disorder or other factor to account for the insomnia. They have primary insomnia.
   5. Anxiety is the most common psychiatric cause of insomnia.
   6. Depression is also a major psychiatric cause of insomnia (Table 13-3).
   7. So-called atypical depression is characterized by vegetative reversal of

TABLE 13-3. **SLEEP IN MAJOR DEPRESSION**

Short REM latency
Long first REM period
Increased REM density
Nocturnal restlessness
Early morning awakening
Daytime lethargy

symptoms, so that patients exhibit hypersomnia along with increased appetite.

8. Treatment of insomnia consists of first identifying the underlying cause of the symptom and then providing specific intervention.

9. Drugs and alcohol frequently produce fragmented sleep, as do caffeinated beverages. Poor sleep hygiene may also be the cause of insomnia. Nonpharmacologic measures to improve sleep quality include
   a. Regular bedtime.
   b. Regular arousal time.
   c. Regular morning and afternoon exercise.
   d. Light evening snack.
   e. Comfortable bed.
   f. Cool room temperature.
   g. Use bed only for sleep or sex. (Do not watch television or do work in bed.)
   h. Avoid stimulant drugs or caffeine.
   i. Get out of bed and engage in other activities if you are having trouble falling asleep. (Do not lie in bed ruminating about not being able to sleep.)

10. Any sedative drug can help to induce sleep. Because of the possible risk of dependence, use of these drugs should be for short periods of time or for intermittent periods (see Chapter 22, Organic Therapy, for specific pharmacologic agents).

B. Disorders of excessive somnolence (DOES)
1. General introduction
   a. Most Americans are chronically sleepy owing to inadequate nocturnal sleep duration.
   b. Multiple sleep latency test (MSLT) is used as a diagnostic tool.
   c. DOES tend to be more serious, i.e., life threatening, than DIMS.
   d. The major DOES are (1) narcolepsy, (2) sleep apnea, (3) nocturnal movement disorders (myoclonus and restless legs), (4) drugs and alcohol, (5) atypical depressions, (6) Kleine-Levin syndrome, (7) idiopathic central nervous system (CNS) hypersomnia, and (8) sleep drunkenness.
   e. Primary hypersomnia is diagnosed when the symptom is not related to another mental disorder, to a known organic factor, or to a medication.
2. Narcolepsy
   a. **Characterized by symptom tetrad** — (1) excessive daytime somnolence, (2) cataplexy, (3) sleep paralysis, and (4) hypnagogic hallucinations.

i. Excessive daytime somnolence
  (a) Considered to be the primary symptom of narcolepsy; others are auxiliary.
  (b) Distinguished from fatigue by irresistible sleep attacks of short duration—less than 15 minutes.
  (c) Sleep attacks may be precipitated by monotonous or sedentary activity.
  (d) Naps are highly refreshing—effects last 30–120 minutes.
ii. Cataplexy
  (a) Reported by 70–80% of narcoleptics.
  (b) Brief (seconds to minutes) episodes of muscle weakness and/or paralysis.
  (c) No loss of consciousness, if episode is brief.
  (d) When attack is over, patient is completely normal.
  (e) Often triggered by
    (1) Laughter. ⎫
    (2) Anger.   ⎬ most common
    (3) Athletic activity.
    (4) Excitement/elation.
    (5) Sexual intercourse.
    (6) Fear.
    (7) Embarrassment.
  (f) Some patients may develop flat affect or lack of expressiveness as attempt to control emotions.
  (g) May manifest as partial loss of muscle tone (weakness, slurred speech, buckled knees, dropped jaw).
iii. Sleep paralysis
  (a) Reported by 25–50% of patients.
  (b) Temporary partial or complete paralysis in sleep/wake transitions.
  (c) Most commonly occurs upon awakening.
  (d) Conscious but unable to move.
  (e) Generally lasts less than 1 minute.
iv. Hypnagogic hallucinations
  (a) Dream-like experience during transition from wakefulness to sleep.
  (b) Patient aware of surroundings.
  (c) Vivid auditory or visual hallucinations or illusions.
  (d) Appear several years after the onset of sleep attacks.
b. Sleep onset REM periods (SOREMPs)
  i. Narcolepsy can be distinguished from other disorders of excessive daytime sleepiness by SOREMPs.
  ii. Defined as appearance of REM within 10–15 minutes of sleep onset.
  iii. More than one SOREMP/MSLT is considered diagnostic.
  iv. Seen in 70% of narcoleptic MSLTs (seen in fewer than 10% of patients with other hypersomnias).

    c. **Increased incidence of other clinical findings in narcolepsy**
       i. Periodic leg movement.
      ii. Sleep apnea—predominantly central.
     iii. Short sleep latency.
     iv. Memory problems.
      v. Ocular symptoms—blurring, diplopia, flickering.
     vi. Depression.

    d. **Onset and clinical course**
       i. Insidious onset before age 15. Once established, is chronic without major remissions.
      ii. Typically, full syndrome emerges in late adolescence or early 20s.
     iii. There may be long delay between the earliest symptoms (excessive somnolence) and the late appearance of cataplexy.

    e. **Human lymphocyte antigen (HLA)-antigen DR$_2$ and narcolepsy**
       i. Strong association between narcolepsy and HLA-antigen DR$_2$.
      ii. Some experts maintain that the presence of HLA-antigen DR$_2$ is necessary for the diagnosis of idiopathic narcolepsy.

    f. **Treatment**
       i. Regular bedtime.
      ii. Daytime naps.
     iii. Safety considerations, such as caution in driving or avoiding sharp edges on furniture.
     iv. Stimulants for daytime sleepiness. High dose propranolol (Inderal) may be effective.
      v. Tricyclics and monoamine oxidase inhibitors (MAOIs) for REM-related symptoms, mainly cataplexy (Table 13-4).

TABLE 13-4. **NARCOLEPSY DRUGS CURRENTLY AVAILABLE**

Drug	Maximal Dosage (All Drugs Administered Orally)
Treatment of excessive daytime somnolence (EDS)	
Stimulants	
Amphetamine	≤ 40 mg/day
Methylphenidate	≤ 60 mg/day
Pemoline	≤150 mg/day
Adjunct effect drugs (i.e., improve EDS if associated with stimulant)	
Protriptyline	≤ 10 mg/day
Treatment of cataplexy, sleep paralysis, and hypnagogic hallucinations	
Tricyclic antidepressants (with atropinic side effects)	
Protriptyline	≤ 20 mg/day
Imipramine	≤200 mg/day
Clomipramine	≤200 mg/day
Desipramine	≤200 mg/day
Antidepressants (without major atropinic side effects)	
Bupropion	≤300 mg/day

Table adapted from Guilleminault C: Narcolepsy syndrome. In *Principles and Practice of Sleep Medicine*, MH Kryger, T Roth, WC Dement, eds. WB Saunders, Philadelphia, 1989, p 344.

3. Sleep apnea. The three types of sleep apnea are (1) obstructive, (2) central, and (3) mixed.

   a. Obstructive sleep apnea

      i. Main symptoms—loud snoring with intervals of apnea.

      ii. Extreme daytime sleepiness with long and nonrefreshing daytime sleep attacks.

      iii. Patients unaware of apneas.

      iv. Other symptoms include severe morning headaches, morning confusion, depression, and/or anxiety.

      v. Findings include hypertension, arrythymias, right heart failure, and peripheral edema; progressively worsens without treatment.

      vi. Sleep lab evaluation reveals cessation of airflow in the presence of continued thoracic breathing movements.

      vii. In severe cases, persons have over 500 apneas/night.

      viii. Each lasts 10–20 seconds.

      ix. Treatment consists of nasal continuous positive airway pressure (CPAP), uvulopharyngopalatoplasty, weight loss, or protriptyline (Vivactil). If specific upper airway abnormality if found, surgical intervention is indicated.

   b. Central sleep apnea

      i. Rare.

      ii. Cessation of air flow secondary to lack of respiratory effort.

      iii. Treatment consists of mechanical ventilation or nasal CPAP.

   c. Mixed sleep apnea — central apnea followed by an obstructive phase.

4. Kleine-Levin syndrome

   a. Periodic disorder of hypersomnolence.

   b. Usually young males who sleep excessively for several weeks.

   c. Awaken only to eat (voraciously).

   d. Associated with hypersexuality and extreme hostility.

   e. Amnesia following attacks.

   f. May resolve spontaneously after several years.

   g. Patients normal between episodes.

   h. Treatment consists of stimulants (amphetamines, methylphenidate [Ritalin], and pemoline [Cylert]) for hypersomnia and preventive measures for other symptoms. Lithium also has been used successfully.

5. Idiopathic CNS hypersomnia

   a. Almost constant need to sleep.

   b. In contrast to most other DOES, patient is able to resist sleep.

   c. Extended periods of spontaneous sleep (12–20 hours).

   d. Difficulty awakening.

   e. Sleep and naps not refreshing.

   f. Confusion and disorientation upon awakening.

   g. Onset in late adolescence or early adulthood.

   h. No specific treatment. Stimulants may be of limited value.

6. Sleep drunkenness

   a. Inability to become fully alert for sustained period after awakening.

   b. Most commonly seen with sleep apnea or after sustained sleep deprivation.
   c. Can occur as an isolated disorder.
   d. No specific treatment. Stimulants may be of limited value.
7. **Nocturnal myoclonus**
   a. Stereotypical leg movements—periodic every 30 seconds.
   b. No seizure activity.
   c. Most prevalent in patients over age 55.
   d. Frequent awakenings.
   e. Unrefreshing sleep.
   f. Daytime sleepiness a major symptom.
   g. Patient unaware of the myoclonic events.
   h. Various drugs have been reported to help. These include clonazepam (Klonopin), opiates, and L-dopa (levodopa [Dopar, Larodopa]).
8. **Restless legs syndrome**
   a. Uncomfortable sensations in legs at rest.
   b. Not limited to sleep, but can interfere with falling asleep.
   c. Relieved by movement.
   d. May have associated sleep-related myoclonus.
   e. Benzodiazepines, e.g., clonazepam, are the treatment of choice. In severe cases, L-dopa or opiates may be used.
9. **Atypical depressions**
   a. Hyperphagia and hypersomnia.
   b. Two major subtypes are hysteroid dysphoria and seasonal affective (mood) disorder.
   c. Treatment of the underlying depression with antidepressants should also resolve the hypersomnia.
C. **Disorders of the sleep-wake schedule**
   1. Transient disturbances associated with jet lag and work shift changes.
      a. Self-limited. Resolve as body readjusts to new sleep-wake schedule.
      b. Adjusting to advance of sleep time more difficult than to delay.
   2. Persistent disturbances include (1) delayed sleep-phase syndrome, (2) advanced sleep-phase syndrome, and (3) non-24-hour sleep-wake syndrome.
      a. Quality of sleep basically normal, but timing is off.
      b. Can adjust through gradual delay of sleep time until new schedule is achieved.
   3. Most effective treatment of sleep-wake schedule disorders is a regular schedule of bright light therapy to entrain the sleep cycle. More useful in transient than in persistent disturbances.
D. **Disorders associated with sleep stages**
   1. **General introduction**
      a. Also known as the parasomnias.
      b. Often have poor recall.
      c. Include a group of diverse, sometimes bizarre, conditions.
      d. Different parasomnias may occur in same person.
   2. **Somnambulism**
      a. Also known as sleepwalking disorder.
      b. Most common in children; generally disappears spontaneously with age.

   c. Often have familial history of other parasomnias.

   d. Complex activity—leaving bed and walking about without full consciousness.

   e. Episodes brief.

   f. Amnesia for the event—no later memory for the episode.

   g. Stage 4 mainly.

   h. Initiated in first third of the night.

   i. In adults and elderly, may reflect psychopathology—rule out CNS pathology.

   j. Can sometimes initiate by standing a child in stage 4 sleep.

   k. Potentially dangerous.

   l. Drugs that suppress stage 4 sleep, such as benzodiazepines, can be used to treat somnambulism.

   m. Precautions include window guards and other measures to prevent injury.

3. Night terrors

   a. Also known as sleep terror disorder.

   b. Sudden awakening with intense anxiety.

   c. Autonomic overstimulation.

   d. Movement.

   e. Crying out.

   f. No memory for the event.

   g. Stage 4.

   h. Often within first hour or two of sleep.

   i. Treatment rarely needed in childhood.

   j. Awakening child prior to regular night terror for several days may eliminate terrors for extended periods.

4. Nightmares

   a. Also known as dream anxiety disorder (nightmare disorder).

   b. REM sleep.

   c. Can occur at any time of night.

   d. Good recall (quite detailed).

   e. Long, frightening dream in which one awakens frightened.

   f. Less anxiety, vocalization, motility, and autonomic discharge than night terrors.

   g. No specific treatment.

5. Enuresis. See Chapter 18, Child and Adolescent Disorders.

6. Paroxysmal nocturnal hemoglobinuria

   a. Sleep-related hemolysis.

   b. Weakness, pallor, anemia.

   c. Dark morning urine.

7. Sleep-related painful erections

   a. Rare.

   b. Painful erections during REM, not during wakefulness.

   c. Cause arousal.

8. Nocturnal headaches (cluster headaches and paroxysmal hemicrania)

   a. Vascular headaches.

   b. Similar to cluster headaches; unilateral.

   c. Cause awakening with agonizing pain.

    d. Associated with REM.

    e. Avoid alcoholic beverages.

    f. Treatment may include ergotamine preparations, amitriptyline (Elavil), or indomethacin (Indocin).

9. Familial sleep paralysis

    a. Isolated symptom.

    b. Not associated with narcolepsy.

    c. Episode terminates with touch or noise (some external stimulus).

10. Impaired sleep-related penile tumescence

    a. Full erections normal during REM sleep.

    b. Full erections during REM sleep suggest that impotence is psychogenic.

    c. Severely depressed males may not have REM erections.

11. Head banging (Jactatio capitis nocturnus)

    a. Rhythmic head or body rocking just before or during sleep; may extend into light sleep.

    b. Usually limited to childhood.

    c. Mainly in stages 1 and 2.

    d. No treatment required in most infants and young children. Crib padding or helmets may be used. Behavior modification, benzodiazepines, and tricyclic antidepressants may be effective.

12. Bruxism

    a. Primarily in stages 1 and 2 or during partial arousals or transitions.

    b. No EEG abnormality (no seizure activity).

    c. Treatment consists of bite plates to prevent dental damage.

13. REM sleep behavior disorder

    a. Chronic and progressive, chiefly in older men.

    b. Loss of atonia during REM sleep with emergence of complex and violent behaviors.

    c. Potential for serious injury.

    d. Neurologic cause in many cases.

    e. May follow during withdrawal REM rebound.

    f. Treat with clonazepam 0.5–2.0 mg/day.

14. Asthma

    a. More common and severe during the night.

    b. Most attacks occur toward the end of the night (when REM is more abundant).

    c. Death from asthma most common during the night and in the early morning.

    d. Oral theophyllines and long-acting oral β_2 agonists can reduce nocturnal symptoms.

15. Sleep-related epileptic seizures

    a. Peak during first and last 2 hours of sleep.

    b. May masquerade as enuresis, night terrors, or sleepwalking.

    c. Difficult to diagnose.

    d. Need to use full clinical EEG, not polysomnogram.

    e. Treatment consists of appropriate use of anticonvulsant drugs.

For more detailed discussion of this topic, see Karacan I, Williams RL, Moore CA: Sleep Disorders, Chap. 22, pp 1105–1135, in *CTP/V*.

14
Impulse Control and Adjustment Disorders

I. **Adjustment disorders**
  A. **Definition.** Pathologic behavioral response to a psychosocial stressor that results in impaired social or vocational functioning. Stressors are within range of normal experience, e.g., birth of baby, going away to school, marriage, job loss, divorce, illness.
  B. **Diagnosis, signs and symptoms.** Onset usually within 3 months of the stressor and persists for no longer than 6 months. Eight patterns of maladaptive behavior can occur.
    1. Depression.
    2. Anxiety.
    3. Mixed emotional features (anxiety, depression, emotional lability).
    4. Work or academic inhibition or impaired performance.
    5. Withdrawal.
    6. Physical complaints—backache, fatigue, headache.
    7. Disturbance of conduct.
    8. Mixed disturbance of emotions and conduct.
  C. **Epidemiology.** Most frequent in adolescence, but can occur at any age.
  D. **Etiology**
    1. **Genetic.** High anxiety temperament more prone to overreacting to stressful event and subsequent adjustment disorders.
    2. **Biologic.** Greater vulnerability with history of serious medical illness or disability.
    3. **Psychosocial.** Greater vulnerability in persons who lost parent during infancy or who had poor mothering experiences. Ability to tolerate frustration in adult life correlates with gratification of basic needs in infant life.
  E. **Differential diagnosis**
    1. **Post-traumatic stress disorder.** Psychosocial stressor determines diagnosis. Stressor is outside the range of normal human experience, e.g., war, rape, mass catastrophe, floods, taken hostage.
    2. **Brief reactive psychosis.** Characterized by hallucinations and delusions.
    3. **Uncomplicated bereavement.** Occurs before, immediately, or shortly after death of loved one; impaired occupational and/or social functioning within expected bounds and remits spontaneously.
  F. **Course and prognosis.** Most symptoms diminish over time without treatment, especially after stressor is removed; subgroup maintains chronic course with risk of secondary depression, anxiety, psychoactive substance use disorder.
  G. **Treatment**
    1. **Psychologic.** Psychotherapy is treatment of choice—explore meaning of stressor to patient, provide support, encourage alternative ways of coping, offer empathy. Biofeedback, relaxation techniques, and hypnosis for anxious mood.

2. Pharmacologic. Subtype, e.g., anxiety/depression, can be treated with medication, but be careful not to allow drug dependency to develop (especially if benzodiazepines are used).

II. Impulse control disorders

A. Definition. The inability to resist acting on an impulse or drive that is dangerous to others or to oneself and that is characterized by a sense of pleasure when gratified.

B. Diagnosis, signs and symptoms. The five types of impulse control disorders are outlined in Table 14–1.

C. Etiology. Usually unknown. Some disorders may have abnormal electroencephalogram (EEG), mixed cerebral dominance or soft neurologic signs, e.g., intermittent explosive disorder. Alcohol reduces ability to control impulses (disinhibition).

D. Psychodynamics. Acting out of impulses related to need to express sexual or aggressive drive. Gambling often associated with underlying depression representing unconscious need to lose and experience punishment.

E. Differential diagnosis

1. Temporal lobe epilepsy. Characteristic temporal lobe abnormal EEG foci are found that account for aggressive outbursts, kleptomania, pyromania.

2. Head trauma. Residual signs of trauma with brain imaging techniques will be found.

3. Bipolar disorder, manic (mania). May have gambling or associated feature.

4. Psychoactive substance abuse. Will reveal history of drug use, alcohol.

5. Rule out **organic disorder, brain tumor, degenerative disease, endocrine disorder** on basis of characteristic findings for each.

6. Schizophrenia shows delusions or hallucinations to account for acting out of impulse.

F. Course and prognosis

1. Usually chronic course for all impulse control disorders. Intermittent explosive disorder may increase in severity with time.

2. Kleptomaniacs frequently arrested for shoplifting.

3. Pathological gambling is progressive with increasing financial losses, writing bad checks, total deterioration.

4. Pyromaniacs often produce increasingly larger fires over time.

5. Trichotillomania associated with remissions and exacerbations.

G. Treatment

1. Intermittent explosive disorder. Combined pharmacotherapy and psychotherapy. May have to try different medications before result achieved: phenothiazine, imipramine (Tofranil), lithium. If EEG abnormality present, carbamazepine (Tegretol) may be used. Benzodiazepines can aggravate condition because of disinhibition. Propranolol (Inderal) can be of help in selected cases. Supportive psychotherapy, limit-setting, family therapy if patient is child or adolescent. Group therapy used cautiously if patient is liable to attack fellow group member.

2. Kleptomania. Insight-oriented psychotherapy to understand motivation,

TABLE 14–1. **TYPES OF IMPULSE CONTROL DISORDERS**

Type	Definition	Diagnosis	Other Features
Intermittent Explosive Disorder	Episodes of aggression resulting in harm to others	Discrete episodes of violence; may have aura before attack	Males > Females; first-degree relative often affected
Kleptomania	Repeated stealing or shoplifting	Stealing of objects not generally needed; pleasure at time of commiting theft	Females > Males; worse during times of stress
Pathological Gambling	Repeated gambling episodes that result in socioeconomic disruption, indebtedness, illegal activities	Restless or irritable if unable to gamble; continues even with mounting debts; need to increase amount wagered; constant gambling preoccupation	Males > Females; affects 2-3% of U.S. population; may be part of bipolar disorder, manic
Pyromania	Deliberate setting of fires	Irresistible impulse to set fire, which relieves inner tension state; no personal gain involved	Males > Females; differentiate from arson, which is setting fires for money, insurance, to destroy evidence
Trichotillomania	Compulsive hair pulling producing bald spots (alopecia areata)	Hair pulling occurs repeatedly with sense of gratification when pulling out hair, followed by agitation	Females > Males

e.g., guilt, need for punishment, and to control impulse. Behavior therapy to learn new patterns of behavior. Underlying depression responds to antidepressants.

3. **Pathological gambling.** Insight-oriented psychotherapy coupled with peer support groups, especially Gamblers Anonymous (GA). Total abstinence is goal. Treat associated depression, mania, substance abuse, sexual dysfunction.

4. **Pyromania.** Insight-oriented therapy, behavior therapy. Patients require close supervision because of repeated fire-setting behavior and danger to others as a result. May need inpatient facility, night hospital, or other structured setting.

5. **Trichotillomania.** Supportive and insight-oriented psychotherapies of value, but medications may also be required: benzodiazepines with high anxiety level, antidepressants with depressed mood. Although fluoxetine (Prozac) is approved only for major depressive disorder, there are reports in the literature that it may diminish compulsive behavior and can be used as adjunct to psychotherapy. Consider hypnosis and biofeedback in some cases. Clomipramine (Anafranil) 25–250 mg/day reported to be useful.

For more detailed discussion of this topic, see Popkin MK: Adjustment Disorder, Sec. 24.1, pp 1141–1145; Popkin MK: Impulse Control Disorders Not Elsewhere Classified, Sec. 24.2, pp 1145–1154, in *CTP/V*.

15

Psychosomatic Disorders (Psychological Factors Affecting Physical Condition)

I. Psychosomatic disorders

  A. Definition. The term "psychosomatic disorder" refers to physical conditions caused or aggravated by psychological factors. Although most physical disorders are influenced by stress, conflict, or generalized anxiety, some disorders are more affected than others. In DSM-III-R, psychosomatic disorders are subsumed by the classification known as psychological factors affecting physical condition.

  B. Etiology

   1. Specificity theory. This theory postulates specific stresses or personality types for each psychosomatic disease and is typified by the work of the following investigators:

   a. Flanders Dunbar — described personality traits that are specific for a psychosomatic disorder, e.g., coronary personality. Type A personality is hard-driving, aggressive, irritable, and susceptible to heart disease.

   b. Franz Alexander — described unconscious conflicts that produce anxiety, are mediated through the autonomic nervous system, and result in a specific disorder, e.g., repressed dependency needs result in peptic ulcer.

   2. Nonspecific theory. This theory states that any prolonged stress can cause physiologic changes, which result in a physical disorder. Each person has a "shock organ" that is genetically vulnerable to stress: some patients are cardiac reactors, gastric reactors, skin reactors. Persons who are chronically anxious or depressed have a greater vulnerability to physical and/or psychosomatic disease.

   3. Pathophysiology. Hans Selye described the general adaption syndrome (GAS), which is the sum of all nonspecific systemic reactions of the body that follow prolonged stress. The hypothalamic-pituitary-adrenal axis is affected with excess secretion of cortisol, producing structural damage to various organ systems. George Engel postulated that in the stressed state, functional changes occur in all neuroregulatory mechanisms that depress the body's homeostatic mechanisms, leaving the body vulnerable to infection and other disorders.

   Neurophysiologic pathways thought to mediate stress reactions include the cerebral cortex, limbic system, hypothalamus, adrenal medulla, and sympathetic and parasympathetic nervous systems. Neuromessengers include such hormones as cortisol, thyroxin, and epinephrine.

C. Diagnosis. To meet the diagnostic criteria known as psychological factors affecting physical condition, the following two criteria must be fulfilled: (1) The psychologically meaningful environmental stimulus is temporally related to the initiation or exacerbation of the specific physical condition or disorder. (2) The physical condition must show either demonstrable organic pathology, e.g., rheumatoid arthritis, or a known pathophysiologic process, e.g., migraine headache. A number of physical disorders meet these criteria and are listed in Table 15-1.

TABLE 15-1. **PHYSICAL CONDITIONS AFFECTED BY PSYCHOLOGICAL FACTORS**

Disorder	Observations/Comments/Theory Approach
Angina, Arrhythmias, Coronary spasms	Type A person is aggressive, irritable, easily frustrated, and prone to coronary artery disease. Arrhythmias common in anxiety states. Sudden death from ventricular arrhythmia in some patients who experience massive psychological shock or catastrophe. Life-style changes: cease smoking, curb alcohol intake, lose weight, lower cholesterol to limit risk factors. Propranolol (Inderal) prescribed for patients who develop tachycardia as part of social phobia—protects against arrhythmia and decreases coronary blood flow.
Asthma	Attacks precipitated by stress, respiratory infection, allergy. Examine family dynamics, especially when child is the patient. Look for overprotectiveness and try to encourage appropriate independent activities. Propranolol and β-blockers contraindicated in asthma patients for anxiety. Psychological theories: strong dependency and separation anxiety; asthma wheeze is suppressed cry for love and protection.
Connective tissue diseases: Systemic lupus erythematosus, Rheumatoid arthritis	Disease can be heralded by major life stress, especially death of loved one. Worsens with chronic stress, anger, or depression. Important to keep patient as active as possible to minimize joint deformities. Treat depression with antidepressant medications or psychostimulants, and treat muscle spasm and tension with benzodiazepines.
Headaches	Tension headache results from contraction of strap muscles in neck constricting blood flow. Associated with anxiety, situational stress. Relaxation therapy, antianxiety medication useful. Migraine headaches are unilateral and can be triggered by stress, excercise, high tyramine foods. Manage with ergotamine (Cafergot). Propranolol prophylaxis can produce associated depression.
Hypertension	Acute stress produces catecholamines (epinephrine), raising systolic blood pressure. Chronic stress associated with essential hypertension. Look at life-style. Prescribe exercise, relaxation therapy, biofeedback. Benzodiazepines of use in acute stress if blood pressure rises as shock organ. Psychological theories: inhibited rage, guilt over hostile impulses, need to gain approval from authority.
Hyperventilation syndrome	Accompanies panic disorder, generalized anxiety disorder with associated hyperventilation, tachycardia, vasoconstriction. May be hazardous in patients with coronary insufficiency. Antianxiety agents of use; some patients respond to monoamine oxidase inhibitors, tricyclic antidepressants, or serotonergic agents.
Inflammatory bowel diseases: Crohn's disease, Irritable bowel syndrome, Ulcerative colitis	Depressed mood associated with illness; stress exacerbates symptoms. Onset after major life stress. Patients respond to stable doctor-patient relationship and supportive psychotherapy in addition to bowel medication. Psychological theories: passive personality, childhood intimidation, obsessive traits, fear of punishment, masked hostility.
Metabolic and endocrine disorders	Thyrotoxicosis following sudden severe stress. Glycosuria in chronic fear and anxiety. Depression alters hormone metabolism, especially adrenocorticotropic hormone (ACTH).

TABLE 15–1.   PHYSICAL CONDITIONS AFFECTED BY PSYCHOLOGICAL FACTORS (Continued)

Disorder	Observations/Comments/Theory Approach
Neurodermatitis	Eczema in patients with multiple psychosocial stressors—especially death of loved one, conflicts over sexuality, repressed anger. Some respond to hypnosis in symptom management.
Obesity	Hyperphagia reduces anxiety. Night-eating syndrome associated with insomnia. Failure to perceive appetite, hunger, and satiation. Psychological theories: conflicts about orality and pathologic dependency. Behavioral techniques, support groups, nutritional counseling, and supportive psychotherapy useful. Treat underlying depression.
Osteoarthritis	Life-style management induces weight reduction, isometric exercises to strengthen joint musculature, maintenance of physical activity, pain control. Treat associated anxiety or depression with supportive psychotherapy.
Peptic ulcer disease	Increased gastric acid and pepsin relative to mucosal resistance; both sensitive to anxiety, stress, coffee, alcohol. Life-style changes. Relaxation therapy. Psychological theories: strong frustrated dependency needs, cannot express anger, superficial self-sufficiency.
Raynaud's disease	Peripheral vasoconstriction associated with smoking, stress. Life-style changes: cessation of smoking, moderate exercise. Biofeedback can raise hand temperature by increased vasodilation.
Syncope, Hypotension	Vaso-vagal reflex with acute anxiety or fear produces hypotension and fainting. More common in patients with hyperreactive autonomic nervous system. Aggravated by anemia, antidepressant medications (produces hypotension as side effect).
Urticaria, Angioedema	Idiopathic type not related to specific allergens or physical stimulus. May be associated with stress, chronic anxiety, depression. Pruritis worse with anxiety; self-excoriation associated with repressed hostility. Some phenothiazines have antipruritic effect. Psychological theories: conflict between dependence-independence, unconscious guilt feelings, itching as sexual displacement.

D. **Medical, surgical, and neurologic conditions that primarily present with psychiatric symptomatology.** A host of medical and neurologic disorders, summarized in Table 15–2, may present with psychiatric symptomatology, which must be differentiated from primary psychiatric disorders.

E. **Differential diagnosis.** As outlined in Table 15–3, various psychiatric syndromes and disorders can be confused with psychosomatic disorders. Each lacks a demonstrable organic pathologic lesion or known pathophysiologic process.

F. **Treatment**

1. **Combined approach** necessary; work in collaboration with internist or surgeon who manages physical disorder, with psychiatrist attending to psychiatric aspects.

2. **Supportive psychotherapy** of great value, especially when psychiatrist forms therapeutic alliance with patient. Psychiatrist allows patient to ventilate most fears of illness, especially death fantasies. Many patients have strong dependency needs, which are partially gratified in treatment.

3. **Dynamic insight-oriented psychotherapy.** Explore unconscious conflicts regarding sex and aggression. Anxiety associated with life stresses examined with new, more mature defenses established.

4. **Group therapy** of use with patients who have similar physical disorders or problems, e.g., colitis patients, hemodialysis patients.

TABLE 15–2. **MEDICAL PROBLEMS THAT PRESENT WITH PSYCHIATRIC SYMPTOMS**

Disease	Sex and Age Prevalence	Common Medical Symptoms	Psychiatric Symptoms and Complaints	Impaired Performance and Behavior	Diagnostic Problems
Acquired immune deficiency syndrome (AIDS)	Males>Females: IV drug abusers, homosexuals, female sex partners of bisexual men	Lymphadenopathy, fatigue, opportunistic infections, Kaposi's sarcoma	Depression, anxiety, disorientation	Dementia with global impairment	Seropositive human immunodeficiency virus (HIV) is diagnostic when clinical signs are present
Hyperthyroidism (thyrotoxicosis)	Females 3:1, 20 to 50	Tremor, sweating, loss of weight and strength, heat intolerance	Anxiety, depression	Occasional hyperactive or grandiose behavior	Long lead time; rapid onset resembles anxiety attack
Hypothyroidism (Myxedema)	Females 5:1, 30 to 50	Puffy face, dry skin, cold intolerance	Lethargy anxiety with irritability, thought disorder, somatic delusions, hallucinations	Myxedema madness; delusional, paranoid, belligerent behavior	Madness can mimic schizophrenia; mental status is clear, even during most disturbed behavior
Hyperparathyroidism	Females 3:1, 40 to 60	Weakness, anorexia, fractures, calculi, peptic ulcers			Anorexia and fatigue of slow-growing adenoma resemble involutional depression
Hypoparathyroidism	Females, 40 to 60	Hyperreflexia, spasms, tetany	Either state can cause anxiety, hyperactivity, and irritability or depression, apathy, and withdrawal	Either state can proceed to a toxic psychosis: confusion, disorientation, and clouded sensorium	None: rare condition except after surgery
Hyperadrenalism (Cushing's disease)	Adults, both sexes	Weight gain, fat alteration, easy fatigability	Varied; depression, anxiety, thought disorder with somatic delusions	Rarely produces aberrant behavior	Bizarre somatic delusions caused by bodily changes resemble schizophrenia
Adrenal cortical insufficiency (Addison's disease)	Adults, both sexes	Weight loss, hypotension, skin pigmentation	Depression—negativism, apathy; thought disorder—suspiciousness	Toxic psychosis with confusion and agitation	Long lead time; weight loss, apathy, despondency resemble involutional depression
Porphyria—acute intermittent type	Females, 20 to 40	Abdominal crises, paresthesias, weakness	Anxiety—sudden onset, severe; mood swings	Extremes of excitement or withdrawal; emotional or angry outbursts	Patients often have truly neurotic life-styles; crises resemble conversion reactions or anxiety attacks

TABLE 15–2. **MEDICAL PROBLEMS THAT PRESENT WITH PSYCHIATRIC SYMPTOMS (Continued)**

Disease	Sex and Age Prevalence	Common Medical Symptoms	Psychiatric Symptoms and Complaints	Impaired Performance and Behavior	Diagnostic Problems
Pernicious anemia (Addisonian anemia)	Females, 40 to 60	Weight loss, weakness, glossitis, extremity neuritis	Depression—feelings of guilt and worthlessness	Eventual brain damage with confusion and memory loss	Long lead time, sometimes many months; easily mistaken for involutional depression; normal early blood studies may give false reassurance
Hepatolenticular degeneration (Wilson's disease)	Males 2:1, adolescence	Liver and extrapyramidal symptoms	Mood swings—sudden and changeable; anger—explosive	Eventual brain damage with memory and I.Q. loss; combativeness	In late teens, can resemble adolescent storm, incorrigibility, or schizophrenia
Hypoglycemia (islet cell adenoma)	Adults, both sexes	Tremor, sweating, hunger, fatigue, dizziness	Anxiety—fear and dread, depression with fatigue	Agitation, confusion; eventual brain damage	Can mimic anxiety attack or acute alcoholism; bizarre behavior may draw attention away from somatic symptoms
Intracranial tumors	Adults, both sexes	None early; headache, vomiting, papilledema later	Varied: depression, anxiety, personality changes	Loss of memory, judgment, self-criticism; clouding of consciousness	Tumor location may not determine early symptoms
Pancreatic carcinoma	Males 3:1, 50 to 70	Weight loss, abdominal pain, weakness, jaundice	Depression, sense of imminent doom but without severe guilt	Loss of drive and motivation	Long lead time; exact age and symptoms of involutional depression
Pheochromocytoma	Adults, both sexes	Headache, sweating during elevated blood pressure	Anxiety, panic, fear, apprehension, trembling	Inability to function during an attack	Classic symptoms of anxiety attack, intermittently normal blood pressures may discourage further studies
Multiple sclerosis	Females, 20 to 40	Motor and sensory losses, scanning speech, nystagmus	Varied: personality changes, mood swings, depression; bland euphoria uncommon	Inappropriate behavior due to personality changes	Long lead time; early neurologic symptoms mimic hysteria or conversion disorders
Systemic lupus erythematosus	Females, 8:1, 20 to 40	Multiple symptoms of cardiovascular, genitourinary, gastrointestinal, other systems	Varied; thought disorder, depression, confusion	Toxic psychosis unrelated to steroid treatment	Long lead time, perhaps many years; psychiatric picture variable over time; thought disorder resembles schizophrenia, steroid psychosis

Adapted from table prepared by Maurice J. Martin, M.D.

TABLE 15–3.   CONDITIONS MIMICKING PSYCHOSOMATIC DISORDERS

Diagnosis	Definition and Example
Conversion disorder	There is an alteration of physical function that suggests a physical disorder but is an expression of psychological conflict, e.g., psychogenic aphonia. These symptoms are falsely neurologic-anatomic in distribution, are symbolic in nature, and allow much secondary gain.
Body dysmorphic disorder	Preoccupation with an imagined physical defect in appearance in a normal appearing person, e.g., preoccupation with facial hair.
Hypochondriasis	Imagined overconcern about physical disease when objective examination reveals none to exist, e.g., angina pectoris with normal heart functioning.
Somatization disorder	Recurrent somatic and physical complaints with no demonstrable physical disorder despite repeated physical examinations and no organic basis.
Physical complaints associated with classical psychological disorders	Somatic accompaniment of depression, e.g., weakness, asthenia.
Physical complaints with substance abuse disorder	Bronchitis and cough associated with nicotine and tobacco dependence.

5. Flexibility is key.   With patient's permission, may see families, spouses, friends.

6. Behavior therapy, relaxation techniques, and biofeedback useful when there is strong autonomic nervous system component, e.g., asthma, allergies, hypertension.

7. Pharmacotherapy

a.   Use in limited way so as not to create dependency.

b.   Antipsychotic drugs when there is associated psychosis.

c.   Antianxiety drugs diminish harmful anxiety during period of acute stress.

d.   Antidepressants used with depression secondary to organic illness.

II. Consultation-liaison (C-L) psychiatry.   The C-L psychiatrist serves as a consultant to other fellow medical specialists and usually operates directly in a surgical or medical setting, providing psychiatric consultation and management. Because 65% of medical inpatients have psychiatric problems and 50% are management problems, the C-L psychiatrist has an important role in the hospital setting. Table 15–4 lists the most common C-L problems encountered in a general hospital and includes comments about management.

III. Special medical settings.   Besides the usual medical wards in a hospital, special settings produce uncommon, distinctive stress.

A. Intensive Care Unit (ICU).   The ICU contains seriously ill patients who have life-threatening illnesses. Coronary care units (CCUs) are good examples of this. Among the defensive reactions encountered are fear, anxiety, acting out, signing out against medical advice, hostility, dependency, depression, grief, and delirium.

B. Hemodialysis.   Hemodialysis patients have lifelong dependency on machines and health care providers: 3 times/week for 6 hours for dialysis. They have problems with prolonged dependency, regression to childhood states, hostility, and negativism to following the doctors' directions.

TABLE 15–4.   **COMMON CONSULTATION-LIAISON PROBLEMS**

Reason for Consultation	Comments
Suicide attempt or threat	High-risk factors are males over 45, no social support, alcoholism, previous attempt, incapacitating medical illness with pain, and suicidal ideation. If risk is present, transfer to psychiatric unit or start 24-hour nursing care.
Depression	Suicidal risks must be assessed in every depressed patient (see above); presence of cognitive defects in depression may cause diagnostic dilemma with dementia (pseudodementia); check for history of substance abuse or depressant drugs, e.g., reserpine, propranolol; use antidepressants cautiously in cardiac patients because of conduction side effects, orthostatic hypotension.
Agitation	Often related to organic mental disorder, withdrawal from drugs, e.g., opioids, alcohol, sedative-hypnotics; haloperidol most useful drug for excessive agitation; use physical restraints with great caution; examine for command hallucinations or paranoid ideation to which patient is responding in agitated manner; rule out toxic reaction to medication, e.g., cortisol paranoia, anticholinergic delirium.
Hallucinations	Most common cause in hospital is delirium tremens; onset 3–4 days after hospitalization. In intensive care units, check for sensory isolation; rule out brief reactive psychosis, schizophrenia, organic mental disorder. Treat with antipsychotic medication.
Sleep disorder	Common cause is pain; early morning awakening associated with depression; difficulty falling asleep associated with anxiety. Use antianxiety or antidepressant agent depending on cause. These drugs have no analgesic effect, so prescribe adequate pain killers. Rule out early drug withdrawal reaction.
No organic basis for symptoms	Rule out conversion disorder, somatization disorder, factitious disorder or malingering; glove and stocking anesthesia with autonomic nervous system symptoms seen in conversion; multiple body complaints seen in somatization; wish to be hospitalized seen in factitious disorder; obvious secondary gain in malingering, e.g., compensation case.
Disorientation	Delirium versus dementia; review metabolic status, neurologic findings, drug history. Prescribe small dose of antipsychotics for major agitation; benzodiazepines may worsen condition and cause sundowner syndrome (ataxia, confusion); modify environment so patient does not experience sensory deprivation.
Noncompliance or refusal to consent to procedure	Explore relationship of patient and treating doctor; negative transference is most common cause of noncompliance; fears of medication or procedure require education and reassurance. Refusal to give consent is issue of judgment; if impaired, patient can be declared incompetent, but only by court; organic mental disorder is main cause of impaired judgment in hospitalized patients.

Dialysis dementia is a disorder characterized by loss of cognitive functions, dystonias, and seizures, which usually ends in death. It tends to occur in patients who have been on dialysis for long periods of time.

C. Surgery. Patients who have had severe surgical procedures have a variety of psychological reactions, depending on their premorbid personality and the nature of the surgery. These reactions are summarized in Table 15–5.

IV. Pain. Pain is a complex symptom consisting of a sensation underlying potential disease and an associated emotional state. Acute pain is a reflex biologic response

TABLE 15–5.   **TRANSPLANTATION AND SURGICAL PROBLEMS**

Organ	Biological Factor	Psychological Factor
Kidney	50-90% success rate. May not be done if patient over age 55. Increasing use of cadaver kidneys rather than those from living donors.	Living donors must be emotionally stable; parents are best donors, siblings may be ambivalent; donors are subject to depression. Patients who panic before surgery may have poor prognosis; altered body image with fear of organ rejection is common. Group therapy for patients is helpful.
Bone marrow	Used in aplastic anemias and immune system disease.	Patients are usually very ill and must deal with death and dying; compliance important. Commonly done in children who present problems of prolonged dependency; siblings are often donors who may be angry or ambivalent about procedure.
Heart	End-stage coronary artery disease and cardiomyopathy.	Donor is legally dead; relatives of deceased may refuse permission or be ambivalent. No fall-back position if organ rejected; kidney rejection can go on hemodialysis. Some patients seek transplant hoping to die. Postcardiotomy delirium in 25 percent of patients.
Breast	Radical mastectomy versus lumpectomy.	Reconstruction of breast at time of surgery leads to better postoperative adaptation; veteran patients used to counsel new patients; lumpectomy patients more open about surgery and sex than are mastectomy patients; group support helpful.
Uterus	Hysterectomy performed on 10% of women over 20.	Fear of loss of sexual attractiveness with sexual dysfunction may occur in small percentage of women; loss of childbearing capacity upsetting.
Brain	Anatomic location of lesion determines behavioral change.	Environmental dependency syndrome in frontal lobe tumors characterized by inability to show initiative; memory disturbances involved in periventricular surgery; hallucinations in parieto-occipital area.
Prostate	Cancer surgery has more negative psychobiological effects and is more technically difficult than is surgery for benign hypertrophy.	Sexual dysfunction common except in transurethral prostatectomy (TUP). Perineal prostatectomy produces absence of emission, ejaculation, and erection; penile implant may be of use.
Colon and Rectum	Common outcome is colostomy, especially for cancer.	One-third of patients with colostomy feel worse about themselves than before bowel surgery; shame and self-consciousness about stoma can be alleviated by self-help groups that deal with those issues.
Limbs	Amputation performed for massive injury, diabetes, or cancer.	Phantom limb phenomenon occurs in 98% of cases; experience can last for years; sometimes sensation can be painful, and neuroma at stump should be ruled out; no known cause or treatment, can stop spontaneously.

to injury. By definition, chronic pain consists of pain of a minimum of 6 months' duration. A physiologic classification of pain is listed in Table 15–6, and characteristics of pain are listed in Table 15–7.

V. Somatoform pain disorder
   A. Definition. Somatoform pain disorder is a preoccupation with pain in the absence of physical disease to account for its intensity. It does not follow a

TABLE 15–6. **PHYSIOLOGIC CLASSIFICATION OF PAIN**

Type	Subtypes	Example	Comment
Nociceptive	Somatic Visceral	Bone metastasis Intestinal obstruction	Due to activation of pain-sensitive fibers; usually aching or pressure
Deafferentiation	Peripheral Central Somatic Visceral Sympathetic dependent Nonsympathetic dependent	Causalgia Thalamic pain Causalgia Visceral pain in paraplegics Postherpetic pain Phantom pain	Due to interruption of afferent pathways. Pathophysiology poorly understood, with most syndromes probably involving both peripheral and central nervous system changes. Usually dysesthetic, often burning and lancinating
Psychogenic	Somatization disorder Psychogenic pain Hypochondriasis Specific pain diagnoses, with organic contribution	Failed low back Atypical facial pain Chronic headache	Does not include factitious disorders; i.e., malingering or Munchausen's syndrome

Table from Berkow R, ed: *Merck Manual*, ed 15. Merck Sharp & Dohme Research Laboratories, Rahway, NJ, 1987, p 1341, with permission.

TABLE 15–7. **CHARACTERISTICS OF SOMATIC AND NEUROPATHIC PAIN**

Somatic pain:
  Nociceptive stimulus usually evident.
  Usually well localized; visceral pain may be referred.
  Similar to other somatic pains in patient's experience.
  Relieved by anti-inflammatory or narcotic analgesics.

Neuropathic pain:
  No obvious nociceptive stimulus.
  Often poorly localized.
  Unusual, dissimilar from somatic pain.
  Only partially relieved by narcotic analgesics.

Table from Braunwald E, Isselbacher K, Petersdorf RG, Wilson JD, Martin JB, Fauci AS: *Harrison's Principles of Internal Medicine-II, Companion Handbook.* McGraw-Hill, New York, 1988, p 1, with permission. Modified from Maciewicz R, Martin JB: HPIM-11, p. 15.

neuroanatomic distribution. There may be a close correlation between stress and conflict and the initiation or exacerbation of the pain.

B. Diagnosis, signs and symptoms.   Pain may be accompanied by localized sensorimotor symptoms, such as anesthesia, paresthesia (Table 15-8). Symptoms of depression are common.

TABLE 15–8. **DSM-III-R DIAGNOSTIC CRITERIA FOR SOMATOFORM PAIN DISORDER**

A. Preoccupation with pain for at least 6 months.

B. Either (1) or (2):

   (1) appropriate evaluation uncovers no organic pathology or pathophysiologic mechanism (e.g., a physical disorder or the effects of injury) to account for the pain
   (2) when there is related organic pathology, the complaint of pain or resulting social or occupational impairment is grossly in excess of what would be expected from the physical findings.

Used with permission, APA.

C. Epidemiology.   Any age of onset, especially from 30–40s. More common in women than in men. Some evidence of first-degree biologic relatives having a higher incidence of pain, depression, and alcoholism.

D. Etiology. Psychogenic.

E. Differential diagnosis. Rule out organic factors. If presentation of symptoms are dramatic, consider histrionic personality disorder. Also, differentiate from somatization disorder, depressive disorder, and schizophrenia. In malingering, symptoms are invented for secondary gain, such as drug-seeking behavior.

F. Treatment. Use analgesic medications cautiously, if at all. Behavior modification, biofeedback of use. Antidepressant medication useful, e.g., imipramine (Tofranil) 25–100 mg/day. Pain clinics bring multispeciality staffs to bear on the complex cases. Drugs used to relieve pain are listed in Table 15–9.

TABLE 15–9. **DRUGS USED TO RELIEVE PAIN**

Nonnarcotic analgesics: equivalent doses and intervals

Generic name	Dose, mg	Interval
Aspirin	750–1250	q 3 h
Phenacetin	750–1000	q 3 h
Acetaminophen	600–800	q 3 h
Phenylbutazone	200–400	q 4 h
Indomethacin	50–75	q 4 h
Ibuprofen	200–400	q 4 h
Naproxen	250–500	q 4 h

Narcotic analgesics compared to 10 mg morphine sulfate (MS)

Generic name	IM dose, mg	PO dose, mg	Differences from MS
Oxymorphine	1	6	None
Hydromorphine	1.5	7.5	Shorter acting
Levorphanol	2	4	Good PO-IM potency
Heroin	4		Short-acting
Methadone	10	20	Good PO-IM potency
Morphine	10	60	
Oxycodone	15	30	Short-acting
Meperidine	75	300	None
Pentazocine	60	180	Agonist-antagonist
Codeine	130	200	More toxic

Anticonvulsants

Generic name	PO dose, mg	Interval
Phenytoin	100	q 6–8 h
Carbamazepine	200	q 6 h
Clonazepam	1	q 6 h

Antidepressants

Generic name	PO dose, mg	Range, mg/day
Doxepin	200	75–400
Amitriptyline	150	75–300
Imipramine	200	75–400
Nortiptyline	100	40–150
Desipramine	150	75–300
Amoxapine	200	75–300
Trazodone	150	50–600

Table from R Maciewicz, Martin JB: Pain: Pathophysiology and management. In Braunwald E, Isselbacher K, Petersdorf RG, Wilson JD, Martin JB, Fauci AS: *Harrison's Principles of Internal Medicine-11*. McGraw-Hill, New York, 1988, p. 16, with permission.

VI. Analgesia. Analgesia is the loss or absence of pain. Most effective are the narcotics (drugs derived from opium or an opium-like substance that relieves pain, alters mood and behavior, and produces the potential for dependence and tolerance). Opioids is a generic term that includes drugs that bind to opioid receptors and produce a narcotic effect. They are most useful in acute short-term serious pain. A goal should be to lower pain level so that the patient can eat and sleep with minimal upset. A guideline should be to give the drug at the request of the patient but not more than hourly for the two first doses. It can then be reduced to a frequency of every 3 hours. Self-administration of measured amounts of narcotics through an intravenous pump by patients with pain, when carried out in a hospital, is a new approach to pain control which is proving quite effective. The major opioid analgesics are

(1) **Morphine**—10 mg intramuscularly; 60 mg orally.

(2) **Meperidine** (Demerol)—75 mg intramuscularly; 300 mg orally; is a synthetic opioid analgesic.

(3) **Methadone**—10 mg intramuscularly; 20 mg orally. Is used as short-term treatment for heroin withdrawal and long-term maintenance of opioid addiction and for analgesia in cancer patients. Methadone has a long duration of action, oral effectiveness, and less sedation than morphine.

A. Nonnarcotic analgesics. Typical of this group is aspirin or acetylsalicylic acid (ASA). Unlike narcotic analgesics that act on the central nervous system, salicylates act at the peripheral or local level—the site of the origin of the pain. Usually prescribed every 3 hours for pain.

650 mg of ASA = 32 mg of codeine = 65 mg of propoxyphene (Darvon) = 50 mg of oral pentazocine (Talwin). Peak analgesia occurs in 45 minutes, with analgesic effects lasting 3–4 hours. Nonsteroidal antiinflammatory drugs (NSAIDs) have analgesic use: ibuprofen 200–400 mg every 4 hours.

B. Placebos. Substances with no known pharmacological activity that act through suggestion rather than biological action. It has recently been demonstrated, however, that naloxone (Narcan), an opioid antagonist, can block the analgesic effects of a placebo, thus suggesting that a release of endogenous opioids may explain some placebo effects.

Chronic treatment with placebos should never be undertaken when patients have clearly stated an objection to such treatment. Furthermore, deceptive treatment with placebos seriously undermines patients' confidence in their physicians. Finally, placebos should not be used when an effective therapy is available.

For more detailed discussion of this topic, see Kaplan HI: History of Psychosomatic Medicine, Sec. 25.1, pp 1155–1160; Oken D: Current Theoretical Concepts in Psychosomatic Medicine, Sec. 25.2, pp 1160–1169; Lipsitt DR: Gastrointestinal Disorders, Sec. 25.3, pp 1169–1179; Lomax JW: Obesity, Sec. 25.4, pp 1179–1186; Hackett TP, Rosenbaum JF, Cassem NH: Cardiovascular Disorders, Sec. 25.5, pp 1186–1198; Vachon L: Respiratory Disorders, Sec. 25.6, pp 1198–1209; Droba M, Whybrow PC: Endocrine and Metabolic Disorders, Sec. 25.7, pp 1209–1221; Strauss GD: Skin Disorders, Sec. 25.8, pp 1221–1225; Ananth J: Rheumatoid Arthritis, Sec. 25.9, pp 1225–1231; Pasnau RO, Fawzy FI: Stress and Psychiatry, Sec. 25.10, pp 1231–1239; Locke SE, Gorman JR: Behavior and Immunity, Sec. 25.11, pp 1240–1249; Lederberg MF, Holland JC: Psycho-oncology, Sec. 25.12, pp 1249–1264; Blackwell B: Chronic Pain Sec. 25.13, pp 1264–1271; Strain JJ, Taintor Z: Consultation-Liaison Psychiatry, Sec. 25.14, pp 1272–1279, in *CTP/V*.

16
Personality Disorders

I. General introduction
A. Definition. Pervasive, persistent maladaptive patterns of behavior that are deeply ingrained, that are not attributable to Axis I disorders, Axis III disorders, or cultural role difficulties. Disorders of trait, rather than state. Maladaptive traits can be behavioral, emotional, cognitive, perceptual, or psychodynamic.

B. Diagnosis, signs and symptoms
1. Requires history of long-term difficulties in various spheres of life.
2. Ego syntonic, i.e., acceptable to the ego.
3. Rigidity.
4. Underneath protective armor—anxiety.
5. Lacks empathy with others.
6. Developmental fixation; immature.
7. Interpersonal difficulties in love and work.

C. Epidemiology
1. Prevalence—6–9%.
2. Early analog is a disorder of temperament. Usually, personality disorder is first evident in late adolescence or early adulthood.
3. Overall, male = female.
4. Family history—frequently nonspecific history of psychiatric disorders is present. With some personality disorders, a partial genetic transmission is established.

D. Etiology
1. Multifactorial.
2. Biologic determinants are sometimes evident (genetics, perinatal injury, encephalitis, head trauma). High concordance rate in monozygotic twins.
3. Developmental histories frequently reveal individual difficulties and family problems, sometimes severe (abuse, incest).

E. Psychological tests
1. Neuropsychological test can reveal organicity (electroencephalogram [EEG], computed tomography [CT] scan, and electrophysiologic mapping can be useful).
2. Projective tests can reveal preferred personality patterns and styles (Minnesota Multiphasic Personality Inventory [MMPI], Thematic Apperception Test [TAT], Rorschach, Draw-A-Person [DAP]).

F. Pathophysiology
1. Frontal lobe—impulsivity, poor judgment, abulia.
2. Temporal lobe—Klüver-Bucy traits, religiosity, possible violence.
3. Parietal lobe—denial or euphoric features.

G. Psychodynamics. Vary with different disorders.

H. Course and prognosis. Variable—usually stable or deteriorating but some patients improve.

I. Treatment. Usually, patients are not motivated. Otherwise, multiple and mixed modalities are employed: psychoanalysis, psychoanalytic psychotherapy, supportive psychotherapy, group therapy, family therapy, milieu therapy, hospitalization (short- and long-term), pharmacotherapy.

J. Classification. DSM-III-R groups the personality disorders into three clusters. The first cluster is the **odd, eccentric cluster** and consists of the paranoid, schizoid, and schizotypal personality disorders; the second cluster is the **dramatic, emotional, and erratic cluster** and includes the histrionic, narcissistic, antisocial, and borderline personality disorders; the third cluster is the **anxious, fearful cluster** and includes the avoidant, dependent, and passive aggressive personality disorders.

II. Odd and eccentric cluster
A. Paranoid personality disorder
1. Definition. Tendency to attribute malevolent motives to others.

2. Diagnosis, signs and symptoms

TABLE 16–1.   **DSM-III-R DIAGNOSTIC CRITERIA FOR PARANOID PERSONALITY DISORDER**

A pervasive and unwarranted tendency, beginning by early adulthood and present in a variety of contexts, to interpret the actions of people as deliberately demeaning or threatening, as indicated by at least *four* of the following:

(1) expects, without sufficient basis, to be exploited or harmed by others
(2) questions, without justification, the loyalty or trustworthiness of friends or associates
(3) reads hidden demeaning or threatening meanings into benign remarks or events, e.g., suspects that a neighbor put out trash early to annoy him or her
(4) bears grudges or is unforgiving of insults or slights
(5) is reluctant to confide in others because of unwarranted fear that the information will be used against him or her
(6) is easily slighted and quick to react with anger or to counterattack
(7) questions, without justification, fidelity of spouse or sexual partner

Used with permission, APA.

3. Epidemiology
   a. Increased incidence in families of probands with schizophrenia and delusional disorders.
   b. More common in men than in women.

4. Etiology
   a. Genetic component.
   b. Nonspecific early family difficulties; childhood abuse.
   c. Rule out drug abuse, e.g., amphetamine.

5. Psychodynamics
   a. Projection, denial, rationalization.
   b. Shame.
   c. Defensive, masochistic, hypochondriacal features.
   d. Unresolved separation and autonomy issues.
   e. Identification with aggressor.

6. Differential diagnosis
   a. Paranoid psychosis—shows loss of reality testing.

      b. Schizoid and avoidant personality disorders—do not show similar active involvement with others.

  7. Course and prognosis. Variable, depending on individual ego strengths and life circumstances; possible complications of delusional disorders, schizophrenia, depression, anxiety disorders.

  8. Treatment

      a. Rarely low-dose antipsychotics, e.g., haloperidol (Haldol) 2 mg/day.

      b. Usually supportive psychotherapy.

        1. Openness, consistency, avoidance of humor.

        2. Support healthy parts of the ego.

        3. Emphasize reality.

      c. Does not do well in group psychotherapy.

B. Schizoid personality disorder

  1. Definition. Isolated life-style without overt longing for others.

  2. Diagnosis, signs and symptoms

TABLE 16–2. **DSM-III-R DIAGNOSTIC CRITERIA FOR SCHIZOID PERSONALITY DISORDER**

A pervasive pattern of indifference to social relationships and a restricted range of emotional experience and expression, beginning by early adulthood and present in a variety of contexts, as indicated by at least *four* of the following:

  (1) neither desires nor enjoys close relationships, including being part of a family
  (2) almost always chooses solitary activities
  (3) rarely, if ever, claims or appears to experience strong emotions, such as anger and joy
  (4) indicates little if any desire to have sexual experiences with another person (age being taken into account)
  (5) is indifferent to the praise and criticism of others
  (6) has no close friends or confidants (or only one) other than first-degree relatives
  (7) displays constricted affect, e.g., is aloof, cold, rarely reciprocates gestures or facial expressions, such as smiles or nods

Used with permission, APA.

  3. Epidemiology

      a. Increased incidence among family members of schizophrenic probands.

      b. Greater incidence among men than women.

  4. Etiology

      a. Genetic factors likely.

      b. Theories regarding etiology of schizophrenia apply.

      c. Disturbed early family relationships often elicited.

  5. Psychodynamics

      a. Social inhibition.

      b. Restriction of affect and denial are defenses used most prominently against aggression.

  6. Differential diagnosis

      a. Paranoid personality disorder—involved with others.

      b. Schizotypal personality—oddities and eccentricities of manners.

      c. Avoidant personality disorder—isolated but want to be involved with others.

  7. Course and prognosis

      a. Variable.

      b. Possibility of complications of delusional disorder, schizophrenia, other psychoses.

8. **Treatment**
   a. Low-dose antipsychotics may be of some benefit in some patients, e.g., haloperidol (Haldol) 2 mg/day.
   b. Supportive psychotherapy—focus on relatedness, identification of emotions.
   c. Group psychotherapy.
   d. Possible milieu therapy in some patients.

C. **Schizotypal personality disorder**
   1. **Definition.** Multiple oddities and eccentricities of behavior, thought, affect, speech, appearance.
   2. **Diagnosis, signs and symptoms**

TABLE 16–3. **DSM-III-R DIAGNOSTIC CRITERIA FOR SCHIZOTYPAL PERSONALITY DISORDER**

A pervasive pattern of deficits in interpersonal relatedness and peculiarities of ideation, appearance, and behavior, beginning by early adulthood and present in a variety of contexts, as indicated by at least *five* of the following:

(1) ideas of reference (excluding delusions of reference)
(2) excessive social anxiety, e.g., extreme discomfort in social situations involving unfamiliar people
(3) odd beliefs or magical thinking, influencing behavior and inconsistent with subcultural norms, e.g., superstitiousness, belief in clairvoyance, telepathy, or "sixth sense," "others can feel my feelings" (in children and adolescents, bizarre fantasies or preoccupations)
(4) unusual perceptual experiences, e.g., illusions, sensing the presence of a force or person not actually present (e.g., "I felt as if my dead mother were in the room with me")
(5) odd or eccentric behavior or appearance, e.g., unkempt, unusual mannerisms, talks to self
(6) no close friends or confidants (or only one) other than first-degree relatives
(7) odd speech (without loosening of associations or incoherence), e.g., speech that is impoverished, digressive, vague, or inappropriately abstract
(8) inappropriate or constricted affect, e.g., silly, aloof, rarely reciprocates gestures or facial expressions, such as smiles or nods
(9) suspiciousness or paranoid ideation

Used with permission, APA.

3. **Epidemiology**
   a. 3% prevalence.
   b. Increased prevalence in families of schizophrenic probands.
   c. More common in men than in women.
4. **Etiology.** Etiologic models of schizophrenia apply.
5. **Psychological tests.** Thought disorder is often evident.
6. **Pathophysiology**
   a. Possible diminished monoamine oxidase (MAO).
   b. Possible impairments in smooth pursuit eye tracking.
   c. Possible diminished brain mass, especially temporal.
7. **Psychodynamics.** Dynamics of psychosis and schizophrenia apply.
8. **Differential diagnosis**
   a. Paranoid personality disorder—no eccentricities.
   b. Schizoid personality disorder—no eccentricities.
   c. Borderline personality disorder—prominent affect, anger, impulsiveness.
   d. Schizophrenia—reality testing lost.
9. **Course and prognosis**
   a. Prognosis probably guarded.
   b. Possible schizophrenic decompensation.

10. Treatment

a. Pharmacologic treatment—use guidelines for treating residual schizophrenia (low dose antipsychotics, e.g., haloperidol 2–5 mg/day; pimozide [Crap] 2–5 mg/day; adjunctive benzodiazepines, e.g., diazepam [Valium] 2–10 mg/day).

b. Supportive psychotherapy.

c. Group psychotherapy.

d. Milieu therapy.

III. Dramatic, emotional, and erratic cluster

A. Antisocial personality disorder

1. Definition. Maladaptive behavior that does not recognize the rights of others.

2. Diagnosis, signs and symptoms

TABLE 16–4. **DSM-III-R DIAGNOSTIC CRITERIA FOR ANTISOCIAL PERSONALITY DISORDER**

A. Current age at least 18.

B. Evidence of conduct disorder with onset before age 15, as indicated by a history of *three* or more of the following:

(1) was often truant

(2) ran away from home overnight at least twice while living in parental or parental surrogate home (or once without returning)

(3) often initiated physical fights

(4) used a weapon in more than one fight

(5) forced someone into sexual activity with him or her

(6) was physically cruel to animals

(7) was physically cruel to other people

(8) deliberately destroyed others' property (other than by fire-setting)

(9) deliberately engaged in fire-setting

(10) often lied (other than to avoid physical or sexual abuse)

(11) has stolen without confrontation of a victim on more than one occasion (including forgery)

(12) has stolen with confrontation of a victim (e.g., mugging, purse-snatching, extortion, armed robbery)

C. A pattern of irresponsible and antisocial behavior since the age of 15, as indicated by at least *four* of the following:

(1) is unable to sustain consistent work behavior, as indicated by any of the following (including similar behavior in academic settings if the person is a student):

(a) significant unemployment for 6 months or more within 5 years when expected to work and work was available

(b) repeated absences from work unexplained by illness in self or family

(c) abandonment of several jobs without realistic plans for others

(2) fails to conform to social norms with respect to lawful behavior, as indicated by repeatedly performing antisocial acts that are grounds for arrest (whether arrested or not), e.g., destroying property, harassing others, stealing, pursuing an illegal occupation

(3) is irritable and aggressive, as indicated by repeated physical fights or assaults (not required by one's job or to defend someone or oneself), including spouse- or child-beating

(4) repeatedly fails to honor financial obligations, as indicated by defaulting on debts or failing to provide child support or support for other dependents on a regular basis

(5) fails to plan ahead, or is impulsive, as indicated by one or both of the following:

(a) traveling from place to place without a prearranged job or clear goal for the period of travel or clear idea about when the travel will terminate

(b) lack of a fixed address for a month or more

(6) has no regard for the truth, as indicated by repeated lying, use of aliases, or "conning" others for personal profit or pleasure

(7) is reckless regarding his or her own or others' personal safety, as indicated by driving while intoxicated, or recurrent speeding

(8) if a parent or guardian, lacks ability to function as a responsible parent, as indicated by one or more of the following:

TABLE 16–4. DSM-III-R DIAGNOSTIC CRITERIA FOR ANTISOCIAL PERSONALITY DISORDER (Continued)

(a) malnutrition of child
(b) child's illness resulting from lack of minimal hygiene
(c) failure to obtain medical care for a seriously ill child
(d) child's dependence on neighbors or nonresident relatives for food or shelter
(e) failure to arrange for a caretaker for young child when parent is away from home
(f) repeated squandering, on personal items, of money required for household necessities
(9) has never sustained a totally monogamous relationship for more than one year
(10) lacks remorse (feels justified in having hurt, mistreated, or stolen from another)

Used with permission, APA.

3. Epidemiology
a. Prevalence—3% men, 1% women.
b. Increased incidence of antisocial personality disorder, somatization disorder, and alcoholism in families.
c. Adoptive studies demonstrate genetic factors.
d. More common in lower socioeconomic groups.
e. Predisposing conditions—attention-deficit hyperactivity disorder (ADHD), conduct disorder.

4. Etiology
a. Genetic factors.
b. Organicity can be due to perinatal brain injury, head trauma, encephalitis, etc.
c. Parental abandonment or abuse.
d. Repeated, arbitrary, or harsh punishment by parents.

5. Pathophysiology
a. If organicity is present, impulsivity usually due to frontal lobe injury.
b. Other brain lesions, e.g., amygdala or possibly other temporal lesions, can predispose to violence.

6. Psychodynamics
a. Impulse-ridden with associated ego deficits in planning, judgment.
b. Superego deficits or lacunae; primitive or poorly formed conscience.
c. Object relation deficits—failure in empathy, love, basic trust.
d. Prominence of aggression.
e. Features of sadomasochism, narcissism, depression.

7. Differential diagnosis
a. Adult antisocial behavior—does not meet all criteria in Table 16–4.
b. Psychoactive substance use disorders—exhibit antisocial behavior as a consequence of substance abuse and dependence; may coexist.
c. Mental retardation—may exhibit antisocial behavior as a consequence of impaired intellect and judgment; may coexist.
d. Psychoses—may exhibit antisocial behavior as a consequence of psychotic delusions; may coexist.
e. Borderline personality disorder—usually show suicide attempts, self-loathing, and intense, ambivalent attachments.
f. Narcissistic personality disorder—remains law abiding in the service of narcissistic needs.
g. Sadistic personality disorder—less impulsive and more directed specifically toward sadistic cruelty; may coexist.

8. Course and prognosis
a. Begins by age 15.
b. Diagnosis not made before age 18.
c. Course is variable.
d. Often significantly improves after early or middle adulthood.
e. Complications include death by violence, substance abuse, suicide, physical injury, legal and financial difficulties.

9. Treatment
a. Difficult.
b. Often treatment of substance abuse effectively treats antisocial traits.
c. Long-term hospitalization or therapeutic community can be effective in some cases.
d. Usually, when effective, treatment is behavioral, i.e., legal sanctions, fear of punishment.

B. Borderline personality disorder
1. Definition
a. Multiple complexities and controversies in defining this disorder. Often confused with neurosis, psychosis, mood disorders, other personality disorders, organic mental disorders.
b. Manifestations of separation-individuation problems, affective control problems, and intense, personal attachments appear central.

2. Diagnosis, signs and symptoms

TABLE 16-5.   **DSM-III-R DIAGNOSTIC CRITERIA FOR BORDERLINE PERSONALITY DISORDER**

A pervasive pattern of instability of mood, interpersonal relationships, and self-image, beginning by early adulthood and present in a variety of contexts, as indicated by at least *five* of the following:

(1) a pattern of unstable and intense interpersonal relationships characterized by alternating between extremes of overidealization and devaluation
(2) impulsiveness in at least two areas that are potentially self-damaging, e.g., spending, sex, substance use, shoplifting, reckless driving, binge eating (Do not include suicidal or self-mutilating behavior covered in [5].)
(3) affective instability: marked shifts from baseline mood to depression, irritability, or anxiety, usually lasting a few hours and only rarely more than a few days
(4) inappropriate, intense anger or lack of control of anger, e.g., frequent displays of temper, constant anger, recurrent physical fights
(5) recurrent suicidal threats, gestures, or behavior, or self-mutilating behavior
(6) marked and persistent identity disturbance manifested by uncertainty about at least two of the following: self-image, sexual orientation, long-term goals or career choice, type of friends desired, preferred values
(7) chronic feelings of emptiness or boredom
(8) frantic efforts to avoid real or imagined abandonment (Do not include suicidal or self-mutilating behavior covered in [5].)

Used with permission, APA.

3. Epidemiology
a. More common in women than in men.
b. Increased prevalence of mood disorders in families.
c. Increased prevalence of borderline personality disorder in mothers of borderlines.

4. Etiology
a. Organicity can be due to perinatal brain injury, encephalitis, head injury, etc.

b. Physical and sexual abuse, abandonment, or overinvolvement.

5. Psychological tests. Projective tests reveal impaired reality testing.

6. Pathophysiology
   a. Frontal lesions can impair judgment and affective control.
   b. Temporal lesions can produce Klüver-Bucy traits.

7. Psychodynamics
   a. Splitting—manifests rage without a consciousness of ambivalent or positive emotions toward someone. Usually transient. Associated ability to divide staff into those who like and those who hate patient.
   b. Primitive idealization.
   c. Projective identification—attributes idealized features to another, then seeks to engage the other in various interactions that may resolve the patient's ambivalence. Also, patient tries, unconsciously, to make the therapist feel as the patient feels.
   d. Both intense aggressive needs and intense object hunger, often alternating.
   e. Fear of abandonment.
   f. Rapprochement subphase of separation-individuation is unresolved; object constancy is impaired.
   g. Turning against the self—self-hate, self-loathing.
   h. Generalized ego dysfunction results in identity disturbance.

8. Differential diagnosis
   a. Psychoses—reality testing impairment persists.
   b. Mood disorders—mood disturbance is usually nonreactive.
   c. Atypical depression. Often a difficult differential. At times, only a treatment trial will tell. But, atypicals often have sustained episodes of depression.
   d. Organic personality syndrome—testing for significant organicity.
   e. Schizotypal personality disorder—affective features are less severe.
   f. Antisocial personality disorder—defect in conscience and attachment is more severe.
   g. Histrionic personality disorder—suicide and self-mutilation are less common. More stable interpersonal relationships.
   h. Narcissistic personality disorder—more stable identity formation.
   i. Dependent personality disorder—attachments are stable.
   j. Self-defeating personality disorder—fewer problems with anger; self-destructive features are usually more pervasive.

9. Course and prognosis
   a. Variable; may improve in later years.
   b. Suicide, self-injury, depression, somatoform disorders, brief reactive psychosis, atypical psychosis, substance abuse are possible.
   c. Identity disorder is diagnosed before age 40.

10. Treatment
   a. Usually mixed supportive and exploratory psychotherapy. Management of transference psychosis, countertransference, acting out, and suicide threats and wishes are problematic. Therapist functions as auxiliary ego and uses limit-setting.
   b. Frequent use of medications—antidepressants; lithium; low-dose an-

tipsychotics, e.g., haloperidol 2 mg/day; carbamazepine (Tegretol) at therapeutic levels.

    c. Hospitalization is usually brief; long-term hospitalization for some patients.

C. Histrionic personality disorder

    1. Definition. Dramatic, emotional, impressionistic style.

    2. Diagnosis, signs and symptoms

TABLE 16–6.   **DSM-III-R DIAGNOSTIC CRITERIA FOR HISTRIONIC PERSONALITY DISORDER**

A pervasive pattern of excessive emotionality and attention-seeking, beginning by early adulthood and present in a variety of contexts, as indicated by at least *four* of the following:

    (1) constantly seeks or demands reassurance, approval, or praise

    (2) is inappropriately sexually seductive in appearance or behavior

    (3) is overly concerned with physical attractiveness

    (4) expresses emotion with inappropriate exaggeration, e.g., embraces casual acquaintances with excessive ardor, uncontrollable sobbing on minor sentimental occasions, has temper tantrums

    (5) is uncomfortable in situations in which he or she is not the center of attention

    (6) displays rapidly shifting and shallow expression of emotions

    (7) is self-centered, actions being directed toward obtaining immediate satisfaction; has no tolerance for the frustration of delayed gratification

    (8) has a style of speech that is excessively impressionistic and lacking in detail, e.g., when asked to describe mother, can be no more specific than, "She was a beautiful person."

Used with permission, APA.

3. Epidemiology

    a. Greater prevalence in women than in men.

    b. Underdiagnosed in men.

4. Etiology.   Suggestion that early interpersonal difficulties were resolved by dramatic behavior.

5. Psychodynamics

    a. Fantasy, emotionality, and dramatic style are typical.

    b. Common defenses—regression, identification, somatization, conversion, dissociation, denial, externalization.

    c. Faulty identification with and ambivalent relationship to opposite sex parent.

    d. Fixation at early genital level.

    e. Prominent oral traits.

    f. Fear of sexuality, despite seductiveness.

6. Differential diagnosis

    a. Borderline personality disorder—more overt despair, suicidal and self-mutilating features; can coexist.

    b. Somatization disorder—physical complaints predominate.

    c. Conversion disorder—apparent physical deficits are present.

    d. Dependent personality disorder—lacks the emotional style.

7. Course and prognosis

    a. Variable.

    b. Possible complications of somatization disorders, conversion disorders, dissociative disorders, sexual disorders, depressive disorders.

8. **Treatment**
   a. Usually individual psychotherapy, insight-oriented or supportive, depending on ego strength.
   b. Psychoanalysis for some.
   c. Group therapy can be useful.
   d. Adjunctive use of medications, usually anxiolytic, for transient emotional states, e.g., diazepam 5–10 mg/day.
D. **Narcissistic personality disorder**
   1. **Definition.** Pervasive pattern of grandiosity and overconcern with issues of self-esteem.
   2. **Diagnosis, signs and symptoms**

TABLE 16–7. **DSM-III-R DIAGNOSTIC CRITERIA FOR NARCISSISTIC PERSONALITY DISORDER**

A pervasive pattern of grandiosity (in fantasy or behavior), lack of empathy, and hypersensitivity to the evaluation of others, beginning by early adulthood and present in a variety of contexts, as indicated by at least *five* of the following:

(1) reacts to criticism with feelings of rage, shame, or humiliation (even if not expressed)
(2) is interpersonally exploitative: takes advantage of others to achieve his or her own ends
(3) has a grandiose sense of self-importance, e.g., exaggerates achievements and talents, expects to be noticed as "special" without appropriate achievement
(4) believes that his or her problems are unique and can be understood only by other special people
(5) is preoccupied with fantasies of unlimited success, power, brilliance, beauty, or ideal love
(6) has a sense of entitlement: unreasonable expectation of especially favorable treatment, e.g., assumes that he or she does not have to wait in line when others must do so
(7) requires constant attention and admiration, e.g., keeps fishing for compliments
(8) lack of empathy: inability to recognize and experience how others feel, e.g., annoyance and surprise when a friend who is seriously ill cancels a date
(9) is preoccupied with feelings of envy

Used with permission, APA.

3. **Epidemiology.** Probably common, but no hard data.
4. **Etiology.** Failure in maternal empathy, early rejection or loss.
5. **Psychodynamics**
   a. Defense versus deficit controversy—are narcissistic traits developmental arrests or defenses?
   b. Grandiosity and empathic failure defend against primitive aggression.
   c. Sense of entitlement.
   d. Fixation at practicing subphase of separation-individuation.
   e. Prominence of shame.
   f. Passivity.
   g. Depressive features.
   h. Discrepancy between self-image and ego-ideal.
6. **Differential diagnosis**
   a. Antisocial personality disorder—more flagrant disregard of the law and the rights of others.
   b. Psychoactive substance use disorders—can manifest narcissistic traits. Can coexist.

    c. Paranoid schizophrenia—overt delusions are present.

    d. Borderline personality disorder—higher anxiety, greater chaos.

7. Course and prognosis. This disorder is chronic and difficult to treat. Possible complications of mood disorders, transient psychoses, somatoform disorders, psychoactive substance use disorders. Guarded prognosis.

8. Treatment

    a. Individual psychotherapy, supportive or insight-oriented, depending on ego strength.

    b. Milieu therapy for severe disorders.

    c. Treatment challenge is preservation of self-esteem, threatened by psychiatric interventions.

IV. Anxious or fearful cluster

A. Obsessive-compulsive personality disorder

    1. Definition. Perfectionism and inflexibility predominate.

    2. Diagnosis, signs and symptoms

TABLE 16–8. **DSM-III-R DIAGNOSTIC CRITERIA FOR OBSESSIVE-COMPULSIVE PERSONALITY DISORDER**

A pervasive pattern of perfectionism and inflexibility, beginning by early adulthood and present in a variety of contexts, as indicated by at least *five* of the following:

  (1) perfectionism that interferes with task completion, e.g., inability to complete a project because own overly strict standards are not met

  (2) preoccupation with details, rules, lists, order, organization, or schedules to the extent that the major point of the activity is lost

  (3) unreasonable insistence that others submit to exactly his or her way of doing things, **or** unreasonable reluctance to allow others to do things because of the conviction that they will not do them correctly

  (4) excessive devotion to work and productivity to the exclusion of leisure activities and friendships (not accounted for by obvious economic necessity)

  (5) indecisiveness: decision making is either avoided, postponed, or protracted, e.g., the person cannot get assignments done on time because of ruminating about priorities (do not include if indecisiveness is due to excessive need for advice or reassurance from others)

  (6) overconscientiousness, scrupulousness, and inflexibility about matters of morality, ethics, or values (not accounted for by cultural or religious identification)

  (7) restricted expression of affection

  (8) lack of generosity in giving time, money, or gifts when no personal gain is likely to result

  (9) inability to discard worn-out or worthless objects even when they have no sentimental value

Used with permission, APA.

    3. Epidemiology

        a. Greater prevalence in men than in women.

        b. Likely familial transmission.

        c. Increased concordance in identical twins.

    4. Etiology. Patients often have backgrounds characterized by harsh discipline.

    5. Psychodynamics

        a. Isolation, reaction formation, undoing, intellectualization, rationalization.

        b. Distrust of emotions.

        c. Issues of defiance and submission.

        d. Fixation during anal period.

6. **Differential diagnosis.** Obsessive-compulsive disorder—has true obsessions or compulsions, compared with obsessive-compulsive personality disorder, which does not. If obsessions and compulsions appear, a diagnosis of obsessive-compulsive disorder should be made.

7. **Course and prognosis.** Possible complications of depressive disorders, somatoform disorders, alcoholism.

8. **Treatment**

   a. Individual psychotherapy, supportive or insight-oriented, depending on ego strengths.

   b. Group therapy can be beneficial.

   c. Therapeutic issues include those of control, submission, intellectualization.

   d. Pharmacotherapy may be useful.

B. **Avoidant personality disorder**

1. **Definition.** Shy or timid personality.

2. **Diagnosis, signs and symptoms**

TABLE 16–9. **DSM-III-R DIAGNOSTIC CRITERIA FOR AVOIDANT PERSONALITY DISORDER**

A pervasive pattern of social discomfort, fear of negative evaluation, and timidity, beginning by early adulthood and present in a variety of contexts, as indicated by at least *four* of the following:

(1) is easily hurt by criticism or disapproval
(2) has no close friends or confidants (or only one) other than first-degree relatives
(3) is unwilling to get involved with people unless certain of being liked
(4) avoids social or occupational activities that involve significant interpersonal contact, e.g., refuses a promotion that will increase social demands
(5) is reticent in social situations because of a fear of saying something inappropriate or foolish, or of being unable to answer a question
(6) fears being embarrassed by blushing, crying, or showing signs of anxiety in front of other people
(7) exaggerates the potential difficulties, physical dangers, or risks involved in doing something ordinary but outside his or her usual routine, e.g., may cancel social plans because she anticipates being exhausted by the effort of getting there

Used with permission, APA.

3. **Epidemiology**

   a. Common; but no hard data.

   b. Possible predisposing factors—avoidant disorder of childhood or adolescence, deforming physical illness.

4. **Etiology.** Possible overt parental deprecation.

5. **Psychodynamics**

   a. Avoidance and inhibition are defensive.

   b. Phobic style of condensation and displacement.

   c. Underlying aggression, either oedipal or preoedipal.

6. **Differential diagnosis**

   a. Schizoid personality disorder—no overt desire for involvement with others.

   b. Social phobia—specific social situations, rather than personal relationships, are avoided. May coexist.

   c. Dependent personality disorder—does not avoid attachments, greater fear of abandonment.

7. Course and prognosis. Function best in protected environment. Possible complication of social phobia.

8. Treatment

   a. Individual psychotherapy, supportive or insight-oriented, depending on ego strength.

   b. Group therapy is often helpful.

   c. Social skills and assertiveness training.

C. Dependent personality disorder

   1. Definition. Predominantly dependent and submissive.

   2. Diagnosis, signs and symptoms

TABLE 16–10.   **DSM-III-R DIAGNOSTIC CRITERIA FOR DEPENDENT PERSONALITY DISORDER**

A pervasive pattern of dependent and submissive behavior, beginning by early adulthood and present in a variety of contexts, as indicated by at least *five* of the following:

(1) is unable to make everyday decisions without an excessive amount of advice or reassurance from others
(2) allows others to make most of his or her important decisions, e.g., where to live, what job to take
(3) agrees with people even when he or she believes they are wrong, because of fear of being rejected
(4) has difficulty initiating projects or doing things on his or her own
(5) volunteers to do things that are unpleasant or demeaning in order to get other people to like him or her
(6) feels uncomfortable or helpless when alone, or goes to great lengths to avoid being alone
(7) feels devastated or helpless when close relationships end
(8) is frequently preoccupied with fears of being abandoned
(9) is easily hurt by criticism or disapproval

Used with permission, APA.

   3. Epidemiology

     a. More prevalent in women than in men.

     b. Common.

     c. Possible predispositions include chronic physical illness, separation anxiety disorder.

   4. Etiology. Early childhood parental loss in some patients.

   5. Psychodynamics

     a. Unresolved separation issues.

     b. Possible defense against aggressive wishes.

   6. Differential diagnosis. Agoraphobia—fear of leaving or being away from home.

   7. Course and prognosis. Variable. Possible depressive complications. With treatment, prognosis is favorable.

   8. Treatment

     a. Insight-oriented psychotherapy.

     b. Behavior therapy, assertiveness training, family therapy, and group therapy also useful.

     c. Pharmacotherapy useful for treating specific symptoms, e.g., anxiety, depression.

D. Passive aggressive personality disorder

   1. Definition. Covert obstructionism, procrastination, stubbornness, and inefficiency.

2. Diagnosis, signs and symptoms

TABLE 16-11.   **DSM-III-R DIAGNOSTIC CRITERIA FOR PASSIVE AGGRESSIVE PERSONALITY DISORDER**

A pervasive pattern of passive resistance to demands for adequate social and occupational performance, beginning by early adulthood and present in a variety of contexts, as indicated by at least *five* of the following:

    (1) procrastinates, i.e., puts off things that need to be done so that deadlines are not met
    (2) becomes sulky, irritable, or argumentative when asked to do something he or she does not want to do
    (3) seems to work deliberately slowly or to do a bad job on tasks that he or she really does not want to do
    (4) protests, without justification, that others make unreasonable demands on him or her
    (5) avoids obligations by claiming to have "forgotten"
    (6) believes that he or she is doing a much better job than others think he or she is doing
    (7) resents useful suggestions from others concerning how he or she could be more productive
    (8) obstructs the efforts of others by failing to do his or her share of the work
    (9) unreasonably criticizes or scorns people in positions of authority

Used with permission, APA.

3. Epidemiology.   Oppositional defiant disorder may predispose.

4. Etiology.   Learned behavior—parental modeling.

5. Psychodynamics
    a. Conflicts regarding authority, submission, and defiance.
    b. Conflicts regarding autonomy and dependence.
    c. Fears of aggression.

6. Differential diagnosis
    a. Antisocial personality disorder—defiance is overt.
    b. Obsessive-compulsive personality disorder—usually involves perfectionism, which limits overt opposition.

7. Course and prognosis.   Possible complications of depressive disorders, alcohol abuse.

8. Treatment
    a. Major difficulty lies in opposition to intervention by psychiatrist.
    b. Supportive psychotherapy may be useful if patient willing.
    c. Assertiveness training.

V. Other personality disorders
A. Sadistic personality disorder
1. Definition.   Relationships dominated by cruel or demeaning behavior.

2. Diagnosis, signs and symptoms

TABLE 16-12.   **DSM-III-R DIAGNOSTIC CRITERIA FOR SADISTIC PERSONALITY DISORDER**

A. A pervasive pattern of cruel, demeaning, and aggressive behavior, beginning by early adulthood, as indicated by the repeated occurrence of at least *four* of the following:

    (1) has used physical cruelty or violence for the purpose of establishing dominance in a relationship (not merely to achieve some noninterpersonal goal, such as striking someone in order to rob him or her)
    (2) humiliates or demeans people in the presence of others
    (3) has treated or disciplined someone under his or her control unusually harshly, e.g., a child, student, prisoner, or patient
    (4) is amused by, or takes pleasure in, the psychological or physical suffering of others (including animals)

TABLE 16-12. **DSM-III-R DIAGNOSTIC CRITERIA FOR SADISTIC PERSONALITY DISORDER (Continued)**

(5) has lied for the purpose of harming or inflicting pain on others (not merely to achieve some other goal)

(6) gets other people to do what he or she wants by frightening them (through intimidation or even terror)

(7) restricts the autonomy of people with whom he or she has a close relationship, e.g., will not let spouse leave the house unaccompanied or permit teen-age daughter to attend social functions

(8) is fascinated by violence, weapons, martial arts, injury, or torture

B. The behavior in A has not been directed toward only one person (e.g., spouse, one child) and has not been solely for the purpose of sexual arousal (as in sexual sadism).

Used with permission, APA.

3. Epidemiology
  a. Common in men.
  b. Clinically rare; common in forensic settings.

4. Etiology. Parental abuse.

5. Psychodynamics. Identification with the aggressor.

6. Differential diagnosis
  a. Sexual sadism—for sexual arousal.
  b. Antisocial personality disorder—has a history of prominent conduct problems in childhood.

7. Course and prognosis. Guarded.

8. Treatment
  a. Very difficult.
  b. Behavioral treatments may help some patients.
  c. Treatments for violence can include low-dose antipsychotics, e.g., haloperidol 2 mg/day; beta blocker, e.g., propranolol (Inderal) 40 mg/day; serotonergic agents, e.g., trazodone (Desyrel) 400 mg/day.
  d. Milieu settings may help some patients.
  e. Homogeneous group therapy may help some patients.

B. Self-defeating personality disorder
1. Definition. Patients direct their lives toward bad outcomes; reject help or good outcomes; have dysphoric responses to good outcomes.

2. Diagnosis, signs and symptoms

TABLE 16-13. **DSM-III-R DIAGNOSTIC CRITERIA FOR SELF-DEFEATING PERSONALITY DISORDER**

A pervasive pattern of self-defeating behavior, beginning by early adulthood and present in a variety of contexts. The person may often avoid or undermine pleasurable experiences, be drawn to situations or relationships in which he or she will suffer, and prevent others from helping him or her, as indicated by at least *five* of the following:

(1) chooses people and situations that lead to disappointment, failure, or mistreatment even when better options are clearly available

(2) rejects or renders ineffective the attempts of others to help him or her

(3) following positive personal events (e.g., new achievement), responds with depression, guilt, or a behavior that produces pain (e.g., an accident)

(4) incites angry or rejecting responses from others and then feels hurt, defeated, or humiliated (e.g., makes fun of spouse in public, provoking an angry retort, then feels devastated)

(5) rejects opportunities for pleasure, or is reluctant to acknowledge enjoying himself or herself (despite having adequate social skills and the capacity for pleasure)

(6) fails to accomplish tasks crucial to his or her personal objectives despite demonstrated ability to do so, e.g., helps fellow students write papers, but is unable to write his or her own

(7) is uninterested in or rejects people who consistently treat him or her well, e.g., is unattracted to caring sexual partners

(8) engages in excessive self-sacrifice that is unsolicited by the intended recipients of the sacrifice

Used with permission, APA.

3. Epidemiology
   a. Probably uncommon.
   b. More common in women than in men.
   c. Increased prevalence among first-degree relatives.

4. Etiology. Parental abuse or abuse of one parent by the other.

5. Psychodynamics
   a. Moral masochism.
   b. Guilt, need for punishment.
   c. Passivity needs.

6. Differential diagnosis
   a. Normal coping responses to abuse—behavior is limited to situations in anticipation of abuse.
   b. Depressive disorders—behavior is limited to times when the patient is depressed.

7. Course and prognosis. Possible complications of depressive disorders, physical injury.

8. Treatment
   a. Individual psychotherapy—supportive or insight-oriented, depending on ego strengths.
   b. Group therapy often is helpful.
   c. Treat underlying depression with psychotherapy or antidepressant medication.

For more detailed discussion of this topic, see Perry JC, Vaillant GE: Personality Disorders, Sec. 27.1, pp 1352–1387; Gunderson JG: Borderline Personality Disorder, Sec. 27.2, pp 1387–1395, in *CTP/V*.

17

Suicide, Violence, and Other Psychiatric Emergencies

I. General introduction

A psychiatric emergency is a disturbance in thoughts, feelings, or actions for which immediate treatment is necessary.

A. Common examples include imminent violence, suicide, self-mutilation, and injury to self or others by errors in judgment or passive neglect.

B. Can occur in any location—home, office, street, medical/psychiatric unit, psychiatric emergency room.

C. General interventions of emergency management:
1. Physical restraint.
2. Pharmacotherapy.
3. Hospitalization.
4. Management of medical problems.
5. Crisis intervention.
   a. Supportive psychotherapy.
   b. Environmental manipulation.
   c. Dealing with support systems—spouse, friends.

D. Social service resources, referral centers, and availability of medical backup are important.

E. General strategy in evaluating the patient:
1. Protect self.
2. Prevent harm.
   a. Prevent suicide and self-injury.
   b. Prevent violence toward others.
3. Rule out organic mental disorders.
4. Rule out impending psychosis.

II. Self-protection

A. Know as much as possible about the patient before meeting him/her.

B. Leave physical restraint procedures to those who are trained.

C. Be alert to risks of impending violence.

D. Attend to the safety of the physical surroundings, e.g., door access, room objects.

E. Have others present during your assessment if needed.

F. Have others in the vicinity.

G. Attend to developing an alliance with the patient, e.g., do not confront or threaten patients with paranoid psychoses.

III. Prevent harm

A. Prevent self-injury and suicide

1. **Self-injury.** Use whatever methods are necessary to prevent the patient

from hurting himself or herself during the evaluation (see section on violence below).

2. **Assessing risk of suicide**
   a. **Incidence** — tend to cluster in the spring, summer, and with media exposure. 30,000 suicides per year in U.S.
   b. **Age**
      i. Risk increases starting at age 40–50; especially high in elderly.
      ii. High risk also in adolescence and early adulthood.
   c. **Sex**
      i. Males commit suicide more often than females.
      ii. Females attempt suicide more often than males.
      iii. Males often use more violent methods than females.
      iv. Increasing risk of successful suicide among females, especially elderly.
      v. High risk among widowers.
   d. **Race**
      i. Minority status tends to protect (but not in Native Americans).
   e. **Nationality**
      i. Eastern Europeans, Scandinavians, Japanese—high rates.
      ii. Immigrants—higher than native born.
   f. **Other risk factors**
      i. Recent attempt or gesture.
      ii. Violence of method, e.g., gun, pills.
      iii. Little possibility of rescue.
      iv. Thoroughness and implementation of plan.
      v. Number of lifetime attempts or gestures: 2% succeed within 1 year of recent attempt; 10% eventually succeed; up to 50% repeat attempt.
      vi. Intent to die.
      vii. Reunion fantasy.
      viii. Bizarre method (suggests psychosis).
      ix. Diagnosis—major depression (15% will succeed); bipolar disorder (10% will succeed); psychosis (greater than 10% of schizophrenic persons will succeed); substance use disorders (15% will succeed); antisocial personality disorder; cyclothymia; borderline personality disorder (10% will succeed); organic disorders, especially early; also common with panic disorder.
      x. Medical history—illness, especially if recent onset; chronic; terminal; painful; debilitating; neoplastic; high drug use.
      xi. Recent stressor, e.g., loss of spouse, especially with impulse control disorder.
      xii. Living situation—urban, isolated, extremes of social class, recent geographic move, in prison.
      xiii. Conjugal status—separated, divorced, widowed, single.
      xiv. Vocational status—unemployed (especially recently), professionals.
      xv. Family history—suicide, early parental loss, mood disorder, chaotic family background.
      xvi. Mental status signs—command auditory hallucinations, hopeless-

ness, suicidal ideation (assess intention, plan, method, means, lethality, implementation, violence).

3. Always err in the direction of caution, e.g., admit when in doubt.

B. **Prevent violence toward others**

1. **During the evaluation, briefly assess the patient for risk of violence.** If risk is deemed significant, consider the following options:

   a. Inform patient that violence is not acceptable.

   b. Approach patient in nonthreatening manner.

   c. Reassure, calm, or assist patient's reality testing.

   d. Offer medication.

   e. Inform patient that restraint (or seclusion) will be used if necessary.

   f. Show of force—have teams ready to restrain.

   g. When patient restrained, always closely observe him/her, and frequently check vital signs. Isolate the restrained patient from surrounding agitating stimuli. Immediately plan a further approach—medication, reassurance, medical evaluation.

2. **Signs of impending violence:**

   a. Very recent acts of violence; also property violence.

   b. Verbal or physical threats (menacing).

   c. Carrying weapons or other objects that might be used as such, e.g., forks, ashtrays.

   d. Progressive psychomotor agitation.

   e. Alcohol or drug intoxication.

   f. Paranoid features in a psychotic patient.

   g. Command violent auditory hallucinations—some, but not all, patients are at high risk.

   h. Organic mental disorders, global or with frontal lobe findings; less commonly with temporal lobe findings (controversial).

   i. Patients with catatonic excitement.

   j. Certain patients with mania.

   k. Certain patients with agitated depression.

   l. Personality disorder patients prone to rage, violence, or impulse dyscontrol.

3. **Assess the risk of violence.**

   a. Consider violent ideation, wish, intention, plan, availability of means, implementation of plan, wish for help.

   b. Consider demographics—sex (male), age (15–24), socioeconomic status (lower), social supports (fewer).

   c. Consider past history: violence, nonviolent antisocial acts, impulse dyscontrol, e.g., gambling, substance abuse, suicide or self-injury, psychosis.

   d. Consider overt stressors, e.g., marital conflict.

4. **Management**

   a. Hospitalization

      i. Locked versus unlocked unit.

      ii. Voluntary versus involuntary.

      iii. 1-to-1 precautions versus no precaution (assault, arson, elopement)

  b. Crisis intervention—requires the following:
    i. Reliable and motivated patient.
    ii. Reliable accessory persons.
    iii. Immediate follow-up.
    iv. Avoidance of provocative situations.
    v. Possible medications, electroconvulsive therapy (ECT).

IV. Other Psychiatric emergencies
A. Organic mental disorders.

A group of psychiatric emergencies present with a variety of signs and symptoms, which include confusion, disorientation, hallucinations, and delusions and which are caused by organic mental disorders. In such cases, it is necessary to determine the offending agent that causes the symptomatology if possible; but more important, to treat medically or neurologically progressive central nervous system (CNS) dysfunction if present.

1. Features requiring a higher index of suspicion for organicity:
  a. Acute onset (within hours or minutes, with prevailing symptoms).
  b. First episode.
  c. Geriatric age.
  d. Current medical illness or injury.
  e. Significant substance abuse.
  f. Nonauditory disturbances of perception.
  g. Neurologic symptoms—loss of consciousness, seizures, head injury, change in headache pattern, change in vision.
  h. Classic mental status signs—diminished alertness, disorientation, memory impairment, impairment in concentration/attention, dyscalculia, concreteness.
  i. Other mental status signs—speech, movement, or gait disorders.
  j. Constructional apraxia—difficulties in drawing clock, cube, intersecting pentagons, Bender-Gestalt design.
  k. Catatonic features—nudity, negativism, combativeness, rigidity, posturing, waxy flexibility, echopraxia, echolalia, grimacing, mutism.
2. Use of amytal interview. Slow intravenous (IV) push of sodium amytal in patient to the point of mild sedation. Assess for more clearly organic features or more floridly functional features. Do not use if patient is at risk for respiratory arrest or if he/she has porphyria.
3. Know the common global CNS disorders that require immediate treatment:
  a. Hypoglycemia—dextrose 50% intravenously or juice orally immediately. Give to all diabetics.
  b. Wernicke's encephalopathy—thiamine, 100 mg IV immediately.
  c. Opiate intoxication—nalaxone (Narcan), 4 mg IV immediately.
4. Know the common focal CNS disorders with behavioral features:
  a. Aphasias—fluent or receptive aphasia results in patient not understanding spoken word, although he/she has fluent, but incoherent, speech.
  b. Frontal lobe syndromes—changes in motor behavior, ability to concentrate, reasoning, thinking, social judgment, and impulse control.

   c. Temporal lobe syndromes—psychosis, seizure, personality and Klüver-Bucy features.

   d. Parietal lobe syndromes—right lesion with denial and hypomania.

   e. Occipital lobe syndromes—Anton's syndrome (cortical blindness with denial).

5. **Know the common intoxication syndromes:**

   a. Opiates—can present with psychotomimetic features.

   b. Alcohol—can present with behavioral changes only, e.g., no nystagmus or gait impairment.

   c. CNS depressants—barbiturates, benzodiazepines.

   d. Psychostimulants, including cocaine and crack—can present with psychotomimetic, manic, agitated, or organic symptoms.

   e. Phencyclidine (PCP)—can present with severe agitation.

   f. Anticholingerics—including antidepressants, phenothiazines.

   g. Hallucinogens—lysergic acid diethylamide (LSD), ecstasy, high dose marijuana, mescaline.

   h. Mixed intoxications—the rule, not the exception. Consequently, all patients suspected of substance intoxication, including drunkenness, require immediate medical evaluation.

6. **Know the withdrawal syndromes:**

   a. Alcohol
      i. Minor withdrawal syndrome.
      ii. Hallucinosis.
      iii. Delirium tremens.

   b. CNS depressants.

   c. Psychostimulants.

   d. Opiates.

   e. Use the pentobarbital challenge test if in doubt. (See Chapter 4, Psychoactive Substance Use Disorders, for this test).

B. Anxiety

   a. Severe anxiety state—use antianxiety medication.

   b. Acute obsessional state—use antianxiety medication.

C. Somatoform disorders

   a. Conversion disorders—assess with hypnosis, amytal interview.

D. Dissociative disorders—consider amytal interview.

   a. Amnesia—evaluate cause, e.g., trauma, transient global amnesia, functional. Hypnosis of use in functional memory loss.

   b. Fugue—for agitation, use benzodiazepine.

E. Rape. A woman presenting to an emergency room after a rape has been through a life-threatening situation. During rape, she experiences shock and panic with the prime motivation to stay alive.

   Psychiatric counseling should help the woman explore and ventilate her emotions of fear, rage, shame, and humiliation. Post-traumatic stress disorder may develop, and the victim fares best when immediate support is given. The woman is helped when she knows that arrest and conviction of the rapist is possible; this may help her to cooperate in obtaining evidence, e.g., speculum examination for sperm, fingernail scrapings, general physical examination. Consider venereal disease, AIDS. The patient may be offered abortion services if necessary.

V. Emergency psychopharmacology

A. Indications—dangerousness, agitation, and anxiety.

B. Agents

1. **Antipsychotics.** For example, haloperidol (Haldol) 5 mg orally or intramuscularly.

   a. Indications—functional psychosis and organic mental disorder.

   b. Side effects of emergency significance

   i. Sedation—airway control and ventilation. Attend to levels of consciousness. Assess level of coma according to Glasgow Coma Scale (Table 17–1).

TABLE 17–1. **GLASGOW COMA SCALE**

Activity	Best Response	
Eye Opening	Spontaneous	4
	To speech	3
	To pain	2
	None	1
Verbal	Oriented	5
	Confused	4
	Inappropriate words	3
	Nonspecific sounds	2
	None	1
Motor	Follows commands	6
	Localizes pain	5
	Withdraws to pain	4
	Abnormal flexion	3
	Extend	2
	None	1

Table from Jennett B, Teasdale G. *Lancet*, 1977, with permission.

   ii. Hypotension—supportive measures to maintain blood pressure above 100 mm Hg. Check for arrhythmias.

   iii. Anticholinergic—especially CNS changes, ileus, urinary retention. May treat with physostigmine (Antilirium) 0.5 mg intravenously, but do so with medical consultation.

   iv. Epileptogenic—risk if alcohol withdrawal, sedative-hypnotic withdrawal, or other primary or secondary CNS disorder is present. Obtain medical or neurologic consultation. Table 17–2 lists drugs

TABLE 17–2. **DRUGS OF CHOICE FOR VARIOUS TYPES OF SEIZURES**

Generalized tonic-clonic (grand mal) seizures:
  Phenobarbital
  Phenytoin (Dilantin)
  Carbamazepine (Tegretol)
Absence (petit mal) seizures:
  Ethosuximide (Zarontin)
  Sodium valproate (Depakene)
  Trimethadione (Tridione)
Simple partial (focal) seizures:
  Phenobarbital
  Phenytoin (Dilantin)
Complex partial (temporal lobe) seizures:
  Phenytoin (Dilantin)
  Carbamazepine (Tegretol)
  Primidone (Mysoline)

Myoclonic, atonic, akinetic, and atypical absence seizures:
  Clonazepam (Klonopin)
  Diazepam (Valium)
Infantile spasms:
  Adrenocorticotropic hormone
  Corticosteroids
Status epilepticus:
  Diazepam (Valium)
  Phenobarbital
  Amobarbital (Amytal)
  Phenytoin (Dilantin)
  Paraldehyde
  Anesthetic agent

that are used in the treatment of epilepsy.

   v. Dystonia—especially laryngeal dystonia with stridor. Treat with anticholinergic, e.g., benztropine (Cogentin) 2 mg.

  vi. Akathesia—if severe, treat with beta blocker, e.g., propranolol (Inderal) 20–40 mg, anticholinergic, or benzodiazepine.

 vii. Neuroleptic malignant syndrome—discontinue antipsychotics, support cardiovascular and renal function. Drugs of use: dantrolene (Dantrium) 0.8–1.0 mg/kg every 6 hours intravenously for up to 2 weeks; bromocriptine (Parlodel) 2.5–5.0 mg total daily dose for up to 2 weeks.

2. **Barbiturates.** May give amytal 200 mg orally or 250 mg intramuscularly.

  a. Indications—severe agitation.

  b. Side effects—sedation, hypotension, and respiratory depression (obtain medical consultation immediately).

3. **Benzodiazepines.** May give lorazepam (Ativan) 1.0 mg orally or intramuscularly.

  a. Indications—agitation and anxiety.

  b. Side effects

    i. Similar to barbiturates.

    ii. Anxiolytic/sedation ratio is greater.

4. **Antihistamines.** May give hydroxyzine (Vistaril) 50 mg orally or intramuscularly.

  a. For agitation and anxiety in abusers of CNS depressants

For the sake of brevity and to avoid repetition, not all psychiatric emergencies are covered in this chapter, e.g., hypertensive crisis, tardive dyskinesia, among others. The reader is referred to the index to find the area of the text that covers these and other emergencies.

For more detailed discussion of this topic, see Roy A: Suicide, Sec. 29.1, pp 1414–1427; Slaby AE: Other Psychiatric Emergencies, Sec. 29.2, pp 1427–1441, in *CTP/V*.

18

Child and Adolescent Disorders

I. Principles of child and adolescent diagnostic assessment

A. Supplement data from patient interviews with information from family members, guardians, teachers, outside agencies.

B. Know first what normal development is in order to fully understand what constitutes abnormality at a given age. See Table 18–1 for developmental milestones.

C. Be familiar with the current diagnostic criteria of disorders to guide anamnesis on mental status examination.

D. Understand family psychiatric history, which is necessary given the genetic predispositions and/or environmental influences of many disorders. See Table 18–1.

II. Child development

A. Development results from the interplay of

1. Maturation of the central nervous system (CNS), neuromuscular apparatus, and endocrine system, and

2. Environmental influences, e.g., parents, teachers, who can either facilitate or thwart the child's attainment of his/her developmental potential. This potential is specific to each person given genetic predispositions to (1) intellectual level and (2) mental disorder, temperament, and probably certain personality traits.

Development is continual and lifelong but most rapid in early life. The neonatal brain weighs 350 grams, almost triples in weight by 18 months, and at 7 years is close to 90% of the adult 1,350 grams. Microscopically, cytogenetic changes, such as neuronal differentiation, axonal growth, synapse formation, and myelination, which begin during embryonic and fetal development, continue after birth.

For decades, the most cited theorists in child development have been Sigmund Freud, Margaret Mahler, Erik Erikson, and Jean Piaget; their work is outlined in Table 18–2.

a. Freud was the first to discover, and submit to theoretical frameworks, the importance of early childhood in the development of personality and psychopathology. His data, however, came from the psychoanalyses of late adolescent or adult patients. He did not systematically observe or treat normal or abnormal children. Those who have done so have made additions and revisions to his theory. Moreover, concerning psychopathonogenesis, Freud focused on the Oedipus complex. According to Freud, neurosis resulted from the inability to resolve rivalries and unconscious libidinal and aggressive feelings toward parents within the oedipal triangle. Today this theory accounts for some, but certainly not all, of psychopathology.

b. Mahler observed children and their mothers and evolved a theory of separation-individuation. This is generally accepted today, with the exception of her theory of phases during the first months of life, which emphasizes that infants lack alertness and responsivity.

TABLE 18–1.   DEVELOPMENTAL MILESTONES/LANGUAGE SKILLS

Age	Gross Motor	Visual Motor	Language	Social
1 mo	Raises head slightly from prone, makes crawling movements, lifts chin up	Has tight grasp, follows to midline	Alerts to sound, e.g., by blinking, moving, startling)	Regards face
2 mos	Holds head in midline, lifts chest off table	No longer clenches fist tightly, follows object past midline	Smiles after being stroked or talked to	Recognizes parent
3 mos	Supports on forearms in prone, holds head up steadily	Holds hands open at rest, follows in circular fashion	Coos (produces long vowel sounds in musical fashion)	Reaches for familiar people or objects, anticipates feeding
4–5 mos	Rolls front to back, back to front, sits well when propped, supports on wrists and shifts weight	Moves arms in unison to grasp, touches cube placed on table	Orients to voice
5 mos—orients to bell (localizes laterally) says "ah-goo," razzes	Enjoys looking around environment
6 mos	Sits well unsupported, puts feet in mouth in supine position	Reaches with either hand, transfers, uses raking grasp	Babbles
7 mos—orients to bell (localizes indirectly)
8 mos—"dada/mama" indiscriminately	Recognizes strangers
9 mos	Creeps, crawls, cruises, pulls to stand, pivots when sitting	Uses pincer grasp, probes with forefinger, holds bottle, fingerfeeds	Understands "no," waves bye-bye
10 mos—"dada/mama" discriminately; orients to bell (directly)
11 mos—one word other than "dada/mama"	Starts to explore environment plays pat-a-cake
12 mos	Walks alone	Throws objects, lets go of toys, hand release, uses mature pincer grasp	Follows one-step command with gesture, uses two words other than "data/mama"
14 mos uses three words	Imitates actions, comes when called, cooperates with dressing
15 mos	Creeps upstairs, walks backwards	Builds tower of 2 blocks in imitation of examiner, scribbles in imitation	Follows one-step command without gesture, uses 4–6 words and immature jargoning (runs several unintelligible words together)	
18 mos	Runs, throws toy from standing without falling	Turns 2–3 pages at a time, fills spoon and feeds himself	Knows 7–20 words, knows one body part, uses mature jargoning (includes intelligible words in jargoning)	Copies parent in tasks (e.g., sweeping, dusting), plays in company of other children

TABLE 18–1. **DEVELOPMENTAL MILESTONES/LANGUAGE SKILLS (Continued)**

Age	Gross Motor	Visual Motor	Language	Social
21 mos	Squats in play, goes up steps	Builds tower of 5 blocks, drinks well from cup	Points to 3 body parts, uses two-word combinations, has 20 word vocabulary	Asks to have food and to go to toilet
24 mos	Walks up and down steps without help	Turns pages one at a time, removes shoes, pants, etc., imitates stroke	Uses 50 words, two-word sentences, uses pronouns, (I, you, me) inappropriately, points to 5 body parts, understands 2 step command	Parallel play
30 mos	Jumps with both feet off floor, throws ball overhand	Unbuttons, holds pencil in adult fashion, differentiates horizontal and vertical line	Uses pronouns (I, you, me) appropriately, understands concept of "one," repeats 2 digits forward	Tells first and last names when asked, gets himself drink without help
3 yrs	Pedals tricycle, can alternate feet when going up steps	Dresses and undresses partially, dries hands if reminded, draws a circle	Uses 3 word sentences, uses plurals, past tense. Knows all pronouns. Minimum 250 words, understands concept of "two"	Group play, shares toys, takes turns, plays well with others, knows full name, age, sex
4 yrs	Hops, skips, alternates feet going downstairs	Buttons clothing fully, catches ball	Knows colors, says song or poem from memory, asks questions	Tells "tall tales," play cooperatively with a group of children
5 yrs	Skips, alternating feet, jumps over low obstacles	Ties shoes, spreads with knife	Prints first name, asks what a word means	Play competitive games, abides by rules, likes to help in household tasks

Table from *The Harriet Lane Handbook*, ed 11, Peter C. Rowe, editor, p 105. Year Book Medical Publishers, Chicago, 1987. Reproduced with permission.

    c. Erikson's work extends development throughout life. At each stage, there is a conflict and resolution, e.g., basic trust versus mistrust in the first stage. His work emphasizes the individual's adaptation to society.

    d. Piaget, a genetic epistemologist, studied the behaviors, from birth, of his three children and evolved a comprehensive, respected theory of cognitive development. His work reveals the infant as an active problem solver.

III. Developmental disorders (Axis II)

  A. Mental retardation (MR) occurs in 3% of live births and 1% of the population. The male-to-female ratio is 2:1.

    1. Diagnosis

      a. Significantly subaverage general intellectual function. Tested intelligence quotient (I.Q.) is 70 or below (Table18–3).

      b. Impaired adaptive skills in areas of work, socializing, daily living, self-sufficiency.

      c. Onset before the age of 18.

    2. Etiology (organic or psychosocial) is known in 50–70% of cases.

      a. Genetic

        i. Inborn errors of metabolism, e.g., phenylketonuria (PKU), Tay Sachs disease.

        ii. Chromosomal abnormalities, foremost: Down syndrome (trisomy 21) 1/1,000 live births. Typical facies, hypotonia, hyperreflexia, cardiac malformations, gastrointestinal anomalies. Fragile-X syndrome 1/1,000–1/2,000 live male births. Postpubertal macroorchidism, large head and ears, long, narrow face. (Some female carriers have facial features and cognitive dysfunction.)

      b. Psychosocial—mild MR often caused by chronic lack of intellectual stimulation.

      c. Other—sequelae of infection, toxin, or brain trauma, intrauterine, perinatal or later, e.g., cogenital rubella or fetal alcohol syndrome (microcephaly, midfacial hypoplasia, short palpebral fissure, pectus escavatum, possible cardiac defects, short stature).

    3. General considerations. There is no typical behavior or personality type. Poor self-esteem is common. Thinking tends to be concrete and egocentric. 30–75% have concomitant mental disorder running the gamut of DSM-III-R disorders.

    4. Treatment

      a. Special schools or classes for MR.

      b. Pharmacologic.

        i. Concomitant mental disorder, such as attention-deficit hyperactivity disorder (ADHD) or depression, may need stimulants or antidepressants, respectively.

        ii. Agitation, aggression, and tantrumming often respond to antipsychotics. High dosage, low potency drugs, e.g., chlorpromazine (Thorazine) or thioridazine (Mellaril), are more cognitively dulling than low dosage, high potency ones, e.g., haloperidol (Haldol). Many institutionalized mentally retarded persons are poorly monitored on medication.

        iii. Lithium is useful for aggressive or self-abusive behaviors.

        iv. Carbamazepine (Tegretol) and propranalol (Inderal) can be tried for aggressive, tantrumming behaviors. Efficacy is less proven than for antipsychotics and lithium.

      c. Psychologic—the following may be indicated.

        i. Individual supportive psychotherapy. Awareness of inadequacies can breed low self-esteem.

        ii. Verbal, mildly retarded may profit from insight-oriented psychotherapy for concomitant disorders.

TABLE 18–2. A SYNTHESIS OF DEVELOPMENTAL THEORISTS

Age (Years)	Margaret Mahler	Sigmund Freud	Erik Erikson	Jean Piaget	Comments
0–1	Normal autistic phase (birth to 4 weeks) • State of half-sleep, half-wake • Major task of phase is to achieve homeostatic equilibrium with the environment Normal symbiotic phase (3–4 weeks to 4–5 months) • Dim awareness of caretaker, but infant still functions as if he and caretaker are in state of undifferentiation or fusion • Social smile characteristic (2–4 months) The subphases of separation-individuation proper First subphase: differentiation (5–10 months) • Process of hatching from autistic shell, i.e., developing more alert sensorium that reflects cognitive and neurological maturation • Beginning of comparative scanning, i.e., comparing what is and what is not mother • Characteristic anxiety: stranger anxiety, which involves curiosity and fear (most prevalent around 8 months)	Oral phase (birth to 1 year) • Major site of tension and gratification is the mouth, lips, tongue – includes biting and sucking activities	Basic trust vs basic mistrust (oral sensory). (birth to 1 year) • Social mistrust demonstrated via ease of feeding, depth of sleep, bowel relaxation • Depends on consistency and sameness of experience provided by caretaker • Second 6-months teething and biting moves infant "from getting to taking" • Weaning leads to "nostalgia for lost paradise" • If basic trust is strong, child maintains hopeful attitude	Sensorimotor phase (birth to 2 years) • Intelligence rests mainly on actions and movements coordinated under "*schemata*," (Schema is a pattern of behavior in response to a particular environmental stimulus.) • Environment is mastered through *assimilation* and *accommodation*. (Assimilation is the incorporation of new environmental stimuli. Accommodation is the modification of behavior to adapt to new stimuli.) • *Object permanence* is achieved by age 2 yrs. Object still exists in mind if it disappears from view: search for hidden object • Reversibility in action begins	In contrast to Mahler, other observers are impressed with a mutuality and complementarity (not autism or fusion) which provides a groundwork for relatedness and language development as if there were a prewiring for these abilities. Piaget and others emphasize the infant actively striving to manipulate the inanimate environment. This supplements Freud's work because the infant and young child's motivation for behavior is not simply to relieve drive tension and attain oral, anal, and phallic gratification.

TABLE 18–2. A SYNTHESIS OF DEVELOPMENTAL THEORISTS (Continued)

Age (Years)	Margaret Mahler	Sigmund Freud	Erik Erikson	Jean Piaget	Comments
1–2	Second subphase, practicing (10–16 months) • Beginning of this phase marked by upright locomotion—child has new perspective and also mood of elation • Mother used as home base • Characteristic anxiety: separation anxiety Third subphase: rapprochement (16–24 months) • Infant now a toddler—more aware of physical separateness, which dampens mood of elation • Child tries to bridge gap between himself and mother—concretely seen as bringing objects to mother • Mother's efforts to help toddler often not perceived as helpful, temper tantrums typical • Characteristic event: rapprochement crisis: wanting to be soothed by mother and yet not be able to accept her help • Symbol of rapprochement: child standing on threshold of door not knowing which	Anal phase (1 year to 3 years) • Anus and surrounding area is major source of interest • Acquisition of voluntary sphincter control (toilet training)	Autonomy *vs.* shame and doubt (muscular-anal) (1–3 years) • Biologically includes learning to walk, feed self, talk • Muscular maturation sets stage for "holding on and letting go" • Need for outer control, firmness of caretaker prior to development of autonomy • *Shame* occurs when child is overtly self-conscious via negative exposure • *Self-doubt* can evolve if parents overly shame child (e.g., about elimination)	Preoperational phase (2–7 years) • Appearance of *symbolic* functions, associated with language acquisition • *Egocentrism*: child understands everything exclusively from own perspective • Thinking is illogical and magical • Nonreversible thinking with absence of convervation – *Animism*: belief that inanimate objects are alive (i.e. have feelings and intentions)	Supplementing the work of Freud and Mahler, theorists have postulated that severe problems in mother-infant/toddler interactions contribute to the formation of pathologic character traits, gender identity disorder, or personality disorders. Angry, frustrating, narcissistic caretakers often produce angry, needy children and adults who cannot tolerate the normal frustrations and disappointments in relationships and whose character formation is grossly deformed.

Age	Psychosexual (Freud)	Separation-Individuation (Mahler) / Psychosocial (Erikson)	Comments
		way to turn in helpless frustration • Resolution of crisis occurs as child's skills improve and child able to get gratification from doing things himself	*"Imminent justice"*: belief that punishment for bad deeds is inevitable
2–3		Fourth subphase: consolidation and object constancy (24–36 months) • Child better able to cope with mother's absence and engage substitutes • Child can begin to feel comfortable with mother's absences by knowing she will return • Gradual internalization of image of mother as reliable and stable • Through increasing verbal skills and better sense of time, child can tolerate delay and endure separations	
3–4	Phallic-oedipal phase (3–5 years) • Genital focus of interest, stimulation, and excitement • Penis is organ of interst for both sexes	Initiative vs. guilt (locomotor genital) (3–5 years) • *Initiative* arises in relation to tasks for the sake of activity, both motor and intellectual	Researchers have amended Freud's work. Children of both sexes explore and are aware of their own genitals during the second year of life and, with proper parental reinforcement, begin to correctly identify themselves as girls or boys. Penis envy is neither universal nor normative.
4–5	• Genital masturbation common • Intense preoccupation with *castration anxiety* (fear of genital loss or injury) • *Penis envy* (discontent with one's own genitals and wish to possess genitals of male)	• *Guilt* may arise over goals contemplated (especially aggressive) • Desire to mimic adult world; involvement in oedipal struggle leads to resolution via social role identification • Sibling rivalry frequent	

TABLE 18–2. **A SYNTHESIS OF DEVELOPMENTAL THEORISTS (Continued)**

Age (Years)	Margaret Mahler	Sigmund Freud	Erik Erikson	Jean Piaget	Comments
5–6		seen in girls in this phase • *Oedipus complex* universal: child wishes to have sex and marry parent of opposite sex and simultaneously be rid of parent of same sex Latency phase (from 5–6 years to 11–12 years) • State of relative quiescence of sexual drive with resolution of Oedipal complex • Sexual drives channeled into more socially appropriate aims (i.e., schoolwork and sports) • Formation of *superego*:			Contrary to Freud, the onset of latency (school age or middle childhood) is now considered primarily due to changes in the central nervous system (CNS) and less dependent on the nondemonstrable quiescence and sublimation of sexual drive. Changes in the CNS are reflected in developmental progress, during the years 6–8, of perceptual-sensory-motor functioning and thought processes. In Piaget's framework, it is the transition from the preoperational to the concrete (operational) phase. Compared with preschoolers, latency children are capable of greater learning, independent functioning, and socialization. Friendships develop with less dependence on parents (and less preoccupation with intrafamilial oedipal rivalries). Superego development is today considered more prolonged, gradual, and less related to oedipal resolution.
6–11		one of three psychic structures in mind which is responsible for moral and ethical development, including conscience • (Other two psychic structures are *ego*, which is a group of functions mediating between the drives and the external environment, and the *id*, repository of sexual and aggressive drives • The id is there at birth and the ego develops gradually from rudimentary structure present at birth)	Industry vs. inferiority (latency) (6–11 years) • Child is busy building, creating, accomplishing • Receives systematic instruction as well as fundamentals of technology • Danger of sense of inadequacy and inferiority if child despairs of his tools/skills and status among peers • Socially decisive age	Concrete (operational) phase (7–11 years) • Emergence of logical (cause-effect) thinking, including reversibility and ability to sequence and serialize • Understanding of part/whole relationships and classifications • Child able to take other's point of view • Conservation of number, length, weight, and volume	

11+	Genital phase (from 11–12 years and beyond)	Identity vs. role diffusion (11 years through end of adolescence)	Formal (abstract) phase (11 years through end of adolescence)
	• Final stage of psychosexual development—begins with puberty and the biological capacity for orgasm but involves the capacity for true intimacy	• Struggle to develop *ego identity* (sense of inner sameness and continuity) • Preoccupation with appearance, hero worship, ideology • *Group identity* (peers) develops • Danger of *role confusion*, doubts about sexual and vocational identity • *Psychosocial moratorium*, stage between morality learned by the child and the ethics to be developed by the adult	• Hypothetical-deductive reasoning, not only on basis of objects but also on basis of hypotheses or of propositions • Capable of thinking about one's thoughts • Combinative structures emerge, permitting flexible grouping of elements in a system • Ability to use two systems of reference simultaneously • Ability to grasp concept of probabilities

Adapted from table by Sylvia Karasu, M.D. and Richard Oberfield, M.D. Comments added by Richard Perry, M.D.

TABLE 18–3. **SEVERITY OF MENTAL RETARDATION BY I.Q. RANGE**

Subtypes	% of Total MR	I.Q. Range
Mild	85%	50–55 to 70 (considered educable, can attain about grade 6)
Moderate	10%	35–40 to 50–55 (considered trainable, can attain about grade 2)
Severe	3–4%	20–25 to 35–40
Profound	1–2%	below 20–25

      iii. Activity groups to improve socialization.
      iv. Parental and family counseling.
      v. Remediation and tutoring.
    d. See Table 18–4 for an overview of pharmacotherapy of children and adolescents.
B. Pervasive developmental disorder. Autistic disorder (also called infantile autism occurs in 4/10,000. The male-to-female ratio is 3–4:1.
  1. Diagnosis, signs and symptoms (Table 18–5).
  2. General considerations. Children with autistic disorder can be high or low functioning depending on I.Q., amount and communicativeness of language, and severity of other symptoms. 70% have I.Q.s below 70, and 50% have I.Q.s below 40–50. Autistic disorder is an organic disorder. Concordance in monozygotic twins is higher than in dizygotic; at least 2% of siblings are afflicted, and language and/or learning problems are increased in families of autistic children. Associated genetic disorders include tuberous sclerosis and fragile-X syndrome. Prenatal and perinatal insults are increased, but these may be insufficient without genetic predisposition. There is no site of organic damage specific to autistic disorder. The cortex, cerebellum, brain stem, and vestibular apparatus have all been implicated. Electroencephalogram (EEG) often shows nonfocal abnormality; brain computed tomography (CT) scan is abnormal in 25%, with ventricular dilitation the most frequent finding. Preliminary magnetic resonance imaging (MRI) and autopsy reports revealed cerebellar abnormalities in some patients, and a positron emission tomography (PET) scan study revealed increased frontal lobe glucose metabolism in a sample of autistic men. Subgroups have abnormal levels of neurotransmitters or their metabolites in blood or cerebrospinal fluid (CSF).
  3. Treatment
    a. Special education is paramount.
    b. Pharmacologic (Table 18–4).
      i. In nonsedating dosages, haloperidol in controlled studies reduced withdrawal, stereotypies, and hyperactivity. In a long-term study, dyskinesia occurred in 27% of children. It resolved after cessation of drug.
      ii. Fenfluramine (Pondimin) lowers serotonin in blood. It is much less effective than haloperidol.
      iii. Opiate antagonists are currently being explored. Major rationale is to reduce interpersonal withdrawal by blocking endogenous opioids as one does in addicts by blocking exogenous opiates.
      iv. Lithium can be helpful for aggressive or self-injurious behaviors. Beta blockers are under investigation.

TABLE 18–4.   OVERVIEW OF COMMON PSYCHOACTIVE DRUGS IN CHILDHOOD AND ADOLESCENCE

Drug	Indications	Dosage	Adverse Reactions and Monitoring
Antipsychotics Also known as major tranquilizers, neuroleptics Divided into (1) high potency, low dosage, e.g., haloperidol (Haldol), trifluoperazine (Stelazine), thiothixene (Navane) and (2) low potency, high dosage (more sedating), e.g., chlorpromazine (Thorazine), thiordiazine (Mellaril).	In general for agitated, aggressive, self-injurious behaviors in mental retardation (MR), pervasive developmental disorder (PDD), conduct disorder (CD), and schizophrenia. Studies support following specific indications: haloperidol-PDD, CD, with severe aggression, Tourette's disorder.	All can be given in 2–4 divided dosages or combined into one dose after gradual build up. Haloperidol—0.5–16 mg/day. Trifluoperazine—1–40 mg/day. Thiothixene—5–42 mg/day. Chlorpromazine and thioridazine—10–400 mg.	Sedation, weight gain, hypotension, lowered seizure threshold, constipation, extrapyramidal symptoms, jaundice, agranulocytosis, dystonic reaction, tardive dyskinesia. Monitor: blood pressure, complete blood count (CBC), liver function tests (LFTs), electroencephalogram, if indicated. With thioridazine, pigmentary retinopathy is rare but dictates ceiling of 800 mg in adults and proportionately lower in children.
Stimulants Dextroamphetamine (Dexedrine) FDA approved for children 3 years and older. Methylphenidate (Ritalin) and pemoline (Cylert) FDA approved for children 6 years and older.	In attention-deficit hyperactivity disorder (ADHD) for hyperactivity, impulsivity, and inattentiveness.	Dextroamphetamine and methylphenidate are generally given at 8 AM and noon (the usefulness of sustained release preparations is not proved). Dextroamphetamine—2.5–40 mg/day up to 0.5 mg/kg/day. Methylphenidate—10–60 mg/day or up to 1.0 mg/kg/day. Pemoline—37.5–112.5 mg given at 8 AM.	Insomnia, anorexia, weight loss (and possibly growth delay), tachycardia, precipitation of exacerbation of tic disorders. With pemoline, monitor LFTs as hepatotoxicity is possible.

TABLE 18–4. OVERVIEW OF COMMON PSYCHOACTIVE DRUGS IN CHILDHOOD AND ADOLESCENCE (Continued)

Drug	Indications	Dosage	Adverse Reactions and Monitoring
Lithium—considered an antipsychotic drug, also has antiaggressive properties.	Studies support use in MR and CD for aggressive and self-injurious behaviors. Can be used for same in PDD. Also indicated for early onset bipolar disorder.	600–2100 mg in 2–3 divided dosages. Keep blood levels to 0.4–1.2 mEq/L.	Nausea, vomiting, headache, tremor, weight gain. Experience with adults suggests thyroid and renal function monitoring.
Antidepressants—Imipramine (Tofranil) has been used in most child studies. Clomipramine (Anafranil) is effective in child obsessive-compulsive disorder (OCD).	Major depressive disorder, separation anxiety disorder, bulimia nervosa, functional enuresis. Sometimes used in ADHD, anorexia nervosa, sonambulism, or sleep terror disorder. OCD—clomipramine.	Imipramine—start with dosage of about 1.5 mg/kg/day; Can build up to not more than 5 mg/kg/day. Start with 2–3 divided dosages; can eventually combine in one dosage. Not FDA approved for children except for functional enuresis where dosage is usually between 50–100 mg before sleep.	Dry mouth, constipation, tachycardia, drowsiness, postural hypotension. Electrocardiogram (EKG) monitoring is needed owing to risk of cardiac conduction slowing. Blood levels of drug sometimes are useful.
Carbamazepine (Tegretol)—an anticonvulsant.	Aggression or dyscontrol in MR or CD.	Start with 10 mg/kg/day and build to 20–30 mg/kg/day. Therapeutic blood level range appears to be 4–12 mg/L.	Drowsiness, nausea, vertigo, psychosis. Monitor: CBC and LFTs for possible blood dyscrasias and hepatotoxicity.
Anxiolytics—have been insufficiently studied in childhood and adolescence.	Sometimes effective in parasomnias: sonambulism or sleep terror disorder. Can be tried in overanxious disorder.	Parasomnias: diazepam (Valium) 2–10 mg before bedtime.	Benzodiazepines can cause drowsiness, dyscontrol, and can be abused.
Fenfluramine (Pondimin)—an amphetamine congener.	Well studied in autistic disorder. Generally ineffective but some show improvement.	Gradually increase to between 1.0 and 1.5 mg/kg/day in divided doses.	Weight loss, drowsiness, irritability, loose bowel movement.

Table by Richard Perry, M.D.

TABLE 18–5.   **DSM-III-R DIAGNOSTIC CRITERIA FOR AUTISTIC DISORDER**

At least eight of the following sixteen items are present, these to include at least two items from A, one from B, and one from C.

Note: Consider a criterion to be met *only* if the behavior is abnormal for the person's developmental level.

A. Qualitative impairment in reciprocal social interaction as manifested by the following:
    (The examples within parentheses are arranged so that those first mentioned are more likely to apply to younger or more handicapped, and the later ones to older or less handicapped persons with this disorder.)

    (1) marked lack of awareness of the existence or feelings of others (e.g., treats a person as if he or she were a piece of furniture; does not notice another person's distress; apparently has no concept of the need of others for privacy)
    (2) no or abnormal seeking of comfort at times of distress (e.g., does not come for comfort even when ill, hurt, or tired; seeks comfort in a steryotyped way, e.g., says "cheese, cheese, cheese" whenever hurt)
    (3) no or impaired imitation (e.g., does not wave bye-bye; does not copy mother's domestic activities; mechanical imitation of others' actions out of context)
    (4) no or abnormal social play (e.g., does not actively participate in simple games; prefers solitary play activities; involves other children in play only as "mechanical aids")
    (5) gross impairment in ability to make peer friendships (e.g., no interest in making peer friendships; despite interest in making friends, demonstrates lack of understanding of conventions of social interaction, for example, reads phone book to uninterested peer)

B. Qualitative impairment in verbal and nonverbal communication, and in imaginative activity, as manifested by the following:
    (The numbered items are arranged so that those first listed are more likely to apply to younger or more handicapped, and the later ones, to older or less handicapped, persons with this disorder.)

    (1) no mode of communication, such as communicative babbling, facial expression, gesture, mime, or spoken language
    (2) markedly abnormal nonverbal communication, as in the use of eye-to-eye gaze, facial expression, body posture, or gestures to initiate or modulate social interaction (e.g., does not anticipate being held, stiffens when held, does not look at the person or smile when making a social approach, does not greet parents or visitors, has a fixed stare in social situations)
    (3) absence of imaginative activity, such as playacting of adult roles, fantasy characters, or animals; lack of interest in stories about imaginary events
    (4) marked abnormalities in the production of speech, including volume, pitch, stress, rate, rhythm, and intonation (e.g., monotonous tone, questionlike melody, or high pitch)
    (5) marked abnormalities in the form or content of speech, including steryotyped and repetitive use of speech (e.g., immediate echolalia or mechanical repetition of television commercial); use of "you" when "I" is meant (e.g., using "You want cookie?" to mean "I want a cookie"); idiosyncratic use of words or phrases (e.g, "Go on green riding" to mean "I want to go on the swing"); or frequent irrelevant remarks (e.g., starts talking about train schedules during a conversation about sports)
    (6) marked impairment in the ability to initiate or sustain a conversation with others, despite adequate speech (e.g., indulging in lengthy monologues on one subject regardless of interjections from others)

C. Markedly restricted repertoire of activities and interests, as manifested by the following:

    (1) steryotyped body movements, e.g., hand-flicking or -twisting, spinning, head-banging, complex whole-body movements
    (2) persistent preoccupation with parts of objects (e.g., sniffing or smelling objects, repetitive feeling of texture of materials, spinning wheels of toy cars) or attachment to unusual objects (e.g., insists on carrying around a piece of string)
    (3) marked distress over changes in trivial aspects of environment (e.g., when a vase is moved from usual position)
    (4) unreasonable insistence on following routines in precise detail (e.g., insisting that exactly the same route always be followed when shopping)
    (5) markedly restricted range of interests and a preoccupation with one narrow interest (e.g., interested only in lining up objects, in amassing facts about meteorology, or in pretending to be a fantasy character)

D. Onset during infancy or childhood.

Used with permission, APA.

c. **Psychologic** — individual psychotherapy is generally useless given language and other cognitive impairments. Family support is often helpful; it is beneficial that parents be told that autistic disorder does not result from faulty upbringing. Parents often require strategies for management and teaching. Associations exist for parents of children with autistic disorder.

C. Specific developmental disorders.   There are seven disorders arranged in three groups in DSM-III-R: (1) academic skills disorders—developmental arithmetic disorder, developmental expressive writing disorder, and developmental reading disorder; (2) language and speech disorders—developmental articulation disorder, developmental expressive language disorder, and developmental receptive language disorder; and (3) motor skills disorder—developmental coordination disorder. Prevalence is 2–10%. The male-to-female ratio is 2–4:1. Criteria are similar and presented here as an amalgam.

1. Diagnosis, signs and symptoms

a. Impairments in a specific developmental area, be it academic (reading, writing, arithmetic), speech and language (articulation, expressive or receptive language), or coordination. Performance in the specific area is below expectation based on chronologic age, schooling, and intellectual level.

b. The impairment significantly interferes with academic achievement and daily activities requiring the skill.

c. The specific developmental disorder is not due to known physical or neurologic disorder, defects in visual or hearing acuity, or disorders of the oral speech mechanism.

2. General considerations.   A specific developmental disorder is often associated with one or several other specific developmental disorders or other disorders. Specific developmental disorders (excluding articulation disorder) are associated with ADHD; reading disorder is associated with disruptive behavior and deliquency. There is increased family incidence.

Little is known about neurobiology. In reading disorder, a few studies (CT scan, MRI, and autopsy) demonstrate lack of normal hemispheric asymmetries in parietal or temporal lobes.

3. Treatment

a. **Educational intervention** depends on severity. No intervention or tutoring in milder cases. With more severity, the specific developmental disorder is addressed in a resource room with fewer children while other subjects are taught in regular class. In severe cases with multiple deficits, a child is placed in a full-day special class. Caretakers are also taught remedial techniques.

b. **Pharmacologic** — only for associated psychiatric disorder, such as ADHD. No evidence that medication directly benefits children with specific developmental disorders.

c. **Psychologic** — lowered self-esteem, school failure, and dropping-out are frequent with specific developmental disorders. School counseling, or individual, group, or family therapy may be indicated.

IV. Disruptive behavior disorders

A. Attention-deficit hyperactivity disorder (ADHD).   Prevalence in studies—1–20%, probably about 5%. The male-to-female ratio is 5–10:1.

1. Diagnosis, signs and symptoms

TABLE 18–6. **DSM-III-R DIAGNOSTIC CRITERIA FOR ATTENTION-DEFICIT HYPERACTIVITY DISORDER**

Note: Consider a criterion met only if the behavior is considerably more frequent than that of most people of the same mental age. Onset before the age of 7.

A disturbance of at least 6 months during which at least eight of the following are present:

    (1) often fidgets with hands or feet or squirms in seat (in adolescents, may be limited to subjective feelings of restlessness)
    (2) has difficulty remaining seated when required to do so
    (3) is easily distracted by extraneous stimuli
    (4) has difficulty awaiting turn in games or group situations
    (5) often blurts out answers to questions before they have been completed
    (6) has difficulty following through on instructions from others (not due to oppositional behavior or failure of comprehension), e.g., fails to finish chores
    (7) has difficulty sustaining attention in tasks or play activities
    (8) often shifts from one uncompleted activity to another
    (9) has difficulty playing quietly
   (10) often talks excessively
   (11) often interrupts or intrudes on others, e.g., butts into other children's games
   (12) often does not seem to listen to what is being said to him or her
   (13) often loses things necessary for tasks or activities at school or at home (e.g., toys, pencils, books, assignments)
   (14) often engages in physically dangerous activities without considering possible consequences (not for the purpose of thrill-seeking), e.g., runs into street without looking

Used with permission, APA.

2. General considerations. ADHD often coexists with conduct disorders or oppositional defiant disorder in which behaviors are less driven and intentionally antagonistic. ADHD also coexists with specific developmental disorders.

ADHD is thought to reflect subtle, yet unclear, neurologic impairments. It is associated with perinatal trauma and early malnutrition. Incidence is increased in male relatives, and concordance is greater in monozygotic than in dizygotic twins. In neurotransmitter systems, the clearest evidence is of noradrenergic dysfunction. Nonfocal (soft) neurologic signs are often present. A cerebral blood flow (CBF) study revealed frontal hypoperfusion, and frontal lobe dysfunction is suspected, allowing for disinhibition. ADHD is probably not related to sugar intake; few (perhaps 5%) are affected by food additives. 20–25% of those with ADHD continue to show symptoms into adolescence, some into adulthood. Some, especially those with concomitant conduct disorder, become delinquent and/or later develop an antisocial personality disorder.

3. Treatment
    a. Pharmacologic (Table 18–4).
        i. Stimulants reduce symptoms in about 75%; improve self-esteem by improving rapport with parent and teacher. Do not appear to work paradoxically—given to normal patients, activity decreases. Plasma levels are not useful.
            (a) Dextroamphetamine (Dexedrine) approved in Physicians' Desk Reference (PDR) for ages 3 years and over.
            (b) Methylphenidate (Ritalin) approved in PDR for 6 years or

older. Sustained release Ritalin does not have proven usefulness.
(c) Pemoline (Cylert).

 ii. Antidepressants if stimulants fail; may be best in ADHD plus symptoms of depression or anxiety. Imipramine (Tofranil) and desipramine (Norpramin) have shown some efficacy in studies.

 iii. Antipsychotics or lithium if other medications fail but only with severe symptoms and aggression (concomitant conduct disorder or oppositional defiant disorder).

 b. **Psychologic** — multimodality treatment is necessary for child and family. May include medication, individual psychotherapy, family therapy, and special education (especially with coexisting specific developmental disorder). These interventions are crucial in moderate or severe cases given risk of deliquency.

B. Conduct disorder. Prevalence ranges from 5–15% in studies. Accounts for many inpatient admissions in urban areas. The male-to-female ratio is 4–12:1. There are three types of conduct disorder depending on whether conduct problems are initiated as part of a group (group type), individually (solitary aggressive type), or both (undifferentiated type).

1. Diagnosis, signs and symptoms

TABLE 18–7. **DSM-III-R DIAGNOSTIC CRITERIA FOR CONDUCT DISORDER**

A. A disturbance of conduct lasting at least 6 months, during which at least three of the following have been present:

 (1) has stolen without confrontation of a victim on more than one occasion (including forgery)
 (2) has run away from home overnight at least twice while living in parental or parental surrogate home (or once without returning)
 (3) often lies (other than to avoid physical or sexual abuse)
 (4) has deliberately engaged in fire-setting
 (5) is often truant from school (for older person, absent from work)
 (6) has broken into someone else's house, building, or car
 (7) has deliberately destroyed others' property (other than by fire-setting)
 (8) has been physically cruel to animals
 (9) has forced someone into sexual activity with him or her
 (10) has used a weapon in more than one fight
 (11) often initiates physical fights
 (12) has stolen with confrontation of a victim (e.g., mugging, purse-snatching, extortion, armed robbery)
 (13) has been physically cruel to people

Note: The above items are listed in descending order of discriminating power based on data from a national field trial of the DSM-III-R criteria for disruptive behavior disorders.

B. If 18 or older, does not meet criteria for antisocial personality disorder.

Used with permission, APA.

2. General considerations. Conduct disorder is associated with family instability, including victimization by physical or sexual abuse. Propensity for violence correlates with child abuse, family violence, and signs of severe psychopathology, e.g., paranoia and cognitive and/or subtle neurologic deficits. It is crucial to explore for these signs; findings can guide treatment.

Conduct disorder often coexists with ADHD and specific developmental disorder. Suicidal thoughts and acts and alcohol and drug abuse correlate with conduct disorder.

No neurobiologic findings are specific to conduct disorder. Findings reveal varied neurologic impairments.

3. Treatment

a. Pharmacologic (Table 18–4) — generally, children are medicated to control aggression. Under current study is whether psychopathologic findings, e.g., depressive tendencies or neurologic impairment, predict response to medications used in conduct disorder.

Lithium or haloperidol are of proven efficacy in many aggressive children with conduct disorder. Carbamazepine has shown success and it, like beta blockers, deserves study. Two reports of coexisting conduct disorder and major depressive illness show response to imipramine.

b. Psychologic — multimodality as in ADHD. May include medication, individual and/or family therapy, tutoring, or special class placement (for cognitive and/or conduct problems). It is crucial to discover and fortify any interests or talents to build resistance to lure of crime. If environment is noxious and/or if conduct disorder is severe, then placement away from home may be indicated.

C. Oppositional defiant disorder

1. Diagnosis, signs and symptoms

TABLE 18–8.   **DSM-III-R DIAGNOSTIC CRITERIA FOR OPPOSITIONAL DEFIANT DISORDER**

Note: Consider a criterion met only if the behavior is considerably more frequent than that of most people of the same mental age.

A. A disturbance of at least 6 months during which at least five of the following are present:

    (1) often loses temper
    (2) often argues with adults
    (3) often actively defies or refuses adult requests or rules, e.g., refuses to do chores at home
    (4) often deliberately does things that annoy other people, e.g., grabs other children's hats
    (5) often blames others for his or her own mistakes
    (6) is often touchy or easily annoyed by others
    (7) is often angry and resentful
    (8) is often spiteful or vindictive
    (9) often swears or uses obscene language

Used with permission, APA.

2. General considerations.   New to DSM-III in 1980, oppositional defiant disorder is little researched, and its validity has been questioned. It can coexist with many disorders, including ADHD and anxiety disorders. It appears to result from parent-child struggles over autonomy; therefore, occurrence increases in families with overly rigid parents and temperamentally active, moody, and intense children.

3. Treatment

a. Pharmacologic — those drugs used for conduct disorder may be necessary, but only after careful consideration of benefit to risk ratio and failure of other interventions.

b. Psychologic — individual and/or family therapy are interventions of choice. Behavior modification can be helpful.

V. Anxiety disorders of childhood and adolescence.   These disorders account for many outpatient referrals. They are little researched, because only overanxious disorder existed prior to DSM-III in 1980. Children and adolescents also can have anxiety disorders described elsewhere in DSM-III-R: simple phobia, obsessive-compulsive disorder, post-traumatic stress disorder, and panic disorder.

A. Separation anxiety disorder. Prevalence is unknown. The male-to-female ratio is equal. Onset is from preschool to adolescence; some children evidence most severe form of disorder when onset is about age 11.

1. Diagnosis, signs and symptoms

TABLE 18–9.　**DSM-III-R DIAGNOSTIC CRITERIA FOR SEPARATION ANXIETY DISORDER**

A. Excessive anxiety concerning separation from those to whom the child is attached, as evidenced by at least three of the following:

  (1) unrealistic and persistent worry about possible harm befalling major attachment figures or fear that they will leave and not return

  (2) unrealistic and persistent worry that an untoward calamitous event will separate the child from a major attachment figure, e.g., the child will be lost, kidnapped, killed, or be the victim of an accident

  (3) persistent reluctance or refusal to go to school in order to stay with major attachment figures or at home

  (4) persistent reluctance or refusal to go to sleep without being near a major attachment figure or to go to sleep away from home

  (5) persistent avoidance of being alone, including "clinging" to and "shadowing" major attachment figures

  (6) repeated nightmares involving the theme of separation

  (7) complaints of physical symptoms, e.g., headaches, stomachaches, nausea, or vomiting, on many school days or on other occasions when anticipating separation from major attachment figures

  (8) recurrent signs or complaints of excessive distress in anticipation of separation from home or major attachment figures, e.g., temper tantrums or crying, pleading with parents not to leave

  (9) recurrent signs of complaints of excessive distress when separated from home or major attachment figures, e.g., wants to return home, needs to call parents when they are absent or when child is away from home

B. Duration of disturbance of at least 2 weeks.

C. Onset before the age of 18.

Used with permission, APA.

2. General considerations. Separation anxiety disorder clusters in families but genetic transmission is unclear. Some data link affected children with parents who have a history of that disorder as well as current panic disorder, agoraphobia, or depression. Neurobiologic data are lacking. Social debilitation is a risk in severe cases.

3. Treatment

  a. Pharmacologic (Table 18–4).

    i. Antidepressants. Imipramine was superior to placebo in one study.

    ii. Anxiolytics. Little researched in childhood anxiety disorders, with little evidence of efficacy.

    iii. Antipsychotics not useful in anxiety disorders. Risk of side effects outweigh potential benefits.

    iv. Antihistamines. Diphenhydramine (Benadryl) is sometimes used to relieve childhood anxiety. Usefulness is limited, and child can have a paradoxical reaction.

  b. Psychologic — these are treatments of choice, although effectiveness has not been shown in rigorous studies.

    i. Individual psychotherapy. Inseparability from parents can result from rageful destructive feelings toward parents, which are repressed and projected onto the environment and then experienced as constant threats to the child and parents' well-being. Relieved only by avoiding separation.

    ii. Family therapy or parent guidance if parents are fostering separation anxiety.

    iii. Behavior modification may be helpful to achieve separation from parents and/or return to school.

B. Overanxious disorder. Prevalence unknown. The male-to-female ratio is equal.

1. Diagnosis, signs and symptoms

TABLE 18–10.   **DSM-III-R DIAGNOSTIC CRITERIA FOR OVERANXIOUS DISORDER**

Excessive or unrealistic anxiety or worry, for a period of 6 months or longer, as indicated by the frequent occurrence of at least four of the following:

(1) excessive or unrealistic worry about future events
(2) excessive or unrealistic concern about the appropriateness of past behavior
(3) excessive or unrealistic concern about competence in one or more areas, e.g., athletic, academic, social
(4) somatic complaints, such as headaches or stomachaches, for which no physical basis can be established
(5) marked self-consciousness
(6) excessive need for reassurance about a variety of concerns
(7) marked feelings of tension or inability to relax

Used with permission, APA.

2. General considerations. Fostered by parents predicating love and approval on high performance and achievement. Rivalries with parents and siblings abound. Genetic transmission is suspected; there are increased anxiety disorders in mothers. No neurobiologic data. These children may remain anxious but generally prognosis is good concerning general adaptation.

3. Treatment

    a. Pharmacologic — usually not necessary. Benzodiazepines can be tried but in adolescence, consider potential for abuse.

    b. Psychologic

        i. Individual psychotherapy accompanied by parent counseling or family therapy.

        ii. Behavioral approaches are not applicable when anxiety-provoking situations are numerous.

C. Avoidant disorder of childhood or adolescence

1. Diagnosis, signs and symptoms

TABLE 18–11.   **DSM-III-R DIAGNOSTIC CRITERIA FOR AVOIDANT DISORDER OF CHILDHOOD OR ADOLESCENCE**

A. Excessive shrinking from contact with unfamiliar people, for a period of 6 months or longer, sufficiently severe to interfere with social functioning in peer relationships.

B. Desire for social involvement with familiar people (family members and peers the person knows well), and generally warm and satisfying relations with family members and other familiar figures.

C. Age at least 2½ years.

Used with permission, APA.

2. **General considerations.** Avoidance can result from any physical or psychic trauma leading to child's belief of inherent worthlessness or inferiority, e.g., chronic medical handicaps, speech and language problems, abuse, or neglect. Temperamentally withdrawing children may be predisposed.

3. **Treatment**

   a. **Pharmacologic** — trial of anxiolytic in conjunction with other therapies.

   b. **Psychologic** — individual therapy, parent counseling, or family therapy and arranging relatively nonthreatening peer interactions. Group therapy can be tried.

VI. Eating disorders

A. **Anorexia nervosa.** Prevalence is 0.5–1.0% of adolescent girls. Onset usually 13–20 years. The male-to-female ratio is 1:9–10.

1. **Diagnosis, signs and symptoms.** **Note:** Actual loss of appetite occurs only late in illness.

TABLE 18–12. **DSM-III-R DIAGNOSTIC CRITERIA FOR ANOREXIA NERVOSA**

A. Refusal to maintain body weight over a minimal normal weight for age and height, e.g., weight loss leading to maintenance of body weight 15% below that expected; or failure to make expected weight gain during period of growth, leading to body weight 15% below that expected.

B. Intense fear of gaining weight or becoming fat, even though underweight.

C. Disturbance in the way in which one's body weight, size, or shape is experienced, e.g., the person claims to "feel fat" even when emaciated, believes that one area of the body is "too fat" even when obviously underweight.

D. In females, absence of at least three consecutive menstrual cycles when otherwise expected to occur (primary or secondary amenorrhea). (A woman is considered to have amenorrhea if her periods occur only following hormone, e.g., estrogen, administration.)

Used with permission, APA.

---

2. **General considerations.** Potentially fatal (5–12% in studies) and complicated physiologically due to starvation and frequently associated symptoms of bulimia nervosa. Many medical or psychiatric disorders can cause anorexia and/or weight loss, e.g., various cancers, gastrointestinal (GI) disorders, drug abuse, depression. As in depression, there is hypercortisolemia and nonsuppression of dexamethasone, but these normalize with weight gain.

Anorexia nervosa is more common in middle and upper socioeconomic groups, models, and ballerinas. Anorexics are rigid, self-debasing, obsessional, and anxious. Anorexia nervosa appears to be a reaction to demands for independence and/or social/sexual functioning in adolescence. There is increased familial depression. Some evidence of increased anorexia nervosa in sisters and a higher concordance in monozygotic than dizygotic twins. Neurobiologically, 3-methoxy-4-hydroxyphenylgylcol (MHPG) in urine and CSF is reduced, suggesting lessened norepinephrine turnover and activity. Endogenous opioid activity appears lessened as a consequence of starving. In one PET scan study, caudate nucleus metabolism was higher during the anorectic state than after weight gain. In long-term follow up, 40% recover, 30% improve, and 30% are chronic.

3. **Treatment**

a. May be outpatient or inpatient pediatric/medical/psychiatric unit, depending on degree of weight loss and physical condition. Psychiatry unit is indicated if physical condition permits, when there is depression, high suicide risk, or family crisis. The inpatient treatment of starvation provides for (1) assured weight gain and (2) the monitoring and treatment of the potentially life-threatening effects of starvation (and metabolic complications of bulimia nervosa, if present). A desired weight is set and a strategy devised, which may include supervised meals, food supplements, and nasogastric feedings for uncooperative patients.

b. **Pharmacologic** (Table 18–4). Anorexics often resist medication, and no drugs are of proven efficacy. Most promising is cyproheptadine (Periactin), and antidepressants are tried if major depression coexists. Serotonergic agents, as well as bupropion (Wellbutrin), may be useful.

c. **Psychologic** — psychotherapy is generally ineffective. Cognitive behavior therapy aimed at changing attitudes and habits concerning food, eating, and body image seems promising. Family therapy also is useful.

B. **Bulimia nervosa.** Prevalence 4–15% of female high school and college students. Onset usually 16½–18 years. The male-to-female ratio is 1:9–10.

1. **Diagnosis, signs and symptoms**

TABLE 18–13. **DSM-III-R DIAGNOSTIC CRITERIA FOR BULIMIA NERVOSA**

A. Recurrent episodes of binge eating (rapid consumption of a large amount of food in a discrete period of time).

B. A feeling of lack of control over eating behavior during the eating binges.

C. The person regularly engages in either self-induced vomiting, use of laxatives or diuretics, strict dieting or fasting, or vigorous exercise in order to prevent weight gain.

D. A minimum average of two binge eating episodes a week for at least 3 months.

E. Persistent overconcern with body shape and weight.

Used with permission, APA.

2. **General considerations.** Self-induced vomiting can result in calluses and lacerations of fingers, dental caries, and salivary gland swelling, as well as potentially life-threatening metabolic alkalosis, hypocholoremia, and hypokalemia. In about 50% there is abnormal dexamethasone suppression, but in bulimia nervosa attitudes and practices about food are different than in depression.

Bulimia nervosa, which is often preceded by dieting, reflects society's premium on thinness. It is most prevalent in the middle and upper socioeconomic groups, where the incidence is rising. Bulimics are perfectionistic and achievement oriented. Bulimia nervosa may be precipitated by fear of leaving family after high school. Anxiety and depressive symptoms are common; suicide is a risk. Alcohol abuse occurs, and approximately one-third shoplift food. There is increased incidence of family mood disorder and obesity; family strife, rejection, and neglect are more common than in anorexia nervosa. Metabolic studies indicate less norepinephrine and serotonin activity and turnover. Course is usually chronic but not debilitating when not complicated by electrolyte imblance and metabolic alkalosis.

3. Treatment

  a. Electrolyte imbalance and metabolic alkalosis may necessitate hospitalization.

  b. Pharmacologic (Table 18–4) — Antidepressants appear to be more beneficial than in anorexia nervosa. Imipramine, trazodone, and the monoamine oxidase inhibitors (MAOIs) phenelzine (Nardil) and isocarboxazid (Marplan) have reduced symptoms in studies. Fluoxetine is also of reported benefit in reducing binging and subsequent purging episodes.

  c. Psychologic — lack of control over eating usually motivates for therapy, which may include individual psychotherapy, cognitive behavioral therapy, and group psychotherapy. Normalization of eating habits, attitudes about food, and the pursuit of the ideal body must be addressed.

C. Pica is the repeated ingestion of a nonnutritive substance for at least 1 month in infants who do not meet criteria for autistic disorder, schizophrenia, or Kleine-Levin syndrome. Prevalence is unclear; studies report 10–32%. It is associated with mental retardation, neglect, and nutritional deficiency, e.g., iron or zinc. Lead or other poisonings can result. It usually stops in early childhood. Treatment involves testing for lead intoxication and treating if necessary. Any iron or zinc deficiency is corrected. Parent guidance may be necessary. Infrequently, aversive conditioning is necessary.

D. Rumination disorder of infancy is the repeated regurgitation, for at least 1 month, following a period of normal eating (in the absence of GI illness) and resulting in weight loss or failure to gain expected weight. Swallowed food is brought back into the mouth, ejected or rechewed, and swallowed. There is no distress. The condition is rare with onset between 3 and 12 months. Immature, ungiving mothers who become further rejecting because of the disorder may be associated with rumination. Little is known of outcome, but it ranges from spontaneous remissions, to malnutrition, to failure to thrive, to death. GI problems, e.g., pyloric stenosis, must be ruled out. Treatment involves parental guidance and behavioral techniques, which may include aversive behavior therapy when the disorder is severe.

VII. Gender identity disorders.   Disorders in which there is discordance between assigned (biologic) sex and gender identity, the subjective experience of gender role. These disorders are separate from those in which biologic sex is ambiguous: Turner's syndrome, Klinefelter's syndrome, adrenogenital syndrome, pseudohermaphroditism, and androgen insensitivity syndrome.

  A. Gender identity disorder of childhood.   Rare; onset is preschool in males, later in females. The male-to-female ratio is 6–30:1 (data from three reports).

   1. Diagnosis, signs and symptoms.   In prepubertal children, there is distress with assigned sex and intense desire to be or insistence that one is of opposite sex. A marked preference exists for the clothing and activities of the opposite sex and/or repudiation of one's sex organs. They may assert that their sex organs will disappear to be replaced by those of the opposite sex.

2. General considerations. Contributing to gender identity disorder of childhood are absence of same-sex role models and explicit or implicit encouragement from caretakers to behave like the opposite sex. Mothers may be depressed or withdrawn. In some, inborn temperamental traits may result in sensitive delicate boys and energetic, aggressive girls. Physical and sexual abuse may predispose. Course is variable. Symptoms may diminish spontaneously or with treatment. In young boys, social ostracism may be intense; in young girls, tomboyism is generally better tolerated. Associated psychopathology varies from none, especially in girls, to severe. Many boys (one-to-two thirds) and some girls become homosexual. A minority go on to transsexualism.

3. Treatment. Improve existing role models or in their absence provide one from the family or elsewhere, e.g., big brother or sister. Caretakers are helped to encourage sex-appropriate behavior and attitudes. Any associated mental disorder is addressed.

B. Transsexualism. Rare; more common in males than females.

1. Diagnosis, signs and symptoms. After puberty, there is distress with assigned sex, and for at least 2 years there is a desire to eliminate one's primary and secondary sex characteristics and acquire those of the other sex. Depending on history of sexual orientation, there are types: asexual, homosexual, heterosexual, or unspecified.

2. General considerations. Most have had gender identity disorder of childhood. Cross dressing is common. Social and occupational functioning is impaired. Associated mental disorder is common, especially borderline personality disorder or depression. Suicide is a risk. Mutilation of sex organs may occur to coerce surgeons to perform sex reassignment surgery.

3. Treatment. Any coexisting mental disorders are addressed. No psychologic treatment is successful in changing desire for sex reassignment. Specialists in this area have established prerequisites to surgery, which include a favorable adaptation during a trial period of at least 1 year of cross-gender living and hormone treatments. After this period, most having had surgery report satisfactory results. Dissatisfaction correlates with the severity of preexisting psychopathology. A reported 2% commit suicide.

C. Gender identity disorder of adolescence or adulthood, nontranssexual type (GIDAANT). Prevalence unknown. More common in males than females.

1. Diagnosis, signs and symptoms. After puberty, distress with assigned sex accompanied by fantasies or episodes of cross dressing. In GIDAANT, cross dressing is not for purpose of sexual arousal, as in transvestic fetishism, and there is no persistent desire for sex reassignment, as in transsexualism.

2. **General considerations.** Most have history of gender identity disorder of childhood. Anxiety and depression coexist, as does conflict with family members over cross dressing. Some develop transsexualism.

3. **Treatment.** For many, treatment not sought; however, psychotherapy can be helpful.

VIII. Tic disorders

A. **Tourette's disorder (TD)** (also known as Gilles de la Tourette's syndrome). Prevalence is 0.1–0.5/1,000; mean age of onset—7. The male-to-female ratio is 3:1.

1. **Diagnosis, signs and symptoms.** Multiple motor and one or more vocal tics occurring many times a day, nearly every day or intermittently, for more than 1 year. Over time, tics vary in location, frequency, and complexity. Onset is before age 21, and tics do not result exclusively from medications, e.g., stimulants, or central nervous system (CNS) disease.

   Motor and vocal tics can be simple or complex. Simple tics generally are the first to appear. **Examples. Simple motor tics:** eyeblinking, head jerking, facial grimacing. **Simple vocal tics:** coughing, grunting, sniffing. **Complex motor tics:** hitting self, jumping. **Complex vocal tics:** coprolalia (use of vulgar words), palilalia (repeating own words), echolalia (repeating other's words).

2. **General considerations.** There is evidence of genetic transmission—increased tic disorders in family; of 30 monozygotic twins, more than half were concordant for TD. Evidence of neurobiologic substrate—EEG abnormalities in about 50%; implication of dopamine abnormality; abnormal levels of homovanillic acid (dopamine metabolite) in CSF: stimulants, which are dopamine agonists, can worsen tics or perhaps cause TD; dopamine antagonists generally improve tics. Associated with TD: ADHD, learning problems, and obsessive-compulsive symptoms, of which there is increased incidence in first-degree relatives. Social ostracism is frequent. Course, untreated, is usually chronic with periods of lessening interspersed with exacerbation of tics.

3. **Treatment**
   a. **Pharmacologic** (Table 18–4).
      i. **Haloperidol (Haldol).** About 85% improve, many markedly. Often require dosages that are sedating.
      ii. **Pimozide (Orap).** Strongly antidopaminergic like haloperidol. Small potential for slowing cardiac conduction.
      iii. **Clonidine (Catapres).** An alpha-2 adrenergic agonist; not as effective as other two drugs, but no risk of tardive dyskinesia. There is little evidence implicating noradrenergic mechanism in TD.
   b. **Psychologic** — counseling or therapy is often necessary for child and/or family. The nature of TD, coping with it, and ostracism must be addressed. Group therapy may reduce social isolation.

B. **Chronic motor or vocal tic disorder.** Similar to TD. Diagnostic criteria are the same except that there are either motor tics *or* vocal tics, not both. Also, its severity and social impairment generally are less. Genetically, chronic motor or vocal tic disorder and TD frequently occur in the same families. The neurobiology appears to be the same, and the treatment is identical to that of TD.

C. **Transient tic disorder.** Prevalence unclear; nonrigorous surveys report 5–24% of school children have some sort of tic. The male-to-female ratio is 3:1.

   1. **Diagnosis, signs and symptoms.** Single or multiple motor and/or vocal tics occur many times a day, nearly every day for at least 2 weeks but not longer than 12 consecutive months. Onset is before age 21. There is no history of TD or chronic motor or vocal tic disorder and the tics do not result from medications or CNS disease.

   2. **General considerations.** In most cases, the tics are psychogenic, increasing during stress and tending to remit spontaneously. In few cases, chronic motor or vocal tic disorder or TD eventually develop.

   3. **Treatment.** In mild cases, treatment may not be needed. In more severe cases, psychotherapy is indicated. Medication, as used in the other two tic disorders, is tried only in very severe cases.

IX. **Elimination disorders**

A. **Functional encopresis.** Prevalence is about 1% of 5-year-old children; more common in boys than in girls.

   1. **Diagnosis, signs and symptoms.** Repeatedly, at least once a month for 6 months, child of at least 4 years mental age passes feces into inappropriate places, e.g., in clothing or on floor. Fecal passage is involuntary or intentional, but is not due to physical disorder, e.g., aganglionic megacolon (Hirschsprung's disease). Specify if primary type if disorder was not preceded by at least 1 year of fecal continence or secondary if it was.

   2. **General considerations.** Inadequate toilet training can result in child-parent power struggles and functional encopresis. Some children appear to have ineffective GI motility, which contributes. Some fear using the toilet. About 25% retain feces and become constipated and impacted. Defecation is painful. Anal fissures can develop. Overflow incontinence develops. Secondary encopresis often has precipitants: birth of a sibling or parental separation. Functional encopresis usually brings embarrassment and social ostracism. Done deliberately, associated psychopathology is usually severe. About 25% also have functional enuresis. Course—can last for years but usually resolves.

   3. **Treatment.** The child may require individual psychotherapy to address the meaning of the functional encopresis as well as any embarrassment or ostracism. Behavioral techniques often are helpful. Parental guidance and/or family therapy often is needed. Impaction, anal fissures, etc. require consultation with a pediatrician.

B. **Functional enuresis.** Prevalence: Age 5—7% male, 3% female; age 10—3% male, 2% female; age 18—1% male, rare–female.

   1. **Diagnosis, signs and symptoms.** Repeatedly, at least twice a month if age 5 or 6 or once a month if older, voiding of urine into bed or clothes, day or night. Chronologic age is at least 5; mental age at least 4. Voiding

is involuntary or intentional but not due to a physical disorder. Specify if primary or secondary type, as in functional encopresis. Specify if nocturnal or diurnal.

2. **General considerations.** Functional enuresis tends to run in families; concordance is greater in monozygotic than in dizygotic twins. In some, bladders tend to be functionally small, requiring frequent voiding. It does not seem to be related to a specific stage of sleep, as do sleepwalking or sleep terror disorders. In many, there is no coexisting mental disorder and impairment reflects only the conflict with caretakers, loss of self-esteem, and social ostracism, if any. Secondary enuresis is more likely to have coexisting disorders and can be precipitated by such events as sibling birth or parental separation. Spontaneous remissions are frequent at ages 6–8 and puberty.

3. **Treatment**
   1. **Pharmacologic** (Table 18–4). Rarely used given rate of spontaneous remissions, success of behavioral approaches, and tolerance to drug. Imipramine often is effective in reducing or even eliminating wetting. Tolerance can develop after about 6 weeks. Mode of action is unclear; considered are effects on bladder or sleep cycle. Desmopressin has shown success.
   2. **Psychologic**
      a. **Behavioral approaches.** Record dry nights on a calendar and reward dry nights with a star and 5–7 consecutive dry nights with a gift. A bell and buzzer apparatus is a successful treatment but is cumbersome to use.
      b. **Psychotherapy.** Not recommended unless coexisting psychopathology or problems, such as reduced self-esteem.
      The exploration of conflicts underlying functional enuresis has met with little success. Parental guidance related to the management of the disorder often is necessary.

X. **Speech disorders not elsewhere classified.**
   A. **Cluttering,** a new category in DSM-III-R, is little studied. Diagnostically, it is a disorder of speech fluency wherein abnormal rate and rhythm affect intelligibility. Speech consists of rapid, jerky spurts resulting in phrases unrelated to the grammatical structure of sentences.
   Cluttering begins in 2–8-year-old children and sometimes coexists with stuttering, other language and academic skills disorders, ADHD, and language problems in the family. Spontaneous resolution is common. Speech therapy is indicated as well as psychotherapy for secondary problems, such as low self-esteem and problems with social adaptation.
   B. **Stuttering.** Prevalence is 5–10%; onset 2–7 years; the male-to-female ratio is 2–4:1.
      1. **Diagnosis, signs and symptoms.** Frequent repetitions or prolongations of sounds or syllables that markedly impair the fluency of speech.
      2. **General considerations.** Evidence exists of abnormal brain lateralization and genetic predisposition. There is increased incidence of stuttering and other language disorders in families and high concordance rate in monozygotic twins.

Course—begins insidiously with two peaks of onset: 2–3 years and 5–7 years. 80% recover, 60% spontaneously by mid-adolescence. Stutterers commonly have other language disorders, ADHD, anxiety disorders, and withdrawing, avoidant behaviors, as stuttering worsens with increased pressure to communicate.

3. Treatment. Specialized speech therapy is paramount. Psychotherapy addresses secondary problems, such as poor self-esteem or withdrawing and avoidant behaviors. Family therapy if family dysfunction contributes.

XI. Other disorders of infancy, childhood, or adolescence

A. Elective mutism. Rare, more common in females.

Diagnostically, the persistent refusal to talk in school and perhaps elsewhere in a child who both speaks and comprehends. Begins between age 3 and 5, usually resolves in weeks to months. Associated with other speech and language disorders, shyness, and oppositional behavior. Treatment can include individual psychotherapy and/or parent counseling.

B. Identity disorder. Little used and studied category describing late adolescents or young adults distressed by the inability to choose a career, develop values, or enter close relationships. A cohesive sense of self is lacking, which results in social and occupational impairments. Duration is at least 3 months, and it does not result from mood or psychotic disorder. Treatment is individual psychotherapy and perhaps family counseling.

C. Reactive attachment disorder of infancy or early childhood. Prevalence and sex ratio are unknown. Often diagnosed and treated pediatrically.

Diagnostically, grossly inadequate caretaking (persistent disregard of physical or emotional needs or repeated change of caretaker) results in pre-5-year-old child's disturbed social relatedness (failure to initiate or respond to interactions or indiscriminate, but shallow, sociability). These failure-to-thrive children are apathetic, passive, and do not track visually. Their disturbance is not due to mental retardation or autistic disorder.

1. General considerations. Physically, head circumference is generally normal; weight, very low; height, somewhat short. Pituitary functioning is normal. Associated with low socioeconomic status and mothers who are depressed, isolated, and have experienced abuse. Course—the earlier the intervention, the more reversible the disorder. "Affectionless character" can develop. Death can occur.

2. Treatment. If caretaker is beyond help, removal of child may be necessary and permanent. Severe malnourishment and other medical problems may require hospitalization of child. Some caretakers become adequate following education, the provision of a homemaker or financial aid, treatment of concomitant mental disorder, among others.

D. Stereotypy/habit disorder. Diagnostically there are intentional, repetitive, nonfunctional stereotypies (e.g., rocking, head banging) or habits (e.g., nail biting, nose picking, hair pulling) that cause physical injury or markedly interfere with normal activities. Pervasive developmental disorder or tic disorder must be absent. Common in mental retardation and blindness. Treatment varies. If movements increase with frustration, boredom, or tension, then these are addressed. Self-abusive behaviors may require medications, such as haloperidol, lithium, or opiate antagonists (which are currently under study) (Table 18–4).

E. Undifferentiated attention-deficit disorder. Validity of this category has not been established. It was meant to describe very inattentive children, similar to those with ADHD, but without the hyperactivity.

XII. Disorders relevant to children and adolescents but appearing in the adult section of DSM-III-R.

A. Schizophrenia in childhood is diagnosed using adult criteria. Several studies indicate that of the children who meet the criteria, many are delusional and/or hallucinating (auditory and/or visual). Nevertheless, few children or young adolescents are schizophrenic because age of onset is typically 15–35 years. Treat with antipsychotic medications, although studies are lacking. Psychotherapy, family therapy, and special schooling may be necessary.

B. Mood disorders in childhood also rely on adult criteria for diagnosis. Some prepubertal children meet criteria for major depression. The efficacy of antidepressant medication has yet to be demonstrated in child depressives. Some anecdotal reports of prepubertal children with manic-like symptoms claim successful treatment with lithium.

C. Other disorders. Some children meet adult criteria for anxiety disorders: simple phobia, obsessive-compulsive disorder, post-traumatic stress disorder, and panic disorder. Clomipramine (Anafranil) appears to benefit children with obsessive-compulsive disorder. Post-traumatic stress disorder can result from physical or sexual abuse.

Substance, somatoform, sleep, and adjustment disorders can also be diagnosed in childhood and adolescence.

XIII. Other childhood issues

A. Child abuse. An estimated 1 million children are abused annually in the U.S., resulting in 2–4,000 deaths/year. The abused are apt to be low birth weight, handicapped, (e.g., MR, cerebral palsy) or troubled (e.g., defiant, hyperactive). The abusing parent is usually the mother who likely was abused herself. Abusing parents often are impulsive, substance abusers, depressed, antisocial, or narcissistic. In 8 out of 10 sexually abused children, the perpetrator, usually male, is known to the child. In 50%, the offender is a parent, parent surrogate, or relative.

B. Suicide. Serious attempts and completed suicides are rare in children younger than 13 years. Suicidal ideation, threats, and less serious gestures are much more frequent and often a precipitant to hospitalization. Suicidal children tend to be depressed (and sometimes preoccupied with death); however, angry, impulsive children, as well as children suffering recent emotional trauma, can be suicidal.

Suicidal behavior is increasing in adolescents and, as with children, often necessitates hospitalization. It correlates with depression, aggressive behavior, and alcohol abuse. Females have more suicidal ideation and make more suicidal gestures or attempts. Serious attempts and successful suicides correlate with the male sex and the availability of alcohol, illicit drugs, or medications (such substances lower impulse control and/or can be used for overdose).

Parents often are unaware of their children's suicidal thoughts and behavior, thus necessitating direct questioning of children and adolescents about suicide.

C. **Firesetting** is associated with other destruction of property, stealing, lying, self-destructive tendencies, and cruelty to animals. The male-to-female ratio is 9:1.

D. **Obesity** is present in 5–20% of children and adolescents. A small percentage present with an obesity-hypoventilation syndrome similar to adult Pickwickian syndrome. These children can have dyspnea and sleep characterized by snoring, stridor, perhaps apnea, and hypoxia with oxygen desaturation. Death can result. Other conditions, such as hypothyroidism or Prader-Willi syndrome, should be ruled out.

E. **Acquired immune deficiency syndrome (AIDS)**

The AIDS epidemic has presented child and adolescent psychiatrists with a multitude of difficult problems. For example, the care of young patients from lower socioeconomic groups, already grossly inadequate due to insufficient resources, is further burdened by AIDS-related illness or the death of parents and relatives. Young psychiatric patients with concomitant non-symptomatic positive serology who are in need of residential treatment are rejected for fear of the disease's transmission. In adolescence, AIDS has added a critical dimension to the area of sexual practices and the problem of drug abuse. See Chapter 25, Acquired Immune Deficiency Syndrome.

For more detailed discussion of this topic, see Chap. 32 through Chap. 44, pp 1689–1997, in *CTP/V* for the entire spectrum of child and adolescent psychiatry.

19
Geriatric Psychiatry

I. Epidemiology

The absolute number of aged persons and their proportion in the world's industrial nations have been increasing throughout this century. In the United States, approximately 4% of the population was age 65 or over in 1900; today, more than 10% of the U.S. population, or approximately 30 million Americans, are in this age group. Life expectancy in industrialized countries has increased by 50%, resulting in a 20–40% increase in the number of persons over age 65. The oldest old segment of the U.S. population (age 85 or older) is frequently cited as the fastest growing population group. There are presently more than 2.5 million persons in the 85 + age range and more than 30,000 persons in the United States have passed their 100th birthday.

II. Medical background

The leading causes of death in the elderly are heart disease, cancer, stroke, Alzheimer's disease, and pneumonia. Central nervous system (CNS) changes and psychopathology are also frequent concomitants of the other major causes of geriatric demise.

Morbidity is a common factor in aging. More than one-half of persons age 65 and over report arthritic and related symptomatology. Benign prostatic hyperplasia is present in three-quarters of men over age 75. Urinary incontinence is believed to occur in as many as one-fifth of the elderly, frequently in association with dementia. These common disorders result in behavior modification. Arthritis, for example, may restrict activity and alter life-style. The cognizant elderly, like other adults, are profoundly embarrassed by urinary difficulties and will restrict activities and hide or deny their disability in order to maintain self-esteem.

Cardiovascular disease is a prominent cause of morbidity and mortality in the elderly. Hypertension may be present in 40% of the elderly, many of whom are receiving diuretics and/or antihypertensive medications. Hypertension itself can result in CNS effects ranging from headaches to stroke, and pharmacotherapy for this condition can result in mood and cognitive disorders either indirectly, e.g., electrolyte disturbances due to diuretic treatment, or more directly, e.g., neurotransmitter changes associated with beta blockers.

Sensory changes also accompany the aging process. One-third of the aged have some degree of auditory disability. In one study, nearly one-half of persons 75 to 85 years of age had lens cataract formation, and more than 70% had glaucoma. Difficulties with convergence, accommodation, and macular degeneration also are sources of visual disability in the aged. These sensory changes frequently interact with psychopathologic disabilities, serving to magnify psychopathologic deficit and color symptomatology.

III. Clinical syndromes
A. Depression
1. Signs and symptoms. The frequency of depression appears to increase with age, although the relapse rate, i.e., time between depressive episodes

appears to decrease. The frequency of suicide also increases markedly with age. Yet, there is good evidence that certain features of depression, namely obsessional and phobic disorders, decrease with age.

Epidemiologic studies of depression in the elderly are confounded by confusion between depression and dementia. Family members of dementia patients commonly bring the patient with the chief complaint of depression in the absence of any true mood disorder. The psychiatrist must recognize that paucity of speech, slowing of gait, flattening of affect, and decreased interest in and involvement with social and personal activities, which are all indicative of depression in a young patient, are, in the absence of clear-cut dysphoria, indicative of early dementia in the elderly patient. Cognitive assessment, which will reveal deficit in the dementia patient, will further clarify the diagnosis of dementia when applicable.

Depression may coexist with dementia and is a common concomitant of the early stages of Alzheimer's disease (Global Deterioration Scale stages 3–5). When depression occurs in the context of Alzheimer's disease, the most common symptom is tearfulness, which is frequently accompanied by early signs of the characteristic sleep disturbance, suspiciousness, anxieties, and agitation, which form the behavioral syndrome of Alzheimer's disease. Other symptoms, reminiscent of depression in other contexts, may occur in the depressive syndrome of Alzheimer's disease, including somatic complaints and obsessive behaviors. Pervasive dysphoria, however, is relatively rare, and Alzheimer's patients with depression rarely, if ever, manifest suicidal behavior. Manneristic statements such as, ''I wish I were dead,'' are common in Alzheimer's disease; however, these statements are not accompanied by suicidal plans, gestures, or actions.

In contrast to psychosis, depression apparently never occurs in the more advanced stages of Alzheimer's disease, although it is commonly the earliest manifestation of the disease and may precede the cognitive symptomatology by many months or years.

Depression is also a common concomitant of infarction or other brain insult, with or without coexisting dementia. Pathology affecting the frontal brain regions is believed to be particularly associated with affective symptomatology. Depression associated with cerebral infarction is characteristically associated with emotional incontinence, i.e., sudden episodes of tearfulness without a pervasive, consistent, or affective dysphoria.

In addition to dementia and overt brain trauma, depression in the elderly is commonly the result of physical pathology with diverse etiology. For example, electrolyte disturbances from diuretics alone, or in combination with other medications, can result in a mood disorder presentation, as can vitamin B_{12} deficiency due to malabsorption perhaps be associated with gastrointestinal surgery.

2. Treatment.   Primary (idiopathic) depressive illness in the elderly is a serious and, in many cases, even life-threatening condition. Treatment modalities that should be given primary consideration include antidepressants, electroconvulsive therapy (ECT), and monoamine oxidase inhibitors (MAOIs).

   a. Antidepressants are an increasingly diverse category of compounds, all of which are of potential utility in the elderly. Among the antidepressants, those most frequently preferred for use in the elderly are the secondary amines, including desipramine (Norpramin) and nortriptyline (Aventyl, Pamelor), in part because they produce less hypotension than the tertiary amines. Desipramine is very low in anticholinergic side effects in comparison with most other antidepressants. This is an advantage because the elderly are known to have decreased cholinergic neurotransmitter functioning and are believed to be particularly sensitive to anticholinergic side effects. Nortriptyline is also frequently considered a drug of choice for the elderly because of the ability to monitor a therapeutic window of blood levels in relation to clinical response. Fluoxetine (Prozac) and bupropion (Wellbutrin) may be especially useful in the aged because of the minimal presence of anticholinergic side effects.

   b. ECT may be the treatment of choice for depression in the elderly, particularly if cardiac factors limit or preclude the use of antidepressant medications or if refusal to eat presents an immediate, perhaps even life-threatening, problem. The risk of ECT is very low and is often less than that of pharmacotherapy. Any risks of treatment must be weighed against the risks of depression, including the patient's mental status and any suicidal risk.

   c. MAOIs are safe for use in the elderly when given with the usual precautions. In the elderly, the treatment of depression that is secondary to other illness entities does not differ markedly from the treatment of idiopathic depression except that treatment of the underlying disorder, if possible, may precede or preclude the necessity to treat the affective symptoms more directly. When depression and dementia occur together, treatment of the depression may or may not result in resolution of the cognitive disturbance. Even if the cognitive disturbance remits in its entirety, in approximately one-half of cases, early symptoms of cognitive loss will be apparent again in approximately 2–3 years.

B. Mania and bipolar disorder. The relapse rate of mania and bipolar disorder increases with age. The mean length of morbid episodes is at least as long in aged patients as in younger adults. The great majority of cases of bipolar illness begin before age 50; onset after age 65 is considered unusual. When a manic episode occurs for the first time after the age of 65, an overt pathophysiologic (organic) etiology should be strongly suspected. Possible etiologies include medication side effects or concomitant dementia.

   The use of lithium in aged patients is more hazardous because of the common occurrence of age-related morbidity and physiologic changes. Lithium is excreted by the kidneys, and decreased renal clearance and/or renal disease can increase the risk of toxicity. Thiazide diuretics decrease renal clearance of lithium and, consequently, the concomitant use of these medications can necessitate adjustment in lithium dosage. Other medications may also interfere with lithium clearance. Lithium may cause CNS effects to which the elderly may be more sensitive. Because of these factors, more frequent serum monitoring of lithium levels is recommended in the elderly.

C. Schizophrenia, paranoid states, and other late-life psychoses

1. Signs and symptoms. Initial admissions to psychiatric hospitals for schizophrenia peak in occurrence from age 25 to 34 and are relatively uncommon after age 65. Paranoid psychoses of diverse etiology, however, commonly occur in aged persons, including many elderly patients without any premorbid history of significant psychopathology. Sensory deficits appear to predispose to paranoid psychoses in some elderly patients. In others, cerebrovascular events or dementia are associated with the onset of pathology. Medications or other pathophysiologic causes should be carefully explored in all cases. Recent findings indicate that paranoid and delusional psychoses in some instances, may be the harbinger of primary degenerative dementia of the Alzheimer type. In other instances, these states may be associated with cerebrovascular factors, which are not always evident on the basis of clinical or neuroimaging findings. Neurotransmitter changes associated with aging may also predispose to psychosis in the elderly. More specifically, in the elderly, decrements in various neurotransmitter systems have been convincingly demonstrated. There are, for example, decrements in dopaminergic functioning associated with age-related cell loss in the substantia nigra, with or without overt parkinsonian symptomatology. There are also age-related changes in noradrenergic functioning associated with physical evidence of cellular loss in the locus ceruleus. Similarly, age-related cholinergic neurotransmitter system changes occur associated with decreased choline acetyltransferase enzyme activity. Collectively, these and other CNS neurochemical changes result in a resetting of the CNS neurotransmitter balance, and in many cases, these changes may predispose to psychosis in the elderly.

2. Treatment. The changes in neurotransmitter systems in the elderly appear to play a major role, both in the etiology and the treatment of psychosis. In general, psychosis in the elderly frequently responds to much lower doses of medication than psychosis in younger patients. The elderly also are much more sensitive to many of the side effects of antipsychotic medications than younger patients.

Specifically, the elderly are very sensitive to extrapyramidal (parkinsonian) side effects. Elderly patients have been known to stop speaking, ambulating, and swallowing as a result of these side effects with doses of medication that would be very unlikely to produce significant problems in younger patients. Partly as a result of age-related autonomic changes, the elderly also are highly susceptible to orthostatic side effects of antipsychotics. Falling may be associated with the aforementioned extrapyramidal side effects, orthostatic side effects, and sedating effects of antipsychotics. These side effects frequently act in conjunction with other medications, arthritis, peripheral vascular disease, arrhythmias, transient ischemic attacks (TIAs), idiopathic parkinsonism, and other age-associated pathologies to further increase the risk of falling. Hip fracture resulting from falls, partly associated with medication usage, is a major cause of morbidity in the elderly and can be a proximal or distal factor associated with demise. Consequently, efforts to minimize potentially deleterious, and even life threatening, side effects of antipsychotics in the elderly must be carefully considered.

Cholinergic neurotransmitter changes also are believed to predispose the elderly to anticholinergic side effects. It should be noted, however, that the antipsychotic with the highest anticholinergic potency, thioridazine (Mellaril), is roughly equivalent in anticholinergic potency to desipramine, the least anticholinergic antidepressant of the commonly used tricyclics and their derivatives. Futhermore, as previously noted, doses of antipsychotics prescribed in elderly patients are frequently much lower than those used in the treatment of younger patients. Consequently, in practice, anticholinergic side effects of antipsychotics in elderly patients are not as serious a concern as extrapyramidal, orthostatic, and sedating effects.

Clinical experience also indicates that therapeutic effects of antipsychotic medications in the elderly may not become evident on a given dose of medication for 4 weeks or longer. Because of these therapeutic factors and risks, the dictum in treating psychosis in the elderly is "start low and go slow." As in younger patients, side effects' profiles should help determine the choice of medication; however, there is no consensus regarding the antipsychotic of choice for the elderly or even whether high potency or low potency antipsychotics are more desirable treatment alternatives. Among the low potency antipsychotics, thioridazine is frequently prescribed for the elderly, and a typical starting dosage is 10 mg 1–3 times daily; among the high potency antipsychotics, haloperidol (Haldol) is frequently prescribed, and a typical starting dosage is 0.25 mg or 0.5 mg 1–3 times daily.

D. **Age-associated memory impairment, Alzheimer's disease, and other dementing disorders.** Changes in cognition are among the most frequent and the most important (in terms of morbidity, mortality, and impact on family members and society in general) age related medical conditions.

1. **Alzheimer's disease.** Cognitive changes in normal aging and in progressive Alzheimer's disease occur in a continuum. Seven major clinically distinguishable stages from normality to most severe Alzheimer's disease have been described in the Global Deterioration Scale by Barry Reisberg, M.D., and associates. These stages and their implications are summarized below.

Stage 1: Normal: No objective or subjective evidence of cognitive decrement.
Current epidemiologic data indicate that only a minority of elderly persons fall within this category, perhaps 20% of persons over age 65.
Stage 2: Normal for age: Subjective complaints of cognitive decrement.
The majority of persons over age 65 have subjective symptoms of not remembering such things as names and locations of objects as well as in the previous 5–10 years.
These symptoms can be very troubling to aged persons. In Europe, they appear to be the leading reason why persons take medications of all forms. In the United States, elderly persons commonly take lecithin, multivitamins, and various nostrums for these complaints.
Present prognostic data do not indicate that these symptoms of age-associated memory impairment are the precursor of further decline in the majority of elderly

with these common, age-associated complaints. Although medications and nostrums are frequently taken, there remains no convincing evidence of their efficacy.

Stage 3: Compatible with incipient Alzheimer's disease: Subtle evidence of objective decrement in complex occupational or social tasks.

Subtle deficits may become evident in various ways. For example, the patient may become hopelessly lost when traveling to an unfamiliar location; decreased performance may be noted by co-workers in a demanding occupation; patients may display overt word- and name-finding deficits; concentration deficits may be evident to family members and/on clinical testing; and/or an overt tendency to forget what has just been said and to repeat oneself may be manifest.

The prognosis associated with these subtle, but identifiable, symptoms varies. In some cases, these symptoms are the result of brain insults, such as small strokes, which may not be evident from the clinical history, neurologic examination, or neuroimaging findings. In other cases, symptoms are due to subtle, and perhaps not clearly identifiable, psychiatric, medical, and neurologic disorders of diverse etiology. In still other cases, these symptoms do represent the earliest symptoms of Alzheimer's disease and may last as long as 7 years. The diagnosis of Alzheimer's disease in this stage, however, can be made with confidence only in retrospect.

Anxiety is a frequent psychiatric concomitant of the cognitive losses at stage 3. Given the frequently benign prognosis, the inability to make a diagnosis with confidence at this stage, and the prolonged duration of these symptoms in those cases when they do, in fact, represent the earliest manifestations of Alzheimer's disease, the most effective treatment for the anxiety is commonly the psychiatrist's recommendation that the patient withdraw from anxiety-provoking activities. For example, withdrawal from a job that is presently beyond the patient's cognitive capacities can eliminate daily stress and humiliation. It can also eliminate, at least temporarily, the patient's problems, since patients at this stage do not have difficulty with routine tasks of daily living.

Stage 4: Mild Alzheimer's disease: Clearly manifest deficits on a careful clinical interview.

Deficits become manifest in concentration, memory, orientation, and/or functional capacity. Concentration deficit may be of sufficient magnitude that not only does the patient display a deficit on the standard subtraction of serial 7s task, but patients also have difficulty subtracting serial 4s from 40. Recent memory may suffer such that some major events of the previous week are not recalled. Detailed questioning may reveal that the spouse's knowledge of the patient's past is superior to the patient's own recall of his/her personal history. The patient may mistake the date by 10 days or more. The spouse (or other family members) may note that the patient no longer is able to balance the checkbook, no longer remembers to pay the rent or other bills properly, has difficulty preparing meals for family dinners, or displays similar deficits in the ability to manage complex occupational and social tasks.

The diagnosis of Alzheimer's disease can be arrived at with confidence in this stage. It is possible to follow patients through the course of this stage, whose mean duration has been estimated to be 2 years. Symptoms may plateau in this stage, and some patients may not manifest a further overt decline for 4 years or longer.

The most prominent psychiatric features of stage 4 are the patient's decreased interest in personal and social activities, accompanied by a flattening of affect. Depressive symptoms also may be noted, but are generally sufficiently mild such that no specific treatment is indicated. In some cases, depressive symptoms are of sufficient severity to warrant treatment, frequently with a low dose of an antidepressant. Patients are still capable of independent community survival if assistance is provided with such complex, but essential, activities as paying the rent and managing the patient's bank account.

Stage 5: Moderate Alzheimer's disease: Deficits of sufficient magnitude that patients can no longer survive without assistance.

Patients at this stage can no longer recall major relevant aspects of their lives; e.g., they may not recall the name of the president, their correct current address, or the name of the school they attended. Patients at this stage frequently do not recall the current year and have sufficient concentration and calculation difficulty as to err in subtracting serial 2s from 20. In addition to their inability to manage complex activities of daily living, patients generally have difficulty choosing the proper clothing to wear for the season and the occasion.

The duration of this stage is approximately 1½ years, although, as with the previous stage, some patients may plateau with these symptoms for many years.

Although generally more overt, the psychiatric symptoms at stage 5 are in many ways similar to those noted in stage 4. Consequently, the patient's denial and flattening of affect tend to be more evident. Depressive symptoms may occur. Anger and some of the more overt behavioral symptoms of Alzheimer's disease also are frequently evident. Depending on the nature and magnitude of the psychiatric symptomatology, treatment with an antidepressant or an antipsychotic medication may be indicated. When the latter is used, the dictum previously stated for the treatment of psychosis in the elderly applies: "start low and go slow."

Patients who are living alone in the community at this stage require at least part-time assistance for continued community survival. When additional community assistance is not feasible or available, institutionalization may be required. Patients who are residing with a spouse frequently resist additional assistance as an invasion of their home.

Stage 6: Moderately severe Alzheimer's disease: Deficits sufficient in magnitude to require assistance with basic activities of daily living.

Patients at this stage may occasionally forget the name of the spouse on whom they are dependent for survival. They frequently do not know their address but can generally recall some important aspects of their domicile, such as the street or the town. Patients have generally forgotten the schools they attended but recall some aspects of their early lives, such as their birthplace, former occupation, or one or both of their parents' names. Patients generally still can state their correct personal name. They may have difficulty counting backward from 10 by 1s.

Over the course of stage 6, which lasts approximately 2½ years, progressively increased deficits in dressing and bathing occur. In the latter part of this stage, toileting and continence become compromised.

Emotional and behavioral problems become most manifest and disturbing. Agitation, anger, sleep disturbances, physical violence, and negativity are examples of symptoms that commonly require treatment at this point in the illness. Although low doses of antipsychotics may be useful, high doses are frequently necessary for many patients, and a satisfactory response is sometimes difficult to obtain.

Patients require full-time assistance in community settings. If the patient lives with his/her spouse, then the spouse will generally require at least part-time additional management assistance.

Stage 7: Severe Alzheimer's disease: Deficits sufficient to require continuous assistance with activities of daily living.

Speech activity is severely circumscribed early in this stage and is eventually lost during this stage. Ambulation and other motor capacities are also lost.

Most patients survive until this stage, when they commonly succumb at approximately the time ambulatory ability is lost. Although some patients survive in this stage for 6 years or longer, most patients succumb approximately 2–3 years after the onset of stage 7. Pneumonia appears to be the most common proximate cause of death.

Although agitation can be a problem for some patients at this stage, psychotropic medication can frequently be discontinued successfully. Nursing homes may be better equipped than spouses for the management of patients. Many devoted spouses, however, prefer to continue to care for their partner, in which case, round-the-clock home health care assistance may be a necessary adjunct as management of incontinence and other basic life activities, such as bathing and feeding, become major concerns. Psychiatrists should be prepared to counsel family members regarding such issues as institutionalization and the continued meaning of life.

2. Multi-infarct dementia. This is the second major cause of dementia in the elderly. It occurs most frequently in conjunction with Alzheimer's disease. Classic pathologic studies have indicated that approximately 50% of dementia cases coming to autopsy are associated with Alzheimer's disease alone, 25% with Alzheimer's disease in association with cerebrovascular factors, and 15% with multi-infarct dementia in the absence of neuropathologic evidence of Alzheimer's disease.

Multi-infarct dementia is believed to be the result of cerebral infarctions of varying size in multiple brain regions. Conditions associated with cerebral infarction, such as cardiac arrhythmias and hypertension, predispose to multi-infarct dementia.

Clinically, multi-infarct dementia is believed to exhibit a more stepwise course than the relatively gradual course of Alzheimer's disease. The time course of decline of multi-infarct dementia is at least as rapid as that of Alzheimer's disease. In mixed cases, the presence of cerebral infarction appears to increase morbidity. Consequently, the rate of dementia and the time of death are relatively rapid in multi-infarct dementia or in mixed dementia in comparison with pure Alzheimer's disease.

The clinical presentation of multi-infarct dementia is more diverse than that of Alzheimer's disease. Speech disturbance or gait disturbance, for example, may occur at varying points in the evolution of multi-infarct dementia pathology, whereas in Alzheimer's disease these deficits tend to occur at a specific point in the evolution of the dementia process.

Psychiatric disturbances occurring in multi-infarct dementia include general dementia-related psychiatric conditions, such as the affective, psychotic, and agitation disturbances described at each stage of Alzheimer's disease. Emotional changes characteristic of stroke-related dementia also occur, e.g., emotional incontinence and other sudden, labile, mood changes. Emotional incontinence generally is not treated with medication. The guidelines for the treatment of dementia-related psychiatric disturbances previously outlined for Alzheimer's disease apply for the treatment of affective, psychiatric, and other behavioral disturbances in multi-infarct dementia.

The treatment for the underlying cause of multi-infarct dementia is stroke prevention and prophylaxis. These include the treatment of hypertension and cardiac arrhythmias and the use of platelet-deaggregating agents for the prevention of stroke. Among the latter, salicylates, such as aspirin, are perhaps the most effective.

3. **Other dementing disorders and differential diagnosis of dementia.** Other causes of dementia include Pick's disease, Creutzfeldt-Jakob disease, Huntington's chorea, alcohol-related dementia (Korsakoff's dementia), normal pressure hydrocephalus, and dementias secondary to diverse physiologic disturbances.

   a. **Pick's disease** is a degenerative dementia that is difficult to distinguish clinically from Alzheimer's disease. Neuropathologically, it differs in that autopsy brain examination reveals so-called Pick bodies and not the characteristic neurofibrillary tangles, senile plaques, or granulovacuolar degeneration of Alzheimer's disease. Pick's disease also tends to affect the frontal region of the brain, whereas Alzheimer's disease is a much more diffuse cerebral process. Pick's disease has a somewhat younger age distribution than Alzheimer's disease, accounting for a significant percentage of dementia patients in the sixth decade. Clinically, Pick's disease appears to be marked by more frontal lobe features than Alzheimer's disease. There is no known treatment for Pick's disease.

   b. **Creutzfeldt-Jakob disease** is a rare condition, occurring in approximately one person per million of population. Onset and course are variable and acute; subacute and chronic forms have been described. Frequently, Creutzfeldt-Jakob disease is distinguished from Alzheimer's disease by its course, which may be more rapid, or by the occurrence of focal and localized neural pathology. The latter includes cranial nerve signs, such as auditory deficits associated with 8th nerve involvement, and gait disturbance, associated with cerebellar involvement. Occasionally, Creutzfeldt-Jakob disease may closely mimic the course of Alzheimer's disease.

   c. **Huntington's chorea** may present with a dementia disturbance prior to the appearance of choreiform pathology and should be considered in the differential diagnosis of dementia. Alcohol-related dementia and the Korsakoff syndrome associated with it are frequently distinguished from Alzheimer's disease by the presence of confabulation and by a memory deficit out of proportion to cognitive and functional disturbances in other areas.

   d. **Normal pressure hydrocephalus** is marked by gait disturbance, urinary incontinence, and dilated cerebral ventricles out of proportion to the magnitude of cortical atrophy and dementia. Urinary incontinence, neuroradiologic findings, and the relatively early appearance of gait disturbance assist in distinguishing this condition clinically from Alzheimer's disease.

   e. **Dementias secondary to diverse physiologic disturbances.** The diagnosis of dementia, which may be secondary to more than 50 possible primary etiologies, and the differentiation of these conditions from the major cause of dementia, Alzheimer's disease, is based on laboratory investigations and knowledge of the clinical course of Alzheimer's disease. The basic laboratory work up for dementia includes a complete blood count and differential, serum electrolytes and serum enzyme studies, serum B_{12} and serum folate levels, thyroid levels, urinalysis, and a cerebral neuroimaging study. Positive findings from any of these studies must be interpreted by the clinician. They may be indicative of a primary etiology of dementia, which may be treatable; they may be indicative of added insult in the context of degenerative dementia; or they may be incidental. A knowledge of the clinical course of Alzheimer's disease can help the clinician in distinguishing these possibilities. A brief guide to the order and time course of the progression of functional loss in Alzheimer's disease can be found in Table 19–1. Table 19–2 shows differential diagnostic considerations when these functional changes occur prematurely in the evolution of the dementia process. Premature deficits should alert the clinician to possible increased morbidity or a possibly remediable underlying process.

TABLE 19–1. **FUNCTIONAL STAGING AND PROGRESSION IN NORMAL AGING AND ALZHEIMER'S DISEASE**

Functional Assessment Stage	Characteristics	Clinical Diagnosis	Estimated Duration in Alzheimer's Disease*
1	No decrement	Normal adult	
2	Subjective deficit in word finding	Normal aged adult	
3	Deficits noted in demanding employment settings	Compatible with incipient Alzheimer's disease	7 years
4	Requires assistance in complex tasks, e.g., handling finances, planning dinner party	Mild Alzheimer's disease	2 years
5	Requires assistance in choosing proper attire	Moderate Alzheimer's disease	18 months
6a	Requires assistance dressing	Moderately severe Alzheimer's disease	5 months
b	Requires assistance bathing properly		5 months
c	Requires assistance with mechanics of toileting (such as flushing, wiping)		5 months
d	Urinary incontinence		4 months
e	Fecal incontinence		10 months
7a	Speech ability limited to about a half-dozen words	Severe Alzheimer's disease	12 months
b	Intelligible vocabulary limited to a single word		18 months
c	Ambulatory ability lost		12 months
d	Ability to sit up lost		12 months
e	Ability to smile lost		18 months
f	Ability to hold head up lost		12 months or longer

Table adapted from Reisberg B: Dementia: A systematic approach to identifying reversible causes. Geriatrics, 41:30, 1986. Developed by Barry Reisberg M.D. Reprinted with permission of the author.
*In subjects who survive and progress to the subsequent deterioration stage.

TABLE 19–2. **DIFFERENTIAL DIAGNOSTIC CONSIDERATIONS OF FUNCTIONAL ASSESSMENT STAGE (FAST STAGE) NONORDINALITY**

FAST Stage	FAST Characteristics	Differential Diagnostic Considerations: particularly if FAST stage occurs early (nonordinally) in the evolution of dementia
1.	No functional decrement, either subjectively or objectively, manifest	
2.	Complains of forgetting location of objects; subjective work difficulties	2. Anxiety neurosis; depression
3.	Decreased functioning in demanding employment settings evident to co-workers; difficulty in traveling to new locations	3. Depression; subtle manifestations of medical pathology
4.	Decreased ability to perform complex tasks, such as planning dinner for guests, handling finances, and marketing	4. Depression; psychosis; focal cerebral process (e.g., Gerstmann's syndrome)
5.	Requires assistance in choosing proper clothing; may require coaxing to bathe properly	5. Depression
6.	(a) Difficulty putting clothes on properly	6. (a) Arthritis; sensory deficit; stroke; depression
	(b) Requires assistance bathing; may develop fear of bathing	(b) Arthritis; sensory deficit; stroke; depression
	(c) Inability to handle mechanics of toileting	(c) Arthritis; sensory deficit; stroke; depression
	(d) Urinary incontinence	(d) Urinary tract infection; other causes of urinary incontinence
	(e) Fecal incontinence	(e) Infection; malabsorption syndrome; other causes of fecal incontinence
7.	(a) Ability to speak limited to 1–5 words	7. (a) Stroke; other dementing disorder (e.g., diffuse space occupying lesions)
	(b) Intelligible vocabulary lost	(b) Stroke; other dementing disorder (e.g., diffuse space occupying lesions)
	(c) Ambulatory ability lost	(c) Parkinsonism; neuroleptic-induced or other secondary extrapyramidal syndrome; Creutzfeldt-Jakob disease: normal pressure hydrocephalus: hyponatremic dementia; stroke; hip fracture; arthritis; overmedication
	(d) Ability to sit up independently lost	(d) Arthritis; contractures
	(e) Ability to smile lost	(e) Stroke
	(f) Ability to hold head up lost	(f) Head trauma; metabolic abnormality; other medical abnormality; overmedication; encephalitis; other causes

Table adapted from Reisberg B: Dementia: A systematic approach to identifying reversible causes. Geriatrics, *41*:30, 1986. Developed by Barry Reisberg, M.D. Reprinted with permission of the author.

IV. Psychotherapy in the elderly

Fundamental psychologic processes do not differ in the elderly from those of younger mature adults. However, the aging process and associated pathologic changes do result in psychologic issues, which are relatively particular to this age group. Common issues in therapy include evolving and changing relationships of the elderly with their adult children. For example, in the presence of pathology, the elderly may have both a desire for independence and, in the present social context, unrealistic expectations with regard to their adult children. Adult children, in turn, may harbor continuing resentments towards their parents from childhood or, conversely, may experience an unrealistic guilt with regard to what they should be doing for their parents in the event of illness or other traumatic events.

Family therapy, consequently, can be of particular value in the elderly, sometimes in conjunction with group and/or individual psychotherapy. Other goals of individual therapy particular to the elderly include the maintenance of self-esteem despite physical, marital, and social change; the meaningful use of unaccustomed leisure time; and clarification of options in the context of more or less overwhelming physical and social change. In general, psychotherapy in the elderly is relatively situation- and problem-oriented and seeks solutions within the established personality framework, rather than overwhelming personality change. Many elderly persons, however, respond remarkably to seemingly overwhelming changes and personal tragedies, such as loss of personal health or a spouse, revealing unseen social strengths and adaptive capacities.

The reader is referred to Chapter 3, Organic Mental Syndromes and Disorders, for additional information.

For more detailed discussion of this topic, see Jarvik LF, Small GW: Introduction and Overview, Sec. 46.1, pp 2013–2014; Butler RN, Psychosocial Aspects of Aging, Sec. 46.2, pp 2014–2019; Plotkin DA: Psychiatric Examination of the Older Patient, Sec. 46.3a, pp 2019–2021; Van Gorp WG, Satz P: Neuropsychological Examination of the Older Patient, Sec. 46.3b, pp 2022–2024; Gerner RH: Mood Disorders, Sec. 46.4a, pp 2024–2026; Post F: Schizophrenia and Delusional Disorder, Sec. 46.4b, pp 2026–2028; Small GW: Alzheimer's Disease and Other Dementing Disorders, Sec. 46.4c, pp 2028–2031; Guterman A, Eisdorfer C: Other Psychiatric Conditions of the Elderly, Sec. 46.4d, pp 2031–2034; Lazarus LW: Psychotherapy with the Elderly, Sec. 46.5a, pp 2035–2037; Shader RI, Kennedy JS: Biological Treatments, Sec. 46.5b, pp 2037–2049; Small GW: Psychiatric Problems of the Medically Ill Geriatric Patient, Sec. 46.6, pp 2049–2053; Adelman RD, Butler RN: Elder Abuse and Neglect, Sec. 46.7a, pp 2053–2056; Schecter M, Butler RN: Long-Term Care, Sec. 46.7b, pp 2056–2059; Eth S, Mills M: Ethical and Legal Considerations, Sec. 46.7c, pp 2059–2062, in *CTP/V*.

20

Bereavement and Death

I. Grief, mourning, and bereavement. Generally are synonymous terms that describe a syndrome precipitated by the loss by death of a loved one. Attempts have been made to characterize the stages of grief, which are listed in Table 20–1.

TABLE 20–1. **GRIEF AND BEREAVEMENT**

Stage	John Bowlby	Stage	C.M. Parkes
1. **Numbness or protest.** Characterized by distress, fear, and anger. Shock may last moments, days, weeks, or months.		1. **Alarm.** A stressful state characterized by physiologic changes, e.g., rise in blood pressure and heart rate; similar to Bowlby's first stage.	
2. **Yearning and searching for the lost figure.** World seems empty and meaningless, but self-esteem remains intact. Characterized by preoccupation with lost person, physical restlessness, weeping, and anger. May last several months or even years.		2. **Numbness.** Person appears superficially affected by loss, but is actually protecting himself/herself from acute distress.	
3. **Disorganization and despair.** Restlessness and aimlessness. Increase in somatic preoccupation, withdrawal, introversion, and irritability. Repeated reliving of memories.		3. **Pining (searching).** Person looks for or is reminded of the lost person. Similar to Bowlby's second stage.	
		4. **Depression.** Person feels hopeless about future, cannot go on living, and withdraws from family and friends.	
4. **Reorganization.** With establishment of new patterns, objects, and goals, grief recedes and is replaced by cherished memories. Healthy identification with deceased occurs.		5. **Recovery and reorganization.** Person realizes that his/her life will continue with new adjustments and different goals.	

Grief can occur for reasons other than the death of a loved one: (1) the loss of a loved one through separation, divorce, incarceration; (2) the loss of an emotionally charged object or circumstance, e.g., loss of a prized possession or of a valued job or position; (3) the loss of a fantasized love object, e.g., death of intrauterine fetus, birth of a malformed infant; and (4) the loss resulting from a narcissistic injury, e.g., amputation, mastectomy.

Grief differs from depression in a number of ways, which are described in Table 20–2.

A. Do's and don'ts of grief management and therapy

1. Encourage ventilation of feelings. Allow person to talk about loved ones. Reminiscing about positive experiences can be helpful.

2. Don't tell bereaved not to cry or get angry.

3. Try to have small group of people who knew the deceased talk about person in presence of grieving person.

TABLE 20–2. **GRIEF VERSUS DEPRESSION**

Grief	Depression
Normal identification with deceased. Little ambivalence toward deceased	Abnormal overidentification with deceased. Increased ambivalence and unconscious anger toward deceased
Crying, weight loss, decreased libido, withdrawal, insomnia, irritability, decreased concentration and attention	Similar
Suicidal ideas rare	Suicidal ideas common
Self-blame relates to how deceased was treated. No global feelings of worthlessness	Self-blame is global. Person thinks he/she is generally bad or worthless
Evokes empathy/sympathy	Usually evokes interpersonal annoyance or irritation
With time, symptoms abate. Self-limited. Usually clears within 6 months	Symptoms do not abate and may worsen. May still be present after years
Vulnerable to physical illness	Vulnerable to physical illness
Responds to reassurance, social contacts	Does not respond to reassurance, pushes away social contacts
Not helped by antidepressant medication	Helped by antidepressant medication

4. Don't prescribe antianxiety or antidepressant medication on regular basis. If person becomes acutely agitated, it is better to offer verbal comfort than a pill. A small dose of medications (diazepam [Valium] 5 mg), however, may be of help in the short term.

5. Frequent short visits better than fewer longer visits.

6. Be aware of delayed grief reaction, which occurs some time after the death and may be marked by behavioral changes, agitation, lability of mood, and substance abuse. May occur close to anniversary of death, an anniversary reaction.

7. Anticipatory grief reaction happens in advance of loss and can mitigate acute grief reaction at actual time of loss. This can be useful process if recognized when it is occurring.

8. Be aware that person grieving about family member who died by suicide may not want to talk about his or her feelings of being stigmatized.

II. Death and dying.   Reaction of patient to being told by physician that he/she has terminal illness that will lead to death is variable. Described as series of stages by thanatologist Elisabeth Kübler-Ross (Table 20–3).

Be aware that stages do not always occur in sequence. There may be shifts from one stage to another. Moreover, children under age 5 do not appreciate death; they see it as a separation similar to sleep. Between the ages of 5 and 10, there is growing awareness of death but as something that occurs in others, particularly parents. After age 10, death is conceptualized as something that can happen to the child.

A. Do's and don'ts with the dying patient

1. Do not have rigid attitude, e.g., "I *always* tell the patient." Let the patient be your guide. Most patients will want to know the diagnosis, whereas others will not. Determine what the patient already knows and understands

TABLE 20–3.   **DEATH AND DYING (REACTIONS OF DYING PATIENTS)**

Elisabeth Kübler-Ross

Stage 1	**Shock and denial.** Patient's initial reaction is shock, followed by denial that anything is wrong. Some patients never pass beyond this state and may go doctor shopping until they find one who supports their position.
Stage 2	**Anger.** Patients become frustrated, irritable, and angry that they are ill; they ask, "Why me?" Patients in this stage are difficult to manage because their anger is displaced onto doctors, hospital staff, and family. Sometimes anger is directed at themselves in the belief that illness has occurred as a punishment for wrongdoing.
Stage 3	**Bargaining.** Patient may attempt to negotiate with physicians, friends, or even god, that in return for a cure, he/she will fulfill one or many promises, e.g., give to charity or attend church regularly.
Stage 4	**Depression.** Patient shows clinical signs of depression: withdrawal, psychomotor retardation, sleep disturbances, hopelessness, and possibly suicidal ideation. The depression may be a reaction to the effects of illness on his/her life, e.g., loss of job, economic hardship, isolation from friends and family, or it may be in anticipation of the actual loss of life that will occur shortly.
Stage 5	**Acceptance.** Person realizes that death is inevitable and accepts its universality.

about the prognosis. Do not stifle hope or break through patient's denial if that is the major defense, as long as patient is able to obtain and accept necessary help. If patient is refusing to obtain help as a result of denial, you need to gently and gradually assist patient to understand that help is necessary and available.

2. Stay with patient for a period of time after telling condition or diagnosis. There may be period of shock. Encourage patient to ask questions and provide truthful answers. Indicate that you will return to answer any questions that patient or family may have.

3. Make return visit after a few hours, if possible, to check on reaction. If there is measure of anxiety, diazepam 5 mg can be prescribed as needed for 24–48 hours.

4. Advise family members of medical facts. Encourage them to visit and allow patient to talk of fears. Family not only has to deal with loss of loved one but also are faced with their own personal mortality, which causes anxiety.

5. Always check for presence of living will or Do Not Resuscitate (DNR) wishes of patient or family.

6. Alleviate pain and suffering. There is no reason for withholding narcotics for fear of dependence in dying patient.

For more detailed discussion of this topic, see Gonda TA; Death, Dying, and Bereavement, Sec. 26.5, pp 1339–1351, in *CTP/V*.

21

Psychotherapy

I. **General introduction.** In psychiatry, a number of different theories or paradigms are used as models to explain human behavior. Each etiologic theory has corresponding therapeutic techniques that are based on the different underlying explanatory models of behavior. Biologic therapies, for instance, postulate a biologic substrate for behavior, and the corresponding interventions involve biologic treatments, such as psychopharmacology and electroconvulsive therapy (ECT). Other therapies view behavior from perspectives other than the biologic; these corresponding treatments are generally termed the psychotherapies. Biologic treatments are covered in Chapter 22, Organic Therapy.

Most psychiatrists believe that the different theories of behavior are not mutually exclusive, but rather, when taken together, provide a complex and integrated picture of a person's thoughts and actions from different perspectives. Certain clinical problems and patients may be more responsive to one therapy than to another; therefore, psychiatrists must be adept at using a number of different therapeutic techniques and interventions in order to treat patients skillfully. This chapter describes each of the psychotherapies in relation to the underlying theory with which it is associated.

II. **Psychoanalysis and psychoanalytic psychotherapy.** These two forms of treatment are based on Sigmund Freud's theories of a dynamic unconscious and psychologic conflict. The major goal of these forms of therapy is to help the patient develop insight into unconscious conflicts, which are based on unresolved childhood wishes and are manifested as symptoms, and to develop more consciously adult patterns of interacting and behaving.

A. **Psychoanalysis** is the most intensive and rigorous of this type of therapy. The patient is seen from 3-5 times/week, generally for a minimum of several hundred hours over a number of years. The patient lies on a couch with the analyst seated behind, out of the patient's visual range. The patient attempts to say freely and without censure whatever comes to mind, to free associate, in order to follow as deeply as possible the train of thoughts to their earliest roots. This includes associating to dream material and to transference feelings that are evoked in the process. The analyst uses interpretation and clarification to help the patient work through and resolve conflicts that have been often unconsciously affecting the patient's life. Psychoanalysis requires that the patient be stable, highly motivated, verbal, and psychologically minded. The patient also must be able to tolerate the stress generated by analysis without becoming overly regressed, distraught, or impulsive.

B. **Psychoanalytically oriented psychotherapy** is based on the same principles and techniques as classical psychoanalysis but is less intense. There are two types: insight-oriented or expressive psychotherapy and supportive or relationship psychotherapy. Patients are seen 1-2 times/week and sit up facing the psychiatrist. The goal of resolution of unconscious psychologic conflict is similar to that of psychoanalysis, but there is a greater emphasis on day-to-day reality issues and a lesser emphasis on the development of transference issues. Patients suitable for this therapy include those suitable for psychoanalysis, as well as those with a wider range of symptomatic and characterologic problems. Patients with personality disorders also are suitable for this therapy.

In supportive psychotherapy the essential element of this therapy is support, rather than the development of insight. This type of therapy often is the treatment of choice for patients with serious ego vulnerabilities, in particular, psychotic patients. Patients in a crisis situation, such as acute grief, also are suitable. This therapy can be long term, lasting many years, especially in the case of chronic patients. Support can take the form of limit-setting, increasing reality testing, reassurance, advice, and help with developing social skills (Table 21–1).

TABLE 21–1. **PSYCHOANALYSIS AND PSYCHOANALYTIC PSYCHOTHERAPY**

Features	Psychoanalysis	Psychoanalytic Psychotherapy	
		Insight-oriented (Expressive)	Supportive (Relationship)
Basic Theory	Psychoanalytic Psychology	Psychoanalytic Psychology	Psychoanalytic Psychology
Frequency and duration	4 to 5 times weekly, 2 to 5 + years. Sessions usually about 50 minutes. New modifications: shorter sessions	1 to 3 times weekly, few sessions to several years. Sessions usually from 20 minutes to 50 minutes	Daily sessions to once every few months, one session to a lifelong process. Sessions may be brief, ranging from a few minutes to an hour
Activity of patient and therapist	Freely hovering attention by the analyst, free association by the patient. Interpretation of transference and resistance. Analyst assumes neutral role	Freely hovering attention by the therapist but with more focusing than in analysis. Less emphasis on free association, more on discussion by the patient. Analyst is more active	Expressive techniques generally avoided except for some cathartic effects. Therapist actively intervenes, advises, fosters discussion, selects focus. Therapist participates as a real person around current issues
Interpretive emphasis	Focus on resistance and transference to the analyst	Greater emphasis on interpersonal events and external events, less on transferences to the analyst than in analysis, but transference interpretation often effective. Transferences to persons other than the therapist often effectively interpreted	Interpretations of transferences by therapist generally avoided unless significantly interfering with the therapeutic relationship. Strong focus on external events. Clarification of interpersonal events
Transference	Transference neurosis fostered on foundation of the therapeutic alliance. Minimal reality orientation to external events	Transference neurosis discouraged; therapeutic alliance fostered. Considerably more reality oriented	Transference neurosis discouraged; real relationship and therapeutic alliance emphasized. Almost totally reality oriented

TABLE 21–1.   **PSYCHOANALYSIS AND PSYCHOANALYTIC PSYCHOTHERAPY (Continued)**

Features	Psychoanalysis	Psychoanalytic Psychotherapy	
		Insight-oriented (Expressive)	**Supportive (Relationship)**
Regression	Fostered in the form of the transference neurosis	Generally discouraged except as necessary to gain access to fantasy material and other derivatives of the unconscious	Regression generally discouraged
Adjuncts	Couch. The use of psychotropic drugs is controversial; some psychoanalysts will not use drugs, others will. Will not see family members or do group psychotherapy	Couch less used. Mostly face-to-face therapy. Psychotropic drugs used as needed. May do combined group and individual therapy	Always face-to-face therapy. Couch contraindicated. Group methods, family therapy, or family contacts on a planned basis. Other therapists and agencies may be involved. Psychotropic drugs used frequently and as needed
Confidentiality	Absolute. May be compromised by third-party payers	Absolute. May be compromised by third-party payers	Absolute. May be compromised by third-party payers
Prerequisites	Relatively mature personality, favorable life situation, motivation for long undertaking, capacity to tolerate frustration, capacity to tolerate frustration, capacity for stable therapeutic alliance, psychological mindedness	Relatively mature personality, capacity for therapeutic alliance, some capacity to tolerate frustration, adequate motivation, and some degree of psychological mindedness	Some capacity for therapeutic alliance, personality capable of growth, reality situation not too unfavorable. Personality organization may range from psychotic to mature
Diagnostic indications	Neuroses, personality disorders, paraphilias, sexual disorders	Neuroses, personality disorders (especially borderline and narcissistic), paraphilias, sexual disorders, latent schizophrenia, cyclothymia, psychosomatic disorders	Psychoses, adjustment disorders, impulse disorders, psychophysiologic conditions, psychosomatic disorders
Goals	Reorganization of character structure, with diminution of pathologic defenses, integration or ultimate rejection of warded-off strivings and ideation. Understanding rather than symptom relief the objective, but symptom relief usually results. Correction of developmental lags in otherwise relatively mature personalities	Resolution of selected conflicts and limited removal of pathologic defenses. Understanding the primary goal, usually with secondary relief of symptoms	Growth of the relatively immature personality through catalytic relationship with therapist counteracts the neurotogenic effects of prior significant relationships. Restoration of prior equilibrium, reduction of anxiety and fear in new situations. Help in tolerating unalterable situations

C. **Brief dynamic psychotherapy** is a short-term treatment, generally consisting of 10–40 sessions for a period of less than 1 year. The goal, based on Freudian theories, is to develop insight into underlying conflicts, which leads to psychologic and behavior changes.

This therapy is more confrontational than the other insight-oriented therapies in that the therapist is very active in repeatedly directing the patient's associations and thoughts to conflictual areas. The number of hours is explicitly agreed on by the therapist and patient prior to the onset of therapy, and a specific, circumscribed area of conflict is chosen to be the focus of treatment. More extensive change is not attempted. Patients suitable for this therapy must be able to define a specific central problem to be addressed and must be highly motivated, psychologically minded, and able to tolerate the temporary increase in anxiety or sadness that this type of therapy can evoke. Patients who are not suitable include those with fragile ego structures, e.g., suicidal or psychotic patients, and those with poor impulse control, e.g., borderline patients, substance abusers, and antisocial personalities.

III. **Behavior therapy.** The basic assumption of this therapy is that change of maladaptive behavior can occur without insight into its underlying causes. Behavioral symptoms are taken at face value and not as manifest symptoms of a deeper problem. Behavior therapy is based on the principles of learning theory, including operant and classical conditioning. Operant conditioning is based on the premise that behavior is shaped by its consequences; that is, if behavior is positively reinforced it will increase, if it is punished it will decrease, and if it elicits no response it will be extinguished. Classical conditioning is based on the premise that behavior is shaped by its being coupled with or uncoupled from anxiety-provoking stimuli. Just as Pavlov's dogs were conditioned to salivate at the sound of a bell once the bell had become associated with meat, a person can be conditioned to feel fear in neutral situations that have come to be associated with anxiety. Uncouple the anxiety from the situation, and avoidant and anxious behavior will decrease. Behavioral techniques include the following:

A. **Token economy.** A form of **positive reinforcement** used with inpatients. A patient is rewarded with various tokens, e.g., food, passes, for performing desired behaviors, e.g., dressing in street clothes, attending group therapy.

B. **Aversion therapy.** A form of conditioning in which an aversive stimulus, e.g., a shock or unpleasant smell, is paired with an undesired behavior. A less controversial form of aversion therapy involves the patient imagining something unpleasant coupled with the undesired behavior.

C. **Systematic densensitization.** A technique in which a patient with avoidant behavior linked to a specific stimulus, e.g., heights or airplane travel, is asked to construct a hierarchy of anxiety-provoking images in his/her imagination from the least to the most fearful, staying at each level of the hierarchy until anxiety diminishes. When this procedure is performed in real life rather than imagined, it is termed graded exposure. These techniques work through a combination of positive reinforcement for confronting anxiety-provoking stimuli and the extinguishing of maladaptive behavior by the realization of an absence of negative consequences. Hierarchy construction often is associated with relaxation techniques, because it is felt that anxiety and relaxation are incompatible, thus leading to an uncoupling of the imagined images from anxiety (reciprocal inhibition).

D. **Flooding.** A technique in which the patient is exposed immediately to the most anxiety-provoking stimulus, e.g., the top of a tall building if afraid of heights, instead of being exposed gradually or systematically to a hierarchy of feared situations. If this technique occurs in the imagination as opposed to real life, it is termed implosion. Flooding is thought to be the most effective behavioral treatment of such disorders as phobias, if the patient can tolerate the anxiety associated with it.

Behavior therapy is believed to be most effective for clearly delineated, circumscribed maladaptive behaviors, e.g., phobias, compulsions, overeating, cigarette smoking, stuttering, and sexual dysfunctions. Treatment of conditions that can be strongly affected by psychologic factors, such as hypertension, asthma, pain, and insomnia, may use behavioral techniques to induce relaxation and decrease aggravating stresses.

IV. Cognitive therapy. Cognitive therapy is based on the theory that behavior is secondary to the way in which individuals think about themselves and their roles in the world. Maladaptive behavior is secondary to ingrained, stereotyped thoughts, which can lead to cognitive distortions or errors in thinking. The theory is aimed at correcting these cognitive distortions and the self-defeating behaviors that result from them. Therapy is short-term, generally 15-20 sessions over 12 weeks, during which patients are made aware of their own distorted cognitions and the assumptions on which the questions are based. Homework is assigned: patients are asked to record what they are thinking in certain stressful situations (such as, "I'm no good" or "No one cares about me") and to ascertain the underlying, often relatively unconscious, assumptions that fuel the negative cognitions. This process has been called "recognizing and correcting automatic thoughts." The cognitive model of depression includes the cognitive triad, which is a description of the thought distortions that occur when an individual is depressed. The triad includes (1) a negative view of the self, (2) a negative interpretation of present and past experience, and (3) a negative expectation of the future.

Cognitive therapy has been most successfully applied to the treatment of mild to moderate, nonpsychotic depressions. It also has been effective as an adjunctive treatment with substance abusers and in increasing compliance with medication.

V. Family therapy. Family therapy is based on the theory that a family represents a system that attempts to maintain homeostasis, regardless of how maladaptive the system may be. This theory has been termed a family systems orientation, and the techniques include focusing on the family rather than on the identified patient. The family therefore becomes the patient, as opposed to the individual family member who has been identified as sick. One of the major goals of a family therapist is to determine what homeostatic role, however pathologic, the identified patient is serving in the particular family system. One example is the triangulated child—the child who is identified by the family as the patient is actually serving to maintain the family system by becoming involved in a marital conflict as a scapegoat, referee, or even surrogate spouse. The therapist's job is to help the family understand the triangulation process and address the deeper conflict that underlies the child's apparent disruptive behavior. Techniques include reframing and positive connotation (a relabeling of all negatively expressed feelings or behaviors as positive); for example, "this child is impossible" becomes "this child is desperately trying to distract and protect you from what he/she perceives is an unhappy marriage."

Other goals of family therapy include changing maladaptive rules that govern a family, increasing awareness of cross-generational dynamics, balancing individuation and cohesiveness, increasing one-on-one direct communication, and decreasing blaming and scapegoating.

VI. Interpersonal therapy (IPT). IPT is a short-term psychotherapy, from 12-16 weeks, developed specifically for the treatment of nonbipolar, nonpsychotic depression. Intrapsychic conflicts are not addressed. Emphasis is on current interpersonal relationships and on strategies to improve the patient's interpersonal life. Antidepressant medication is often used as an adjunct to IPT. The therapist is very active in helping to formulate the patient's predominant interpersonal problem areas, which define the treatment focus.

VII. Group therapy. Groups are based on as many theories as are individual therapies. Groups range from those that emphasize support and an increase in social skills, to those that emphasize specific symptomatic relief, to those that work through unresolved intrapsychic conflicts. Focus may be on an individual within the context of a group, on interactions that occur among individuals in the group, or on the group as a whole. There can be resolution of both individual and interpersonal issues. Therapeutic factors include identification, universalization, acceptance, altruism, transference, reality testing, and ventilation. Groups provide a forum in which imagined fears and transference distortions can be immediately subjected to exploration and correction.

Groups tend to meet 1–2 times/week, usually for 1½ hours. They may be homogenous or heterogeneous, depending on diagnosis. Examples of homogeneous groups include those for weight-reduction and smoking-cessation, as well as groups whose members share the same medical or psychiatric problem, e.g., patients with acquired immune deficiency syndrome (AIDS), post-traumatic stress disorder, or psychoactive substance use disorders. Certain types of patients do not do well in certain types of groups. Psychotic patients who need structure and clear direction do not do well in insight-oriented groups. Paranoid patients, antisocial personalities, and substance abusers can benefit from group therapy but do not do well in heterogeneous insight-oriented groups. In general, acutely psychotic or suicidal patients do not do well in groups.

A. Alcoholics Anonymous (AA) is an example of a large, highly structured, peer-run group that is organized around persons with a similar, central problem. AA emphasizes a sharing of experience, role-modeling, ventilation of feelings, and strong sense of community and mutual support.

B. Milieu therapy is the multidisciplinary therapeutic approach used on inpatient psychiatric wards. The term "milieu therapy" reflects the idea that all activities on a ward are oriented toward increasing a patient's ability to cope in the world and to relate appropriately to others. Milieu therapy generally involves groups and may include art therapy, occupational therapy, activities of daily living groups, community meetings, group passes, and social events.

C. **Multiple family groups (MFGs)** comprises families of schizophrenic patients. The groups discuss issues and problems related to having a schizophrenic person in the family and share suggestions and means of coping. MFGs are an important factor in decreasing relapse rates among schizophrenic patients whose families participate in the groups.

VIII. **Marital therapy.** As many as 50% of patients are estimated to enter psychotherapy primarily because of marital problems; another 25% experience marital problems along with their other presenting problems. Marital therapy is an effective tool for helping each member of the couple to achieve self-knowledge while working on their marital problems. Marital therapy encompasses a wide range of treatment techniques with the goal of increasing marital satisfaction or addressing marital impairment. Like family therapy, in marital therapy the marital relationship, rather than either of the individuals, is viewed as the patient.

For more detailed discussion of this topic, see Chap. 30, pp 1442-1568, in *CTP/V* for the entire spectrum of psychotherapies.

22
Organic Therapy

I. **Basic principles of psychopharmacology.** Whether used alone or in conjunction with other therapies, psychotropic drugs can significantly reduce the severity and duration of mental disorders. Schizophrenia, depression, mania, panic disorder, generalized anxiety disorder, and obsessive-compulsive disorder are some of the drug-responsive psychiatric disorders. Pharmacologic agents also can provide symptomatic relief of anxiety and insomnia that occur as part of normal life crises.

A. **Classification of drugs.** The traditional division of psychotherapeutic drugs is as follows: (1) antipsychotics, (2) antidepressants, (3) antimanics, (4) anxiolytics, and (5) hypnotics.

These divisions are historically determined by their original clinical use. With most psychotropic drugs, however, clinical experience has shown that they have more than one clinical application. In actual practice, psychotropic drugs are used for purposes other than the primary approved indication. In addition, many compounds used for the treatment of endocrine, cardiovascular, and neurologic conditions are now frequently used to augment existing treatment regimens.

It also is common clinical practice for drugs to be used in higher doses than approved by the Food and Drug Administration (FDA). The FDA's view is that it is generally appropriate for clinicians to prescribe within the guidelines of community norms.

Some combination drugs are used with the rationale that they may increase the patient's compliance by simplifying the drug regimen. A problem with combination drugs, however, is that the clinician has less flexibility in adjusting the dose of one of the components and thus minimizing side effects. The use of combination drugs also may cause two drugs to be administered when only one is actually effective.

B. **Pharmacokinetics.** The principal divisions of pharmacokinetics are drug absorption, distribution, metabolism, and excretion.

1. **Absorption.** Orally administered drugs must dissolve in the fluid of the gastrointestinal (GI) tract before the body can absorb them. The absorption depends on the drug's concentration and lipid solubility and the GI tract's local pH, motility, and surface area. Some antipsychotic drugs are available in depot forms that allow the drug to be administered only once every 1-4 weeks. Intravenous (IV) administration is the quickest route to achieve therapeutic blood levels, but it also carries the highest risk of sudden and life-threatening adverse effects.

The Drug Enforcement Administration (DEA) has classified drugs according to abuse potential (Table 22–1), and clinicians are advised to be

TABLE 22–1.   **CHARACTERISTICS OF DRUGS AT EACH DEA LEVEL**

DEA Control Level (Schedule)	Characteristics of Drug at Each Control Level	Examples of Drugs at Each Control Level
I	High abuse potential No accepted use in medical treatment in the United States at the present time and therefore not for prescription use Can be used for research	LSD, heroin, marijuana, peyote, PCP, mescaline, psilocybin, tetrahydrocannabinols, nicocodeine, nicomorphine, and others
II	High abuse potential Severe physical dependence liability Severe psychological dependence liability No refills; no telephonic prescriptions	Amphetamine, methamphetamine, opium, morphine, codeine, hydromorphine, phenmetrazine, cocaine, amobarbital, secobarbital, pentobarbital, methylphenidate, and others
III	Abuse potential less than levels I and II Moderate or low physical dependence liability High psychological liability Prescriptions must be rewritten after 6 months or 5 refills	Glutethimide, methyprylon, nalorphine, sulfonmethane, benzphetamine, phendimetrazine, clortermine, mazindol, chlorphentermine, compounds containing codeine, morphine, opium, hydrocodone, dihydrocodeine, naltrexone, diethylpropion and others
IV	Low abuse potential Limited physical dependence liability Limited psychological dependence liability Prescriptions must be rewritten after 6 months or 5 refills	Phenobarbital, benzodiazepines,[a] chloral hydrate, ethchlorvynol, ethinamate, meprobamate, paraldehyde, and others
V	Lowest abuse potential of all controlled substances	Narcotic preparations containing limited amounts of nonnarcotic active medicinal ingredients

[a]In New York State, benzodiazepines are treated as Schedule II substances, which require a triplicate prescription for a maximum of 1 month's supply.

more cautious when prescribing Class II drugs than when prescribing less controlled substances.

2. **Distribution.**   Drugs can be freely dissolved in the blood plasma, bound to dissolved plasma proteins (primarily albumin), and dissolved within the blood cells. The distribution of a drug to the brain is determined by the blood-brain barrier, the brain's regional blood flow, and the drug's affinity with its receptors in the brain. The volume of distribution can also vary with the patient's age, sex, and disease state.

3. **Metabolism and excretion.**   The four major metabolic routes for drugs are oxidation, reduction, hydrolysis, and conjugation. The liver is the principal site of metabolism, and bile, feces, and urine are the major routes of excretion. Psychoactive drugs also are excreted in sweat, saliva, tears, and milk; therefore, mothers who are taking psychotherapeutic drugs should not nurse their children.

A drug's **half-life** is defined as the amount of time it takes for one-half of a drug's peak plasma level to be metabolized and excreted from the body.

Clearance is a measure of the amount of drug excreted per unit of time. If some disease process or other drug interferes with the clearance of a psychoactive drug, then the drug may reach toxic levels.

C. **Pharmacodynamics.** The major pharmacodynamic considerations include the receptor mechanism; the dose response curve; the therapeutic index; and the development of tolerance, dependence, and withdrawal phenomena. The dose response curve plots the drug concentration against the effects of the drug. The **potency** of a drug refers to the relative dose required to achieve a certain effect. Haloperidol (Haldol), for example, is more potent than chlorpromazine (Thorazine) because generally only 5 mg of haloperidol are required to achieve the same therapeutic effect as 100 mg of chlorpromazine. Both haloperidol and chlorpromazine, however, are equal in their maximal efficacies, i.e., the maximum clinical response achievable by the administration of a drug.

The side effects of most drugs often are a direct result of their primary pharmacodynamic effects and are better conceptualized as adverse effects. The **therapeutic index** is a relative measure of a drug's toxicity or safety.

A person may become less responsive to a particular drug as it is administered over time, which is referred to as **tolerance.** The development of tolerance is associated with the appearance of physical dependence, which may be defined as the necessity to continue administering the drug in order to prevent the appearance of withdrawal symptoms.

D. **Clinical guidelines.** Optimal results with drug therapy are dependent on several factors. Drugs work best when used according to lessons that have been learned from clinical and research experience. Optimizing results of psychotropic drug therapy involve the following five Ds: diagnosis, drug selection, dose, duration, and dialogue.

1. **Diagnosis.** Careful diagnosis is the first step toward optimal drug treatment. Selection of an inappropriate medication based on a mistaken diagnosis may not only delay the ultimate resolution of the underlying disorder but also actually worsen the patient's clinical condition.

2. **Drug selection.** Factors that determine drug selection include diagnosis, past history of drug response to a particular agent, and the overall medical status of the patient. By far the most important reasons to choose a drug are its relative side-effect profile and safety. Although all available drugs are equivalent in overall efficacy, they differ immensely in how well they are tolerated and how lethal they are in overdose. Drugs should not be selected because of their sedative effects.

In the past, there has been a tendency to treat mental disorders with nonspecific sedation. This approach often reduced subjective distress or insomnia for a brief period, but did little to shorten the course of the underlying disorder. It only recently has been recognized that sedation itself can significantly impair cognition and psychomotor performance. Newer, nonsedating antidepressants, such as fluoxetine (Prozac), or anxiolytics, such as buspirone (BuSpar), are preferable to sedating compounds.

3. **Dose.** The two most common causes of treatment failure involving psychotropic drugs are underdosing and an inadequate therapeutic trial of drug. It is well established that antidepressant drugs produce higher rates of improvement when taken at doses above the equivalent of 225 mg/day

of imipramine (Tofranil). The development of side effects at higher dose levels tends to deter patient compliance, and physicians often are reluctant to encourage dose escalations in a patient complaining of these side effects. Once the decision has been made to treat a patient with medication, all effort should be made to achieve therapeutic dose levels.

4. Duration.   For most psychotropic drugs, 3 weeks is the minimum period of treatment needed to determine whether a drug will prove effective. Ideally, a therapeutic trial should continue for 4–6 weeks if clinical conditions permit. It is important to recognize that psychotropic drugs generally produce their effects with chronic administration. Some patients may respond more rapidly than others.

5. Dialogue.   Patients will generally have less trouble with adverse effects if they have previously been told to expect them. But clinicians should distinguish between probable or expected adverse effects and rare or unexpected adverse effects.

Patients often feel that taking a psychotherapeutic drug means that they are really sick or not in control of their lives, or that they may become addicted to the drug and have to take it forever. A simplified approach to these concerns is to describe the psychiatric disorder partially as a disease or chemical imbalance analogous to diabetes as a disease of the pancreas. Psychiatrists should explain the difference between drugs of abuse that affect the normal brain and psychiatric drugs that are used to treat emotional disorders.

F. Special considerations

1. **Children.**   In practice, it is best to begin with a small dose and to increase the dose until clinical effects are observed. The clinician, however, should not hesitate to use adult doses in children if the dose is effective and there are no side effects.

2. **Geriatric patients.**   Psychiatrists should begin treating geriatric patients with a small dose, usually approximately one-half the usual dose. The dose should be raised in small amounts, more slowly than in middle-age adults until either a clinical benefit is achieved or unacceptable adverse effects appear. Although many geriatric patients require a small dose of medication, many others require the usual adult dosage.

3. **Pregnant and nursing women.**   Avoid administering any drug to a woman who is pregnant (particularly during the first trimester) or who is nursing a child. This rule, however, occasionally needs to be broken when the mother's psychiatric disorder is severe. The two most teratogenic drugs in the psychopharmacopeia are lithium and anticonvulsants. Lithium administration during pregnancy is associated with higher incidence of birth abnormalities, including Ebstein's malformation, a serious abnormality in cardiac development.

4. **Medically ill patients.**   Like children and geriatric patients, medically ill patients should receive the most conservative clinical practice, which is to begin with a small dose, increase it slowly, and watch for both clinical and adverse effects. The application of plasma drug levels may be a particularly helpful clinical test in these patients.

II. Antianxiety Drugs.   The drugs of choice for the treatment of anxiety are the benzodiazepines and buspirone. These compounds offer a wide margin of safety compared with older antianxiety drugs, such as chloral hydrate, barbiturates, and meprobamate (Miltown).

A. Benzodiazepines.   There are 14 benzodiazepines available for clinical use in the United States. They are widely prescribed, with at least 10% of the population using one of these drugs each year (Table 22–2).

TABLE 22–2.   **CURRENTLY MARKETED BENZODIAZEPINES ACCORDING TO PRIMARY APPROVED INDICATION**

Anxiety	Insomnia	Other
Diazepam (Valium)	Temazepam (Restoril)	Clonazepam (Klonopin)
Chlordiazepoxide (Librium)	Triazolam (Halcion)	Midazolam (Versed)
Clorazepate (Tranxene)	Flurazepam (Dalmane)	
Halazepam (Paxipam)	Quazepam (Doral)	
Prazepam (Centrax)		
Lorazepam (Ativan)		
Oxazepam (Serax)		
Alprazolam (Xanax)		

Although best known for their role in treating anxiety, these compounds produce other pharmacologic effects (Table 22–3).

TABLE 22–3.   **PHARMACOLOGIC EFFECTS OF BENZODIAZEPINES**

Therapeutic Effects	Clinical Applications
Sedative	Insomnia, conscious sedation, alcohol withdrawal
Anxiolytic	Panic attacks, generalized anxiety
Anticonvulsant	Seizures
Muscle relaxant	Muscle tension, muscle spasm
Amnestic	Adjunct to chemotherapy or anesthesia
Antistress	Mild hypertension, irritable bowel syndrome, angina

In contrast to antipsychotic and antidepressant drugs, the benzodiazepines produce few systemic side effects. Most side effects are the result of central nervous system (CNS) activity. Although extremely safe when taken alone in overdose, benzodiazepines can be lethal when combined with alcohol or other CNS depressants. Most side effects are subtle, but some can produce significant impairment (Table 22–4).

TABLE 22–4.   **SIDE EFFECTS OF BENZODIAZEPINES**

Side Effects	Consequences
Sedative	Daytime sleepiness, impaired concentration
Amnestic	Mild forgetfulness, anterograde memory impairment
Psychomotor	Accidents, falls
Behavioral	Depression, agitation
Decreased CO_2 response	Worsening of sleep apnea and other obstructive pulmonary disorders
Withdrawal syndrome	Dependence

Discontinuation of benzodiazepines can result in symptom recurrence, rebound (e.g., transient worsening of pretreatment symptoms), or withdrawal symptoms (e.g., emergence of new symptoms). Some patients may need to take benzodiazepines for prolonged periods. This is particularly true for patients being treated for panic disorder. Concern about becoming dependent should lead to caution when prescribing, but should not result in avoidance of benzodiazepine use when indicated. Some patients taking benzodiazepines for years do not develop withdrawal reactions, whereas others encounter difficulties after only a few weeks of use. To avoid dependence and withdrawal it is best, when possible, to use benzodiazepines intermittently for a few days at a time or continuously for no more than 2 weeks.

Several factors contribute to the development of benzodiazepine withdrawal symptoms. Drug type and duration of use are the most significant factors, but other considerations are also important.

Apart from being subjectively distressing, withdrawal symptoms can lead to the perception that the symptoms are part of the underlying disorder and thus result in unnecessary continued use of the drug (Tables 22–5 and 22–6).

TABLE 22–5. **BENZODIAZEPINE WITHDRAWAL SYMPTOMS**

Anxiety
Insomnia
Excess sensitivity to light
Excess sensitivity to sound
Tachycardia
Mild systolic hypertension
Tremor
Headache
Sweating
Abdominal distress
Craving
Seizures

TABLE 22–6. **KEY FACTORS IN THE DEVELOPMENT OF BENZODIAZEPINE WITHDRAWAL SYMPTOMS**

Factor	Explanation
Drug type	High potency, short half-life compounds, e.g., alprazolam, triazolam, lorazepam
Duration of use	Risk increases with time
Dose level	Higher doses increase risk
Rate of discontinuation	Abrupt withdrawal instead of taper increases risk of severe symptoms, including seizures
Diagnosis	Panic disorder patients more prone to withdrawal
Personality	Patients with passive-dependent, histrionic, somatizing or asthenic traits are more likely to experience withdrawal

The most important distinction among the benzodiazepines is their **elimination half-life**—the relative rate of drug excretion.

Long half-life compounds tend to accumulate with repeated dosage. This increases the risk of excessive daytime sedation, difficulties with concentration and memory, and increased risk of falls. Rates of hip fractures due to falls are higher in elderly patients taking these drugs than those taking more rapidly eliminated compounds.

The long half-life of these drugs is accounted for by a common long half-life metabolite, desmethyldiazepam. Its elimination half-life ranges from 50–120 hours.

Shorter half-life benzodiazepines have the advantage of producing less impairment with regular use. However, they appear to produce a more severe withdrawal syndrome (Tables 22–7 and 22–8).

TABLE 22–7.   **LONG HALF-LIFE BENZODIAZEPINES**

Diazepam
Chlordiazepoxide
Clorazepate
Halazepam
Prazepam

TABLE 22–8.   **SHORTER HALF-LIFE BENZODIAZEPINES**

Lorazepam
Oxazepam
Alprazolam

Benzodiazepines differ in potency, i.e., the amount of milligrams needed to achieve comparable clinical effects. In general, high potency drugs are used therapeutically at a daily dose range of 1–4 mg; low potency drugs have a typical therapeutic dose range of 10–30 mg.

High potency benzodiazepines appear to be effective in suppressing panic attacks.

Rate of absorption is another major consideration in benzodiazepine selection. All benzodiazepines are rapidly and completely absorbed from the GI tract, although the presence of food somewhat delays the process. Subtle differences in absorption rate among these drugs may become clinically significant. Diazepam (Valium) and triazolam (Halcion), for example, have a rapid onset; chlordiazepoxide (Librium) and oxazepam (Serax) work more slowly. All intramuscularly (IM) injected benzodiazepines except lorazepam (Ativan) are poorly absorbed, resulting in unpredictable plasma levels (Tables 22–9 and 22–10).

TABLE 22–9.   **DRUGS AFFECTING THE RATE OF ELIMINATION OF OXIDIZED BENZODIAZEPINES**

Increase Elimination Half-Life	Decrease Elimination Half-Life
Cimetidine	Chronic ethyl alcohol use
Propranolol	Rifampin
Oral contraceptives (estrogens)	
Chloramphenicol	
Propoxyphene	
Isoniazid	
Disulfiram	
Allopurinol	
Tricyclic antidepressants	
Acute ethyl alcohol use	

TABLE 22–10.   **BENZODIAZEPINE POTENCY**

High	Low
Alprazolam	Diazepam
Lorazepam	Chlordiazepoxide
	Clorazepate
	Halazepam
	Prazepam

The four benzodiazepines used primarily as hypnotics are flurazepam (Dalmane), temazepam (Restoril), quazepam (Doral), and triazolam (Halcion). Benzodiazepines shorten sleep latency and increase sleep continuity, making them useful for the treatment of insomnia. They also have a complex effect on sleep architecture (Table 22–11).

TABLE 22–11.   **EFFECTS OF BENZODIAZEPINES ON SLEEP**

Decreased stages 3–4
Decreased stage 1
Decreased REM sleep
Increased REM latency
Increased stage 2

The most clinically significant of the effects on sleep stages is the reduction of stages 3–4, also known as slow-wave sleep. Disorders such as sleep-walking and night terrors occur in these deep stages of sleep. Benzodiazepines also suppress rapid eye movement (REM)-related disorders, most notably violent behavior during REM (REM behavior disorder).

Ironically, in view of the usefulness of benzodiazepines in the management of sleep-related problems, one sleep disorder—sleep apnea—is probably the most unequivocal contraindication to benzodiazepine use. This disorder can be provoked or worsened by the use of any CNS depressant, including the benzodiazepines.

A summary profile of all currently used oral preparations of benzodiazepines is presented in Tables 22–12 through 22–14. The therapeutic dose range is given in Table 22–15.

B. Buspirone

   1. General introduction.   Buspirone (BuSpar) is the first anxiolytic of the azapirone class. It is pharmacologically unrelated to the benzodiazepines. In some early clinical trials it was found to be comparable to the benzodiazepines in anxiolytic efficacy.

   2. Dosing and basic kinetic considerations.   Buspirone is available in 5 and 10 mg tablets, with a recommended initial dosing schedule of 5 mg tablet TID. The maximum recommended daily dose is 60 mg. The therapeutic dose of buspirone is approximately 30 mg/day.

   3. Clinically significant drug interaction.   Concurrent administration of buspirone produces an increase in haloperidol serum levels. The use of buspirone in combination with monoamine oxidase inhibitors (MAOIs) can result in elevations of blood pressure.

   4. Time course of improvement.   A major consideration in patient com-

TABLE 22-12.   **COMMENTS ON INDIVIDUAL BENZODIAZEPINE ANXIOLYTICS**

Drug	Comments
Diazepam	Rapidly and completely absorbed. Also very lipid soluble. Result is rapid onset of action. May account for some abuse potential. Due to long half-life, accumulates with daily use.
Chlordiazepoxide	Slower onset of action minimizes abuse potential. Main use today is in the management of alcohol withdrawal and, with caution, treatment of anxiety in alcoholics. Due to long half-life, accumulates with daily use.
Clorazepate	Absorption may be delayed when ingested with antacids. Due to long half-life, accumulates with daily use.
Halazepam	Similar to clorazepate but more reliably absorbed. Due to long half-life, accumulates with daily use.
Prazepam	Similar to clorazepate but more reliably absorbed. Due to long half-life, accumulates with daily use.
Lorazepam	Wide range of elimination half-life (8–25 hours) means that duration of effects varies from person to person. Reliably absorbed IM. Metabolized mainly by conjugation. Risk of amnesia present. May be effective in treating panic disorder.
Oxazepam	Narrow range of elimination half-life (5–13 hours) assures short duration of action. Slowly absorbed. Metabolized mainly by conjugation.
Alprazolam	Effective in blocking panic attacks. May need doses up to 8 mg/day for treating panic disorder. Due to short half-life, may need to be given three times/day (TID) or four times/day (QID). Major problem is difficulty discontinuing treatment because of withdrawal syndrome.
Clonazepam	Not officially an anxiolytic, but now widely used in treating panic disorder. Its half-life range of 18–54 hours may permit QID or two times/day (BID) dosing. May carry higher risk of causing depression than other benzodiazepines.

TABLE 22-13.   **CURRENTLY USED BENZODIAZEPINE HYPNOTICS**

Drug	Comments
Flurazepam	Long half-life produces significant residual sedation, particularly with repeated use. Increased risk of falls in the elderly. Only advantage is a less severe withdrawal syndrome.
Quazepam	Similar to flurazepam. Claim by the manufacturer that Quazepam has relative preference for benzodiazepine type-1 receptors in the brain has not been conclusively demonstrated.
Temazepam	Intermediate half-life results in minimal residual sedation. May find some morning sedation. Only hypnotic metabolized by conjugation.
Triazolam	Very short half-life results in virtually no next-day sedation. Extremely potent, so very low doses should be used. At higher doses, amnesia becomes a possibility. Rebound insomnia a potential problem when the drug is stopped.

pliance with buspirone is the gradual onset of efficacy over a period of several days to weeks. Like antidepressants, buspirone is unlikely to cause patients to notice significant improvement in symptoms before 7 days. Maximum therapeutic effects are generally experienced after 3–4 weeks of treatment. The observed lag period in onset of clinical efficacy argues against the utility of buspirone on an as needed (prn) basis.

5. **Lack of sedation or interaction with CNS depressant.** The incidence of drowsiness reported by patients is no greater than with placebo. No enhancement effect between alcohol and buspirone has been discerned.

TABLE 22–14. **PROFILES OF CURRENTLY USED BENZODIAZEPINES**

Drug	Primary Metabolic Pathway	Elimination Half-Life* Hours (Range)	Potency +
Diazepam (Valium)	Oxidation	50 (50–120)	Low
Chlordiazepoxide (Librium)	Oxidation	50 (50–120)	Low
Clorazepate (Tranxene)	Oxidation	50 (50–120)	Low
Halazepam (Paxipam)	Oxidation	50 (50–120)	Low
Prazepam (Centrax)	Oxidation	50 (50–120)	Low
Lorazepam (Ativan)	Conjugation	13 (8–25)	High
Oxazepam (Serax)	Conjugation	7 (5–13)	Low
Alprazolam (Xanax)	Oxidation	12 (6–18)	High
Triazolam (Halcion)	Oxidation	12 (2–4.5)	Low
Temazepam (Restoril)	Conjugation	11 (9.5–12.5)	Low
Flurazepam (Dalmane)	Oxidation	50 (50–120)	Low
Quazepam (Doral)	Oxidation	50 (50–120)	Low
Clonazepam (Klonopin)	Oxidation	25 (18–54)	High
Midazolam	Oxidation	2 (1–3)	High

*Includes parent drug and active metabolites
+ High potency = Typical therapeutic dose of 1–4 mg/day; Low Potency = 15–30 mg/day

6. Lack of functional impairment. Both acute and chronic buspirone treatment have failed to discern any adverse effect on psychomotor skills.

7. Lack of potential for abuse or physical dependence. Buspirone is not a schedule IV controlled drug and is not widely abused. The drug tends to produce dysphoria at doses above therapeutic levels. Single doses of 40 mg or more produce a highly unpleasant subjective sensation.

8. Withdrawal. There is no withdrawal syndrome in buspirone patients, even with abrupt discontinuation. An implication of this finding is to minimize the likelihood of mistaking rebound anxiety or withdrawal symptoms for a return of the original anxiety symptoms.

9. Side-effect profile. Six side effects occur with a statistically significant incidence greater than placebo: (1) dizziness, (2) nausea, (3) headache, (4) nervousness, (5) lightheadedness, and (6) excitement.

10. Overdose. With doses as high as 375 mg/day, the most commonly observed symptoms are nausea, vomiting, dizziness, drowsiness, miosis,

TABLE 22–15. **THERAPEUTIC DOSE RANGE FOR BENZODIAZEPINES**

Drug	Dose Range (mg/day)
Anxiolytics	
Diazepam	2–60
Chlordiazepoxide	15–100
Clorazepate	7.5–60
Halazepam	60–160
Prazepam	20–60
Lorazepam	2–6
Alprazolam	0.75–4
	3–8 (for panic disorder)
Oxazepam	30–120
Clonazepam*	1.5–10 (for panic disorder)
Hypnotics	
Flurazepam	15–30
Quazepam	7.5–15
Temazepam	15–30
Triazolam	0.125–0.5

*Recommended as an anticonvulsant but widely used in the treatment of panic disorder.

and gastric distress. No deaths have been reported either with deliberate or accidental overdose.

11. Concurrent use with benzodiazepines. Buspirone may be used concurrently with benzodiazepines in several circumstances: (1) treatment resistant cases; (2) instances in which severe insomnia merits use of a benzodiazepine hypnotic; and (3) during a switching period, in which buspirone treatment is initiated before the benzodiazepine is discontinued.

III. Antipsychotic drugs

A. **General introduction.** This group of drugs represents the major treatment for some of the most disturbed patients seen by psychiatrists. Antipsychotic drugs are mainly used to treat acute schizophrenic episodes and to prevent reemergence of psychotic symptoms in schizophrenic patients. These compounds also are useful for other psychiatric conditions, including mania, organic psychosis, and Tourette's disorder.

Antipsychotic drugs also have been termed neuroleptics or major tranquilizers. The word "neuroleptic" refers to the effect of antipsychotic drugs in motor activity rather than their clinical effects and is thus inappropriate. The term "major tranquilizer" is misleading because it suggests that these compounds are similar to benzodiazepines and other antianxiety/hypnotic drugs (the minor tranquilizers). Antipsychotic drugs are pharmacologically unrelated to the antianxiety agents, and their clinical effects do not result from nonspecific sedative action.

B. **Therapeutic effects.** The major therapeutic effects of these drugs are seen during their use in acute psychoses. Effects include reduction of the so-called positive symptoms, e.g., hallucinations, delusions, uncooperativeness, and thought disorder. There also is normalization of psychomotor activity (excitement or retardation) and information processing. Positive symptoms of schizophrenia respond more consistently to antipsychotic drugs.

Negative, or deficit, symptoms, e.g., affective flattening, apathy, anhedonia, and blocking, are less responsive to these drugs.

In general, negative symptoms persist over time, even during remissions, and have proved difficult to treat (Table 22–16).

TABLE 22–16. **SCHIZOPHRENIC SYMPTOMS**

Positive	Negative
Hallucinations	Blunted affect
Delusions	Poverty of speech
Thought disorder	Social withdrawal

C. Types of drugs.   In 1952, chlorpromazine was the first drug found to have a major effect on schizophrenic symptoms. Since then, other phenothiazine analogues have been developed along with several other compounds that are similar in their tricyclic structure. Other compounds unrelated to the tricyclics also are available (Table 22–17).

TABLE 22–17. **CURRENTLY USED ANTIPSYCHOTIC DRUGS**

Phenothiazine	*Butyrophenone*
Aliphatic	Haloperidol (Haldol)
Chlorpromazine (Thorazine)	
Triflupromazine (Vesprin)	*Indolone*
Piperidine	Molindone (Moban)
Thioridazine (Mellaril)	
Piperazine	*Dibenzoxazepine*
Perphenazine (Trilafon)	Loxapine (Loxitane)
Trifluoperazine (Stelazine)	
Fluphenazine (Prolixin)	*Diphenybutylpiperidine*
Acetophenazine (Tindal)	Pimozide (Orap)
Thioxanthene	*Diboroxazepine*
Thiothixene (Navane)	Clozapine (Clozaril)
Chlorprothixene (Taractin)	

D. Efficacy.   Despite the structural diversity of these drugs, no one compound is consistently superior to another. All antipsychotic compounds are equally effective when used at optimal doses. They differ in potency and in side effects. Some patients nevertheless respond better to one drug than another. There is no reliable way to predict this in advance.

Although some patients may show some immediate improvement in agitation or anxiety when started on an antipsychotic drug, these effects are mainly the result of nonspecific sedation. The actual impact of these drugs on psychotic symptoms develops with regular administration over a period of several weeks.

E. Mechanism of action.   The mechanism of action of antipsychotic drugs is probably more complex than is currently hypothesized. Their presumed mode of action involves the postsynaptic blockade of CNS dopamine (D2) receptors.

F. Potency.   A major distinction among antipsychotic drugs is their efficacy at a given dose. Some drugs given at high doses, e.g., 200–600 mg/day, are low potency compounds. Others given at lower doses, e.g., less than 80 mg/day, are high potency compounds. As a rule, the lower potency drugs produce more sedation, orthostatic hypotension, and anticholinergic effects than the high potency drugs, which cause more frequent and severe extrapyramidal symptoms. The therapeutic doses are listed in Table 22–18.

TABLE 22–18. ANTIPSYCHOTICS: TYPICAL THERAPEUTIC DOSES

Drug	Chlorpromazine Equivalent (mg)	Relative Potency	Therapeutic Dose (mg/day)*
Chlorpromazine (Thorazine)	100	Low	150–2000
Triflupromazine (Vesprin)	30	Medium	20–150
Thioridazine (Mellaril)	100	Low	100–800
Mesoridazine (Serentil)	50	Medium	10–400
Perphenazine (Trilafon)	10	Medium	8–64
Trifluoperazine (Stelazine)	3–5	High	5–60
Fluphenazine (Prolixin)	3–5	High	5–60
Acetophenazine (Tindal)	15	Medium	20–100
Chlorprothixene (Taractin)	75	Low	100–600
Thiothixene (Navane)	3–5	High	5–60
Loxapine (Loxitane)	10–15	Medium	30–250
Haloperidol (Haldol)	2–5	High	2–100
Molindone (Moban)	5–10	Medium	10–225
Pimozide (Orap)	1–2	High	2–20
Clozapine (Clozaril)	?	?	?

*Extreme range

G. Pharmacokinetics.   Several aspects of antipsychotic drug metabolism are clinically significant. Phenothiazines generally are well absorbed, but there may be significant differences between patients. Rates of metabolism also vary greatly. Because of the complexity of metabolites of phenothiazines, routine plasma level determinations are of limited clinical value. Liquid preparations generally are more completely absorbed than tablets or capsules. Because this route bypasses first-pass metabolism involving the liver, higher blood levels are obtained with intramuscular (IM) than with oral (PO) administration. Because of generally long half-lives, antipsychotic drugs can be given once a day. Drugs that are lipophilic are difficult to dialyze in case of overdose.

H. Side effects.   Antipsychotic drugs produce a broad range of side effects. These are a result of the multiple neurotransmitter systems affected by these drugs. Many patients who might benefit from the use of these drugs refuse to take them because of effects that can be distressing even to highly motivated patients, let alone those who are fearful and mistrustful. An important consideration in drug selection is avoidance of the most uncomfortable or dangerous adverse reactions—tardive dyskinesia and neuroleptic malignant syndrome.

    1. Obstructive jaundice.   Jaundice, which is rare, mainly occurs with chlorpromazine, about 1–5 weeks after start of treatment (symptoms include fever, nausea, right upper quadrant pain, malaise, and puritis). It is not seen with nonphenothiazines. It may resolve spontaneously. If it occurs, consider discontinuing the chlorpromazine.

    2. Endocrine effects.   Side effects related to endocrine changes include weight gain (perhaps with exception of molindone), shift in glucose tolerance, false positive pregnancy test, impotence/decreased sexual desire, amenorrhea, galactorrhea, and gynecomastia (due to increased prolactin level).

3. **Skin and eye effects.** Skin and eye effects include photosensitivity (use sunscreen), maculopapular rash, blue-gray metallic skin discoloration, deposits in anterior lens and posterior cornea, and pigmentary retinopathy with high doses of thioridazine (Mellaril). The anticholinergic activity of these drugs can precipitate narrow-angle glaucoma and blurred vision, particularly cycloplegia.

4. **Sedation.** Sedation is caused mainly by histamine-1 blockade and is seen most often with low-potency drugs, such as chlorpromazine. Some tolerance to sedation develops. If sedation remains a problem, reduce the dose or switch to a high potency drug, such as haloperidol.

5. **Anticholinergic.** Anticholinergic effects consist mainly of dry mouth, constipation, blurred near vision, delayed micturition, and glaucoma. Although mainly annoying, these effects are a major source of noncompliance. These adverse effects can lead to fecal impaction and urinary retention, and can result in central atropine-like psychosis, a delirium related to anticholinergic toxicity.

Management of anticholinergic side effects includes: neostigmine (Prostigmin) (15–30 mg TID) or bethanechol (Urecholine) (25 mg BID or QID) for urinary retention. Physostigmine (Antilirium) eye drops are not practical; reading glasses may help. Laxatives for constipation should be used judiciously.

6. **Orthostatic (postural) hypotension**
   a. Caused by adrenergic alpha-1 blockade.
   b. Seen most often with aliphatic phenothiazines, mainly chlorpromazine (Thorazine), at high doses or when given IM. Can be caused by clozapine, when started at high dose.
   c. Do not treat with epinephrine (is a beta-adrenergic stimulant and thus may worsen orthostasis). Use metariminol (Aramine) or norepinephrine.

7. **Cardiac effects**
   a. Sudden death (rare).
   b. Electrocardiogram (EKG) changes (prolonged QT and PR intervals, ST depression and blunted T-waves).

8. **Hematologic effects.** Can get benign drop in white blood cell count (WBC), thrombocytopenia, pancytopenia, or agranulocytosis. Slow decline in leukocyte count may occur. Stabilizes at about 3,000; not usually symptomatic. Patients should nevertheless be followed to confirm blood count.

Complete loss of granulocytes. Has an incidence of 1 in 500,000. Occurs abruptly less than 8 weeks after start of treatment. Chlorpromazine most often implicated. Symptoms include sudden sore throat and fever. Stop drug immediately and refer for medical treatment (usually antibiotics and reverse isolation).

9. **Neurologic**
   a. **Pseudoparkinsonism.** This is the most common reversible drug-induced movement disorder (15% of patients). Its incidence increases

with age. Like Parkinson's disease itself, this condition is characterized by dysfunction in tone (e.g., generalized rigidity), movement (e.g., bradykinesia, akinesia, tremor, festinating gait), and posture (e.g., flexed posture).

Current theory holds that drug-induced parkinsonism and other extrapyramidal effects, such as tardive dyskinesia, are the result of nigrostriatal dopamine system blockade. Treatment consists primarily of antiparkinsonian medication.

Other interventions include a dose reduction of antipsychotic drug or the use of a phenothiazine with a relatively low liability for producing pseudoparkinsonism, e.g., thioridazine (Table 22–19).

TABLE 22–19. **DRUGS USED TO TREAT DRUG-INDUCED MOVEMENT DISORDERS**

Drug	Usual Adult Dose Mg/day	Usual Adult Single Dose mg
Benztropine (Cogentin)	1–6	1–2
Trihexphenidyl (Artane)	4–15	2–3
Biperiden (Akineton)	2–6	2
Procyclidine (Kemadrin)	10–20	2–5
Diphenhydramine (Benadryl)	50–300	10–50
Orphenadrine (Disipal)	50–150	50
Amantadine (Symmetral)	100–300	100
Ethopropazine (Parsidol)	100–400	50–100

b. **Acute dystonic reactions**
   i. Experienced by at least 10% of patients.
   ii. Most common in young males.
   iii. Mechanism may involve excessive stimulation of hypersensitive dopamine receptors.
   iv. Attacks subside spontaneously in hours to days.
   v. Attacks aborted spontaneously with anticholinergics or diazepam.
c. **Akathisia**
   i. Motor and mental restlessness.
   ii. Increasing doses of antipsychotic drugs may only increase restlessness.
   iii. Treated with anticholinergics, benzodiazepines, beta blockers.
d. **Neuroleptic malignant syndrome (NMS)**
   i. Unexplained hyperthermia with increase in muscle tone and involuntary movements after initiating or increasing antipsychotic drugs.
   ii. Pulmonary complications and acute renal failure (secondary to dehydration) are common.
   iii. One-quarter of typical cases culminate in stupor, coma, and death.
   iv. Treat with dantrolene (Dantrium) (200 mg/day) and/or bromocriptine (Parlodel) (up to 60 mg/day).
   v. A medical emergency. Stop antipsychotic drug.

e. Lethal catatonia
  i. Rare syndrome in patients on long-term treatment.
  ii. Prodrome of increasing mental and physical agitation lasting weeks to months.
  iii. May culminate in stupor, coma, and death.
  iv. Differentiate from NMS by absence of extrapyramidal rigidity, involuntary movements, and other clinical features listed in Table 22–20.

TABLE 22–20.   **CLINICAL DIFFERENCES BETWEEN LETHAL CATATONIA AND NEUROLEPTIC MALIGNANT SYNDROME**

Other Stage	Lethal Catatonia	Neuroleptic Malignant Syndrome
	Prodrome lasting 2 weeks–2 months, consisting of behavioral and personality changes or frank schizophrenic symptoms Possible acute onset with no prodrome	Period of prior antipsychotic drug exposure can be hours to months Develops rapidly over a few hours to days No prodromal phase has been described
Initial symptoms	Excitement, intense anxiety, and restlessness lasting a few days Possible self-destructive or assaultive behavior Hallucinatory experiences and delusional thinking usually present Possible fever, tachycardia, and acrocyanosis Sudden death may occur	Tremors and dyskinesias are early signs Muscle hypertonicity described as lead pipe or plastic rigidity Severe excitement and intense anxiety are not major features Autonomic instability with tachycardia, labile hypertension, and possible diaphoresis Fever may not be present initially Acrocyanosis has not been described May occur in nonpsychotic patients treated with antipsychotics No deaths reported during early phase
Full syndrome	Continued increasing excitement with wild agitation and violent, destructive behavior, lasting 3–15 days, and possible choreiform movements Mutism, rigidity, and/or stupor may alternate with excitement Refusal of food and fluids Increasing and fluctuating fever, rapid and weak pulse, profuse, clammy perspiration, hypotension	Appearance of most major symptoms (severe muscle rigidity, persistent autonomic instability, fever) usually occurs after 2–9 days Possible agitation, confusion, and clouding of consciousness
Final stage	Cachexia, convulsions, delirium, coma, exhaustion Death may occur	Severe complications, e.g., rhabdomyolysis with elevated creatine phosphokinase, myoglobinuria, renal failure, and intravascular thrombosis with pulmonary embolism and respiratory failure Possible 20–30% mortality rate with full syndrome
Treatment	Antipsychotic drugs and other treatments to reduce severe psychotic symptoms	Immediate cessation of all dopamine-blocking antipsychotic drugs Dopamine agonists (to reduce central hypodopaminergic state), calcium channel blockers (to reduce muscle rigidity), beta-adrenergic blockers (to reduce tachycardia), other supportive measures as needed Consder using electroconvulsive therapy (ECT)

Table adapted from Castillo E, Rubin RT, Holsboer-Trachsler E: Clinical differentiation between lethal catatonia and neuroleptic malignant syndrome. Am J Psychiat *146*:326, 1989, with permission.

  f. **Tardive dyskinesia**
     i. Symptoms include repetitive lip smacking, masticatory and tongue movements, and choreic movements of the trunk and limbs.
    ii. Occurs during or after discontinuation of long-term antipsychotic drug treatment. More common in women than in men.
   iii. Mechanism probably involves denervation hypersensitivity secondary to long-term dopaminergic blockade.
    iv. Irreversible in the majority of patients.
     v. Anticholinergics do not prevent and may actually exacerbate the disease.
    vi. Treat by substituting responsible drug with a different antipsychotic and then slowly withdrawing the substitute drug.
  g. **Rabbit syndrome**
     i. Late-onset, drug-induced extrapyramidal symptoms.
    ii. Rapid fine rhythmic movements of the lips.
   iii. Unlike buccolingual movements of Tourette's disorder, rabbit syndrome improves with antiparkinsonian drugs.
  h. **Seizures.** All antipsychotic drugs can lower the seizure threshold.

I. **Drug selection.** Factors to be considered in drug selection include characteristics of both the patient and the pharmacologic compound.

The popularity of high potency drugs, such as haloperidol, is largely the result of the low degree of both sedation and anticholinergic effects. Even though the risk of extrapyramidal symptoms is great, most clinicians prefer to treat them as they emerge (Table 22–21).

TABLE 22–21. **CONSIDERATIONS IN THE DRUG SELECTION**

Factor	Comment
Diagnosis	The more clear-cut the diagnosis of schizophrenia, the more important an antipsychotic be used.
Past history of drug response	The success or failure of a particular drug in treating a past episode in the patient or biologic family.
Medical status	Specific conditions, such as prostatic hypertropy, glaucoma, cardiac disease or constipation, argue against use of strongly anticholinergic drugs. In patients with parkinsonism, use low potency agents.
Severe depression	Because thioridazine and mesoridazine are more lethal in overdose, they should be avoided in potentially suicidal patients.
Organic mental syndrome	Although used to treat behavioral disturbances associated with organic mental syndrome, the more anticholinergic drugs can worsen mental status and cause delirium.

1. **Phenothiazines**
   a. **Aliphatic (e.g., chlorpromazine [Thorazine], triflupromazine [Vesprin]).** Chlorpromazine is the most widely used of the low potency drugs. Usually these drugs are associated with marked sedation, postural hypotension, and an intermediate profile with respect to frequency of extrapyramidal symptoms.
   b. **Piperazine (e.g, perphenazine [Trilafon], trifluoperazine [Stelazine], fluphenazine [Prolixin], acetophenazine [Tindal]).** Drugs from this group have a higher potency than the aliphatics. One advantage of

the piperazine drugs is the decreased likelihood of causing sedation and orthostatic hypotension. A disadvantage is a high incidence of extra-pyramidal side effects.

   i. **Perphenazine** has less extrapyramidal symptoms than other pi-perazines, but more sedation and cardiovascular effects. It seems to be the pharmacologic middle of antipsychotic drugs.

   ii. **Trifluoperazine** is associated with low sedative effects and mod-erate degrees of hypotension and anticholinergic activity. Apart from extrapyramidal effects, it is generally well tolerated.

   iii. **Fluphenazine** is one of two antipsychotic drugs available in a long-acting injectable preparation. Fluphenazine comes in a dec-anoate form, which is generally administered as an IM injection every 2 weeks. In some cases, an injection can last up to 6 weeks. Fluphenazine decanoate is indicated over oral drugs in patients who are noncompliant with oral regimens and who have absorption problems. Fluphenazine also is available as an enanthate prepa-ration, but this formulation is less frequently used because of its shorter duration and slower onset of action. All patients should take a trial dose of oral fluphenazine before being started on depot preparations.

 c. **Piperidine (e.g., thioridazine [Mellaril], mesoridazine [Serentil]).**

   i. **Thioridazine** is the more commonly used of these two piperidines. It has the advantage of producing a low incidence of extrapyramidal symptoms; consequently, concurrent antiparkinsonian medication is rarely needed. Sedation, hypotension, and anticholinergic effects are similar to the aliphatics. Thioridazine has significant calcium channel-blocking activity, which is thought to be the cause for inhibition of ejaculation in about 5% of male patients taking the drug as well as more pronounced EKG changes than other phe-nothiazines. In addition to an increased QR interval, thioridazine causes broadened, flattened, or clove T-waves. Thioridazine is the only antipsychotic drug with an absolute upper dose limit of 800 mg/day. This restriction is based on the finding that pigmentary retinopathy occurs at doses of 1,600 mg/day or over.

   ii. **Mesoridazine** is similar to thioridazine in most side effects but does not cause retinal or ejaculatory disturbances. It is approxi-mately 2–3 times as potent as thioridazine.

2. **Thioxanthenes**
 a. **Thiothixene (Navane)** has high extrapyramidal effects, but low se-dative and low hypotensive effects. It is similar to trifluoperazine and haloperidol in properties.
 b. **Chlorprothixene (Taractin)** is the thioxanthene analog of chlor-promazine, with similar sedative and hypotensive effects, but min-imal extrapyramidal symptoms.

3. **Butyrophenones**
 Haloperidol (Haldol) is rapidly absorbed from GI tract—highest plasma level in 2–5 hours and is slowly excreted. Half-life is 24–36

hours. IM haloperidol (5–20 mg every 2 hours) is considered by many to be the drug of choice in acutely agitated psychotics because of minimal sedation and hypotension. Extrapyramidal symptoms are common, but there are less anticholinergic and cardiovascular side effects, liver damage, ocular damage, blood disorders, and phototoxicity than with chlorpromazine and other antipsychotics. Long-acting depot form available.

4. **Dihydroindolines**

   Molindone (Moban), the only available dihydroindoline, is structurally unrelated to other antipsychotic drugs. It is equal in efficacy to other antipsychotic drugs and produces similar side effects. Studies, nevertheless, suggest that molindone produces a generally lower incidence of anticholinergic effects, orthostatic hypotension, seizures, and weight gain than other antipsychotic agents. Despite this possibly favorable profile, it is not widely used.

5. **Dibenzodiazepines**

   Clozapine (Clozaril) has been used in Europe for many years for treatment-resistant schizophrenic patients. Unlike other antipsychotic drugs, it does not appear to cause extrapyramidal symptoms. This may be due to the fact that clozapine does not have an affinity for striatal dopamine receptors. Between 30 and 40% of treatment-resistant patients benefit from a trial of clozapine. The drug also appears to have a greater effect on negative symptoms than conventional antipsychotics.

   A special concern with use of clozapine is agranulocytosis, which occurred in about 1–2% of patients during clinical trials in the United States. No cases were fatal because of careful monitoring. The agranulocytosis is reversible if detected within a week or two.

   A controversial patient management system is used to monitor and control clozapine use. A national laboratory monitors the blood count and case managers control dispensing of the drug. A patient does not receive the next weeks' dosages of clozapine until a WBC is done.

   Side effects of clozapine include hypotension, tachycardia, sedation, hypersalivation, and fever. Seizures may occur at high doses.

   The mean dosage is about 200 mg/day.

6. **Pimozide (Orap).** Pimozide is a highly potent and pure dopamine antagonist. It is approved for the treatment of Tourette's disorder, but is equally effective as standard antipsychotic drugs in the treatment of schizophrenia.

   Compared with other high potency compounds, pimozide appears to carry a greater risk of arrhythmias than standard anticonvulsant drugs. Several reports suggest that pimozide is effective in treating monosymptomatic hypochondriasis and the delusions of delusional disorder.

J. **Clinical use.** Because of the various side effects of antipsychotic drugs, all patients have a complete blood count (CBC) and liver profile at the outset of treatment. Older patients should be given an EKG. In ambulatory patients, it is advisable to initiate antipsychotic drug treatment at low doses (the equivalent of 100 mg/day of chlorpromazine) and titrate the dosage upward as the patient's condition warrants and side effects permit. Two different antipsychotics should not be given concurrently; combined therapy does not enhance drug effectiveness and increases the risk of side effects.

Certain factors may interfere with intestinal absorption of antipsychotic drugs and thus decrease the amount of active drug that reaches the CNS. Since absorption is delayed by food and decreased by antacids, patients should receive their medication between meals and about 2 hours after using antacids. An important fact to keep in mind is that anticholinergic antiparkinsonism drugs also delay gastric emptying, resulting in increased degradation of antipsychotics in the stomach. One of the advantages of injectable forms of antipsychotic drugs is that they tend to provide higher plasma levels than oral preparations.

Patients may be given their medication in divided doses early in treatment. After several days, however, plasma levels of the drug become stable, and administration of the total daily dose at bedtime is advisable. Giving medication at bedtime may be necessary if sedating antipsychotic drugs, such as chlorpromazine or thioridazine, are used. One disadvantage of giving the total daily dose at bedtime is the increased risk of orthostatic hypotension if the patient gets out of bed during the night.

Antipsychotic drugs typically take days to weeks to provide maximal therapeutic effect. Improvement usually occurs in the third or fourth week of treatment, assuming adequate doses are used. Unless side effects preclude continued use of the drug, a 6–8 week trial period with the proper dosage is advisable.

Some patients react to initial doses of antipsychotic medication with dysphoria, usually leading to noncompliance. Anticholinergic medications are effective in reducing antipsychotic-induced dysphoria and, consequently, in improving compliance.

Because antipsychotic drugs are nonaddicting, some practitioners prefer to prescribe low doses of these compounds instead of antianxiety medications. This practice is not advisable in view of the potentially serious side effects of antipsychotic drug use.

In monitoring a patient's response to treatment, it is helpful to focus on specific target symptoms, such as auditory hallucinations or suspiciousness. Any reduction or lack of improvement in these symptoms can provide a frame of reference for the degree of success of the drug regimen.

Patients who have responded well to a specific drug during earlier treatment should receive the same drug during subsequent psychotic episodes. When a family member has been treated successfully with a specific drug and the patient has never been treated before, it is best to prescribe the same or similar drug for the patient.

Other factors that influence the selection of a drug include the person's medical status and life-style. For example, patients with conduction disturbances of the heart should not be treated with thioridazine because it produces nonspecific EKG changes that may confound the monitoring of the cardiac condition and may increase the risk of arrhythmias (Table 22–22).

Dosage during the acute phase of a psychotic illness should be higher than maintenance doses. For example, the equivalent of 400 mg of chlorpromazine is considered the average effective dose in the treatment of acute schizophrenia; by comparison, the effective range for prevention of relapse is between 150 and 300 mg. In some cases, it may be necessary to exceed the conventional dose by a wide margin, so that the patient receives 1,000 mg or even 1,600 mg of chlorpromazine. However, it is advisable to avoid megadoses routinely, and when they are used, the reasons should be scru-

TABLE 22–22. **ANTIPSYCHOTIC DRUG INTERACTIONS**

Drug	Consequence
Tricyclic antidepressants	Increased concentrations of both
Anticholinergics	Anticholinergic toxicity, decreased absorption of antipsychotics
Antacids	Decreased absorption of antipsychotics
Cimetidine	Decreased absorption of antipsychotics
Food	Decreased absorption of antipsychotics
Buspirone	Elevation of haloperidol levels
Barbiturates	Increased metabolism of antipsychotics, excessive sedation
Phenytoin	Decreased phenytoin metabolism
Guanethidine	Reduced hypotensive effect
Clonidine	Reduced hypotensive effect
Alpha-methyldopa	Reduced hypotensive effect
Levodopa	Decreased effects of both
Succinylcholine	Prolonged muscle paralysis
Monoamine oxidase inhibitors	Hypotension
Halothane	Hypotension
Alcohol	Potentiation of CNS depression
Cigarettes	Decreased plasma levels of antipsychotics
Epinephrine	Hypotension
Propranolol	Increased plasma concentrations of both
Warfarin	Decreased plasma concentrations of warfarin

pulously considered and treatment should be conducted in an inpatient setting.

It is always best to use the lowest effective dose, because this reduces the incidence and severity of side effects. It is well established, however, that there is no minimal effective dose for each antipsychotic drug, below which it does not exhibit clinical efficacy. The use of such homeopathic doses of medication represents a disservice to the patient exposed to the risks of drug treatment without the possibility of its benefits.

Long-acting injectable (depot) antipsychotics are effective in preventing psychotic relapse and rehospitalization among schizophrenic patients. Patients who benefit most from long-acting preparations are those who are partially or completely noncompliant in taking medication. Noncompliance is a common problem with oral antipsychotic therapy; 40–50% of schizophrenic outpatients and nearly 40% of day hospital patients fail to take medication as prescribed. The usual dose of the most widely used long-acting antipsychotic, fluphenazine decanoate, is 12.5–50.0 mg every 2 weeks. The use of lower doses, such as 1.25–5.0 mg every 2 weeks, is associated with increased relapse rates. Rates of adverse effects are no higher among patients receiving fluphenazine decanoate than among patients taking standard oral antipsychotics.

Abrupt discontinuation of medication increases the risk of withdrawal symptoms, including sweating, nausea, diarrhea, tremor, restlessness, and insomnia. In differentiating the withdrawal syndrome from a return of psychotic symptoms, it is noted that withdrawal symptoms appear within several days of the last dose, then diminish by the second week, whereas relapse begins after several weeks and becomes progressively more severe.

Other drugs that are used to treat psychotic conditions are listed in Table 22–23.

TABLE 22–23.   OTHER DRUGS USED IN TREATMENT OF PSYCHOSIS

Reserpine	Acts as a presynaptic dopamine depleter. Slow onset, marginal efficacy, and risk of depression and suicide. No longer used in schizophrenia.
Lithium	Apart from reducing manic symptoms, lithium also has been reported to be useful in treating refractory schizophrenic patients when given in conjunction with antipsychotic drugs.
Carbamazepine	Some patients get worse with antipsychotic drugs. It is thought they may have atypical psychoses that respond to carbamazepine and other anticonvulsants. Manic psychosis also responds to carbamazepine.
Benzodiazepines	IM lorazepam is useful for acute agitation with psychosis of uncertain cause. There are reports of adjunctive use of benzodiazepines with antipsychotic drugs, producing an improvement in negative symptoms and reducing required dose levels of antipsychotic.
Beta-adrenergic blockers	Beta-adrenergic blockers may be effective in treating aggressive behavior or rage in schizophrenic patients.

IV. Antidepressant drugs

A. General introduction. A broad range of structurally diverse compounds produce improvement in depressive disorders. Controlled studies and clinical experience have demonstrated that

1. Proper use of any antidepressant drug results in clinical improvement in at least 60-70% of depressed patients. By comparison, only 30% of placebo-treated patients improve in the same amount of time.
2. All currently marketed drugs are equally effective.
3. There are significant differences in side effects among drugs. These differences are a major consideration in drug selection, determining both safety and compliance.
4. There is no reliable way of predicting who will respond to a particular drug, or who will tolerate a particular side effect.

At the moment, there are five broad categories of antidepressant drugs: the standard tricyclic compounds, the heterocyclic compounds, the selective serotonergic agents, the selective dopamine reuptake blockers, and the MAOIs (Table 22–24).

B. Synaptic pharmacology. The actual mechanism by which these drugs alleviate depression is not known. At best, it is possible to identify the effects of drugs on synaptic activity, and to postulate which pharmacologic effects are linked to therapeutic effects and which are the cause of adverse effects.

Effects believed to be unrelated to antidepressant activity account for many troublesome adverse reactions.

Each of the antidepressants has a different potency in blocking reuptake of one of the major central neurotransmitters: norepinephrine, serotonin, and dopamine. Desipramine (Norpramin) is the most potent norepinephrine reuptake inhibitor, fluoxetine (Prozac) is the most potent serotonin reuptake inhibitor, and bupropion (Wellbutrin) is the most potent dopamine reuptake inhibitor. By comparing the relative potency of an antidepressant in blocking one neurotransmitter with another, it is possible to determine if they are selective. For example, maprotiline (Ludiomil) is relatively selective in blocking

TABLE 22–24. **CURRENTLY USED ANTIDEPRESSANT DRUGS**

TRICYCLICS

Amitriptyline	(Elavil)	
Doxepin	(Sinequan)	Tertiary
Clomipramine*	(Anafranil)	Amines
Imipramine	(Tofranil)	
Trimipramine	(Surmontil)	
Desipramine	(Norpramin)	
Nortriptyline	(Pamelor)	Secondary
Protriptyline	(Vivactil)	Amines

HETEROCYCLICS

Amoxapine	(Asendin)
Maprotiline	(Ludiomil)
Trazodone	(Desyrel)

SEROTONERGIC AGENTS

Fluoxetine	(Prozac)

DOPAMINE REUPTAKE BLOCKERS

Bupropion	(Wellbutrin)

MONOAMINE OXIDASE INHIBITORS

Tranylcypromine	(Parnate)
Phenelzine	(Nardil)
Isocarboxazid	(Marplan)

*Approved in the United States for the treatment of obsessive-compulsive disorder.

reuptake of norepinephrine, whereas trazodone (Desyrel) selectively blocks reuptake of serotonin.

The clinical significance of antidepressant neurotransmitter selectivity is not known. Nevertheless, some patients do well on one type of drug but not another.

Antidepressants produce changes in receptors with chronic administration. For example, most antidepressant drugs produce a down regulation of beta-adrenergic receptors and serotonin (5HT-2) receptors (Tables 22–25, 22–26, and 22–27).

TABLE 22–25. **ACUTE SYNAPTIC EFFECTS POSSIBLY LINKED TO THERAPEUTIC ACTIVITY**

Norepinephrine reuptake blockade
Serotonin reuptake blockade
Dopamine reuptake blockade
Serotonin$_{1A}$ receptor agonism
Serotonin$_2$ receptor agonism
Monoamine oxidase inhibition

TABLE 22–26. **ACUTE SYNAPTIC EFFECTS ASSOCIATED WITH ADVERSE EFFECTS**

Muscarinic blockade
Alpha$_1$ adrenergic blockade
Alpha$_2$ adrenergic blockade
Histamine blockade
Dopamine$_2$ blockade

TABLE 22–27.   **NEURONAL REUPTAKE BLOCKADE POTENCY AND SELECTIVITY**

| Agent | Potency of Blocking Uptake[†] | | | |
	Norepinephrine[‡]	Serotonin[§]	Dopamine[l]	Selectivity
Norepinephrine-Selective Drugs				
Maprotiline (Ludiomil)	14	0.030	0.034	440
Desipramine (Norpramin)	110	0.29	0.019	380
Protriptyline (Vivactil)	100	0.36	0.054	280
Amoxapine (Asendin)	23	0.21	0.053	110
Nortriptyline (Pamelor)	25	0.38	0.059	66
Doxepin (Sinequan)	5.3	0.36	0.018	15
Trimipramine (Surmontil)	0.20	0.040	0.029	5
Imipramine (Tofranil)	7.7	2.4	0.020	3.2
Amitriptyline (Elavil)	4.2	1.5	0.043	2.8
Serotonin-Selective Drugs				
Trazodone (Desyrel)[a]	0.020	0.53	0.0071	26
Fluoxetine (Prozac)	0.36	8.3	0.063	23
Dopamine-Selective Drugs				
Bupropion (Wellbutrin)	0.043	0.0064	0.16	3.7

Table adapted from Richelson E: Synaptic pharmacology of antidepressants: An update. McLean Hosp J *13*:67, 1988, with permission.

[†]Potency $= 10^{-7} \times K_i$: $K_i =$ inhibitor-constant molarity

[‡]Norepinephrine selectivity $= \dfrac{\text{norepinephrine potency}}{\text{serotonin potency}}$

[a]Trazodone is serotonin-selective only in vitro

[§]serotonin selectivity $= \dfrac{\text{serotonin potency}}{\text{norepinephrine potency}}$

[l]dopamine selectivity $= \dfrac{\text{dopamine potency}}{\text{norepinephrine potency}}$

C. **Drug selection.**   Important considerations in choosing an antidepressant drug are its relative sedative effect, anticholinergic effect, effect in seizure threshold, effects in cardiac function, and toxicity in overdose. Some drugs may produce unique side effects and may require special monitoring because of rare but potentially serious adverse reactions.

There is no objective method of determining in advance whether a patient will respond more favorably to treatment with one type of drug than to another. The most reliable indication for choice of a specific drug is a prior history of positive response to that drug. Although not conclusively established as a clinical fact, there is some evidence that some depressive subtypes, such as atypical depression or seasonal affective (mood) disorder, may respond better to MAOIs or fluoxetine. In cases of major depression, however, all drugs appear to be equally effective.

D. **Side effects.**   Available evidence shows that all currently available antidepressants are equally efficacious and possess a similar onset of action. Some, however, are appreciably more toxic when taken in overdose and are likelier to produce side effects. Most side effects are qualitatively similar among the drugs, but differ in frequency and/or severity. Some drugs produce idiosyncratic side effects (Table 22–28).

E. **Tricyclic antidepressants.**   Of the 7 available tricyclics, four (amitriptyline [Elavil], imipramine [Tofranil], trimipramine [Surmontil], and doxepin [Sinequan]) are called tertiary amine compounds because of the demethylated

TABLE 22–28. **SIDE EFFECTS OF ANTIDEPRESSANTS**

Anticholinergic
• Dry mouth
• Constipation
• Loss of visual accommodation
• Urinary retention
• Paralytic ileus (absent bowel sounds)
• Precipitation of narrow angle glaucoma
• Memory disturbances
• Central anticholinergic toxicity
—Confusion
—Disorientation
—Delirium
—Auditory and visual hallucinations
—Agitation
—Hyperpyrexia
—Concommitant anticholinergic symptoms

Sedative
• Fatigue
• Decreased energy
• Lassitude
• Hypersomnia

Cardiovascular*
Effects on heart rate, EKG, rhythm, and contractility
• Palpitations
• Mild tachycardia
• Delayed conduction (like quinidine, may be antiarrhythmic)
—Prolonged PR, QRS, and QT intervals
—Flattened T-waves
• Clinical significance
—Depends on underlying condition of cardiovascular system
—At therapeutic levels, negligible effect on mechanical performance
• Overdose
—QRS duration greater than 100 msec indicates severe toxicity
—Aggravation of existing conduction defects
• Special cautions
—Post-myocardial infarction when atroventricular (A-V) block develops
—Coadministration of quinidine, lidocaine, phenytoin, thyroid medication

Orthostatic hypotension
• About 20% of patients experience up to a 25 mm Hg reduction in systolic pressure
• Clinical predictor: pretreatment change greater than 15 mm Hg
• Greatest risk: elderly and patients with congestive heart failure
• Unrelated to dose or plasma level

Behavioral effects
• Mania, excitement, agitation
• Central anticholinergic syndrome
• Nervousness

Neurologic effects
• Tremor
• Paresthesias
• Peripheral neuropathy
• Parkinson's syndrome (with amoxapine)
• Generalized seizures
• Myoclonus

Effects on sleep
• Normalization of depressed sleep
—REM suppression
—Increased stage 4
—Reduced nocturnal awakening
• Interference with sleep
• Night terrors
• Nightmares
• Nocturnal myoclonus

Sexual disturbances
• Decreased libido
• Erectile and ejaculation dysfunction

Miscellaneous
• Weight gain
• Sweating
• Skin rash
• Flushing
• Agranulocytosis, leukopenia, eosinophilia

Withdrawal reactions
• (Occur within first postdrug week, last for several days)
• GI symptoms
• Anxiety
• Agitation
• Shakiness

Overdose
• Myoclonic jerks
• Agitation, delirium, coma
• Metabolic acidosis
• Hyperpyrexia, neuromuscular irritability, seizures
• Ophthalmopegia with intact pupillary responses
• Paralytic ileus
• Cardiovascular manifestations (hypotension, QRS prolongation, arrhythmia)
• Respiratory depression

*For details of cardiovascular effects of individual antidepressants, see Table 22–29.

terminal nitrogen in their side chain. As a group, the tertiary compounds produce significantly more sedation, dry mouth, constipation, and orthostatic hypotension than secondary amine tricyclics (nortriptyline [Pamelor], desipramine, and protriptyline [Vivactil]), those with monomethylated terminal nitrogens. Although the increased side-effect profile of the tertiary compounds makes them troublesome to use in depression, they are increasingly being used for other conditions. Doxepin, trimipramine, and amitriptyline, for example, are potent H_1- and H_2-receptor blockers, making them useful as antipruritic agents and in the treatment of gastric ulcer. It is worth remembering that the tricyclics were originally synthesized as antihistamines.

From a purely clinical perspective, two of the secondary amine tricyclics—nortriptyline and desipramine—represent better choices as first-line antidepressants than the tertiary compounds. They are markedly less sedating, have less anticholinergic activity, and are thus better tolerated by patients. Desipramine has the least anticholinergic effect of any tricyclic. Nortriptyline has been reported to produce less orthostatic hypotension in patients with congestive heart failure (Table 22–29).

TABLE 22–29 **CARDIOVASCULAR EFFECTS OF INDIVIDUAL ANTIDEPRESSANTS**

STANDARD TRICYCLICS
* Increased heart rate
* Slowed conduction as reflected by prolonged PR and QRS intervals
* Orthostatic hypotension a serious problem, particularly in patients with congestive heart failure (left ventricular function impaired)
* Less of a problem with nortriptyline than with other tricyclics

AMOXAPINE
* Slowed conduction at therapeutic dose
* Fatal in overdose due to heart block
* Orthostatic hypotension

MAPROTILINE
* Slowed conduction at therapeutic dose
* Fatalities in overdose due to heart block
* Orthostatic hypotension

TRAZODONE
* No effect on cardiac conduction at therapeutic doses
* No reported fatalities when taken alone in overdose
* Orthostatic hypotension
* Ventricular irritability (questionable)

FLUOXETINE
* Clinically insignificant decrease in heart rate by 3 beats/minute
* No change in PR and QRS intervals
* One reported fatality when taken alone in overdose
* No known effect in blood pressure or ventricular function
* Minimal anticholinergic, histaminergic, and alpha-adrenergic effects

BUPROPION
* Relatively free of cardiac side effects, with minimal effects in cardiac conduction
* No orthostatic hypotension

F. **Heterocyclic antidepressants.** The three cyclic antidepressants, amoxapine, maprotiline, and trazodone, are tricyclic compounds with minor structural modifications.

The tricyclics produce a broad spectrum of side effects, which are a frequent source of noncompliance. Roughly 25% of patients tolerate initial tricyclic therapy poorly.

The most subjectively distressing of the side effects are autonomic symptoms, such as dry mouth, constipation, and blurred vision; sweating and orthostatic hypotension; and behavioral and CNS symptoms, such as sedation, lethargy, agitation, and tremor. Other adverse effects that cause subjective distress include tachycardia, weight gain, and diminished sexual performance.

In morbidity and mortality, cardiovascular side effects cause the greatest concern. In addition to tachycardia, the tricyclics produce nonspecific ST-T changes, diminished T-wave amplitude, increased PR-QT intervals, and prolongation of QRS complex. In fact, tricyclics produce quinidine-like effects and are considered Type 1a antiarrhythmic drugs.

Although the cardiac effects of tricyclics present little risk to healthy patients, they can prove dangerous to patients with cardiac disease. The most serious risks are heart block and arrhythmias. It is standard practice to obtain an EKG in all patients before initiating tricyclic therapy.

Other side effects that need to be anticipated because of their potential severity are worsening of glaucoma; seizures; and triggering of mania, delirium, and agitation.

1. Amoxapine (Asendin). Amoxapine is an analog of loxapine, a potent antipsychotic drug. Amoxapine has clinically significant dopamine-blocking activity. Each 100 mg of amoxapine is equivalent to about 0.5–1.0 mg of haloperidol in antipsychotic activity. Thus, amoxapine appears to have dual activity in depressive and psychotic symptoms. This combined effect can be put to therapeutic use in cases of severe depression in which psychotic symptoms are present. Use of amoxapine can obviate the need for a separate antipsychotic and antidepressant.

Amoxapine has been shown to relieve symptoms rapidly in some patients, often at doses as low as 100 mg/day; the typical therapeutic dose range is 150–200 mg/day. Amoxapine has a short elimination half-life (8 hours) and should be taken in divided doses. Because it also blocks post-synaptic dopamine receptors, amoxapine produces a side-effect profile characteristic of antipsychotic drugs; specifically, it can produce akathisia, dystonia, acute dyskinesia, and tardive dyskinesia. The overall incidence of amoxapine-induced extrapyramidal symptoms is low, but physicians always should be alert to their emergence during treatment. Apart from its antipsychotic activity, amoxapine is similar to the more norepinephrine-selective drugs, particularly maprotiline and desipramine, in side effects.

2. Maprotiline (Ludiomil). Maprotiline is the most selective inhibitor of norepinephrine reuptake of currently marketed antidepressant drugs. It is structurally and pharmacologically similar to desipramine, the second most selective norepinephrine blocker. The only significant structural difference between the two compounds is a bridge across the central ring of amoxapine; this molecular alteration accounts for maprotiline's being termed a tetracyclic.

The major advantage of maprotiline is its mild to moderate degree of sedative and anticholinergic side effects. The most notable drawback of the drug is the increased incidence of seizures associated with its use. This higher incidence of seizures has been reported both at therapeutic doses and in overdose in patients without a prior history of seizure disorder. The risk of seizures is dose-related, a fact that warrants caution when the upper recommended dose of 225 mg/day is approached or exceeded. Caution should be used when discontinuing benzodiazepines in patients who are receiving maprotiline, because it may result in a lowered seizure threshold.

Maprotiline has an elimination half-life of 43 hours. Its long half-life may require an extended period of observation following an overdose.

3. **Trazodone (Desyrel).** Trazodone is a highly specific serotonin-reuptake blocker in vitro. Its therapeutic effects are due to its activity as a serotonin 2 (5HT-2) agonist. Its efficacy resembles the tricyclic antidepressants.

Cardiovascular effects of trazodone differ from those of the tricyclics. Generally, it produces a low incidence of cardiovascular effects owing to its lack of quinidine-like activity. However, trazodone has been shown to be arrhythmogenic, causing isolated premature ventricular contractions (PVCs), ventricular couplets, and short episodes (3–4 beats) of ventricular tachycardia.

It is suggested that trazodone be taken following a meal or light snack. When taken on an empty stomach, some patients experience dizziness. The incidence of dizziness with trazodone is about 6%.

Trazodone is safer than tricyclic antidepressants when taken alone in overdose. Taken with other CNS depressants and/or alcohol, however, the drug may have synergistic effects. It does not cause seizures in overdose.

About 1 in 800 male patients experience abnormal penile erections; most cases resolve spontaneously. If priapism develops, however, the patient shoud be directed to an emergency room, where treatment with intracorpeal epinephrine injections can be adminstered.

The most common side effect associated with trazodone use is sedation. About 10% of patients taking the drug report significant drowsiness. Many clinicians use trazodone as a hypnotic agent in patients who fail to respond to benzodiazepines or when there is concern about drug abuse. Trazodone is particularly useful in cases of depression with severe insomnia. It also is effective in treating insomnia caused by MAOIs.

G. **Serotonergic agents.** Fluoxetine offers several distinct advantages over the tricyclic agents in side effects and toxicity.

1. **Fluoxetine (Prozac).** Fluoxetine is a potent and relatively selective serotonin-reuptake inhibitor with antidepressant efficacy equivalent to that of the tricyclic antidepressant agents. It also possesses a highly favorable side-effect profile, causing little or no dry mouth, drowsiness, dizziness, excessive sweating, or constipation—side effects that are typical of the tricyclics. Because of its side-effect profile, fluoxetine use is associated with less likelihood of early treatment termination due to drug intolerance. The likelihood of an adequate therapeutic trial is thus increased.

Unique aspects of fluoxetine's side-effect profile include a propensity to cause weight loss rather than weight gain and alertness rather than sedation. To minimize possible sleep disruption, patients are advised to take fluoxetine in the morning. The most common side effects of fluoxetine are insomnia, nervousness, and nausea. These may remit after the first weeks of therapy.

Another unique aspect of fluoxetine is its demonstrated efficacy at a fixed dose of 20 mg/day. Patients initiate therapy at 20 mg/day and remain on that dose without escalation through the full course of treatment. Some patients may do better at a higher dose, but increasing the dose to 40 mg should not occur for at least 3–4 weeks and in many cases as long as 6–8 weeks. Fluoxetine has a half-life of about 3 days and has an active metabolite with a half-life of 7 days. In some cases, the drug can be taken every other day.

Fluoxetine may slightly decrease pulse rate. No significant changes are observed in mean PR, QRS, or QT duration, reflecting fluoxetine's lack of cardiac conduction effects. It does not cause orthostatic hypotension. Adverse cardiovascular effects have not been noted in cases of fluoxetine overdose.

Initial experience with fluoxetine suggests that it is effective in the atypical subgroup of depressions, including seasonal affective disorder. Studies are currently underway using fluoxetine to treat obsessive-compulsive disorder. This effect is independent of its antidepressant action. Because more than 80% of obsessive-compulsive patients experience concurrent depression, fluoxetine provides benefit for the mood disturbances as well.

Some clinicians express a hesitancy to use fluoxetine in depressed patients with anxiety or insomnia. As clinical experience has been gained, fluoxetine also appears to be equally effective in these patients. This demonstrates that sedation is not a necessary feature of antidepressants.

When considering all factors, efficacy, side effects, safety in overdose, and fixed-dose throughout treatment, fluoxetine may be considered an antidepressant drug of first choice.

H. Bupropion (Wellbutrin). Bupropion differs from other available antidepressants in that it has weak reuptake blocking effects on both serotonin and norepinephrine. Its most marked effect is neuronal reuptake of dopamine. The onset of antidepressant response is similar to other antidepressants requiring 2–3 weeks.

The side-effect profile of bupropion differs from that of standard antidepressants. A substantial proportion of patients experience some degree of increased restlessness, agitation, anxiety, and insomnia, especially at the start of treatment (these can be treated by sedative-hypnotic drugs). In only 2% of patients are these symptoms sufficiently severe to require discontinuation of bupropion.

The occurrence of generalized seizures in patients taking bupropion has been reported to be approximately 0.4%, a rate that may exceed that of other antidepressants. Therefore, bupropion is contraindicated in patients with a seizure disorder. Risk of seizure may be minimized if the total daily dose is under 450 mg/day; single doses should not exceed 150 mg.

Advantages of bupropion include the fact that it has no clinically significant effects on cardiac conduction or pulse rate and causes no significant orthostatic hypotension. It also produces few anticholinergic side effects, little or no weight gain, and little or no daytime drowsiness.

I. **Clinical use.** Effective use of antidepressant drugs begins with accurate diagnosis. Diagnosis is important for several reasons. Depression may be mistaken for an anxiety disorder or another condition. Some subtypes, such as atypical depression, may have better response to some drugs. Drug selection involves choosing the drug that presents the fewest risks and best side-effect profile considering a patient's overall medical status. Once depression has been established and a drug chosen, it is crucial to use adequate doses of medication. In most cases, this involves a least the equivalent of 225 mg/day of imipramine.

After a specific drug has been selected, the physician should have a clear treatment plan involving dosage, duration of the therapeutic trial, and alternative treatment strategies should the initial intervention fail. The physician should also assume an active role in communicating with the patient and family members.

Patients should have realistic expectations about therapeutic and adverse effects. Some depressed patients are reluctant to take medication, particularly if it is their first experience with acute depression. The 2-3 week lag in onset of clinical effects, coupled with troublesome side effects, often lead to discouragement and noncompliance. For these reasons, it is helpful to explain the likely time course of improvement, common side effects, and contingency treatments, if necessary. Encouragement and information, provided through frequent communication, can increase the likelihood of compliance and achievement of optimal therapeutic results.

With the exception of fluoxetine, to which most patients respond to a single fixed 20 mg dose throughout the course of treatment, all antidepressant treatment begins with a low test dose. The purpose of starting at lower doses is to determine drug tolerance and to minimize initial side effects. Dosage can be raised to about half the maximum recommended dose by the end of the first week (e.g., 150 mg of imipramine, 50 mg of nortriptyline). Patients stay on this dose until the end of the second treatment week. If there is no response at this point, the dose should be raised to the upper recommended limit.

Higher doses (e.g., 300 mg/day of imipramine) are more effective than lower doses. Up to 50% of patients treated with 200-225 mg/day of imipramine are found to have subtherapeutic blood levels. Lack of clinical response after 4 weeks of treatment is an indication for plasma-level monitoring. Because inadequate dosage is the most common cause of treatment failure, treating physicians should not hesitate to escalate the dosage to the highest tolerated level.

Because of their generally long half-lives, tricyclics can be given in a single bedtime dose.

Most patients who ultimately benefit from antidepressant medication show signs of improvement by the end of the third treatment week. A significant subgroup of patients who are unresponsive after 4 weeks of treatment show a positive response, however, when the antidepressant trial is extended to a sixth week.

There is no absolute rule on how long to continue antidepressant drug therapy after an acute depressive episode remits. Continuation therapy prevents relapse during the period of greatest risk (4–6 months following initial symptomatic recovery). Most experts recommend a 6–9 month course of therapy. During this period, the dose can be reduced by 25%.

The question of long-term maintenance therapy as a means of preventing future depressive episodes remains controversial. Some patients require chronic treatment, but there is little evidence that continuous antidepressant therapy prevents the onset of new episodes. Relapse or recurrence of depressive symptoms in patients treated successfully during an acute episode are about 30% at 1 year, 50% at 2 years, and 70% at 3 years.

Some patients fail to improve even after all appropriate dose and duration criteria have been met. For them, several options are available.

One strategy is to switch to another, chemically unrelated drug. For instance, a patient who has not responded to imipramine might be switched to fluoxetine, trazodone, or one of the MAOIs. Before switching to another drug, however, many psychiatrists prefer to augment the existing drug with a second compound, e.g., lithium and thyroid hormones. Tricyclics also can be combined (with caution) with MAOIs.

When lithium is used in such combination therapy, its dosage is generally 600–900 mg/day, or serum concentrations between 0.6 and 0.8 mg/L. A typical combination of tricyclics with thyroid hormones involves 25–50 mg/day of T_3 or 100 mg/day of T_4.

In some treatment-refractory cases, psychostimulants, alone or in combination with antidepressants, help alleviate depressive symptoms. Psychostimulants, such as amphetamine, may also be useful in patients who are unable to tolerate antidepressant drugs.

An ever-present risk in treating depression with medication is the possibility that the patient will use the drugs to attempt suicide. Many of the antidepressant drugs, particularly the tricyclic and heterocyclic compounds, are lethal in overdose, mainly because of their cardiac effects. In cases in which the risk of suicide is thought to be high and the patient is unable or unwilling to be hospitalized, fluoxetine or trazodone should be prescribed because of their relative safety in overdose.

J. **Monoamine oxidase inhibitors.** The MAOIs have been available for several decades, but concern about potential interactions with tyramine-containing food and stimulant drugs have deterred many clinicians from routinely prescribing them. Nevertheless, they are highly effective in treating depression and often benefit patients who have not responded to treatment with other classes of drugs. Use of MAOIs has increased in recent years mainly because of their effectiveness in treating panic disorder. Studies also suggest that MAOIs are more effective than tricyclics in the treatment of atypical depression, having a more pronounced effect in interpersonal sensitivity; the overall response rate in patients with atypical depression is 71% with MAOIs, 50% with tricyclics, and 28% with placebo.

Three MAOIs are currently prescribed: phenelzine (Nardil), tranylcypromine (Marplan), and isocarboxazid (Parnate). Although equal in general efficacy, it is commonly observed that patients who fail to respond to one MAOI do quite well when switched to another.

Hypertensive reactions may occur spontaneously but usually result from interactions between an MAOI and tyramine in food or sympathomimetic drugs. MAOIs should not be given to patients who cannot understand or comply with dietary and medication prescriptions. MAOIs should only be used as drugs of last resort in patients with asthma, who may need treatment with epinephrine during an attack.

MAOIs also may pose problems for patients undergoing procedures that require anesthesia or analgesia. They interact with narcotics to produce a potentially lethal syndrome characterized by agitation, fever, headache, seizures, and coma. They also may cause respiratory depression and coma. Meperidine (Demerol) has been implicated in fatal excitatory reactions. If analgesia is necessary, morphine may be used, but only if the dose is titrated and the patient closely monitored. Local anesthetics containing cocaine and epinephrine should be avoided.

Patients taking MAOIs should be given 50 mg tablets of chlorpromazine in the event they feel symptoms of an hypertensive crisis. Should this happen, immediate medical attention is warranted.

In cases of MAOI-related emergencies, chlorpromazine, phentolamine (Regitine), or other alpha-blocking agents are effective. Peripheral vasodilators also may prove useful.

MAOI therapy should be discontinued 3 weeks prior to elective surgery.

A major side effect of MAOIs is orthostatic hypotension. By comparison, the hypertensive reaction, which is the result of an interaction with certain foods or drugs, is rare. Almost all patients taking MAOIs experience postural hypotension. Other troublesome side effects include an inability to ejaculate or reach orgasm, paresthesias, anorexia, and pedal edema. Severe weight gain may occur with use of phenelzine.

Patients already on MAOIs should not be started on another type of antidepressant. Instead, a 2-week interval should separate the last dose of an MAOI and initiation of a tricyclic, cyclic, or serotonin-reuptake blocker therapy. Patients already on a tricyclic can be started on an MAOI; those on fluoxetine should not be switched directly to an MAOI, but should have a 2-week period without medication.

The currently used antidepressant drugs and their dose range are summarized in Table 22–30.

V. Antimanic drugs

A. Lithium.
Antipsychotic drugs are used in the treatment of mania to achieve rapid symptom control. ECT can also produce dramatic improvement of acute manic symptoms. The mainstay of treatment for mania, however, is lithium. It not only helps to control acute episodes of mania, but it also reduces the risk of relapse. Several anticonvulsants and calcium channel blockers can serve as alternatives to lithium.

Must have baseline thyroid function test, CBC, electrolytes, blood urea nitrogen/creatinine (BUN/Cr). If BUN/Cr are abnormal progress to 2-hour creatinine clearance and then to 24-hour creatinine clearance. Must follow with regular serum lithium levels, electrolytes (especially in patients also on diuretics). Must monitor thyroid and renal status—lithium can cause renal insufficiency, hypothyroidism, and, rarely, hyperthyroidism.

Renal clearance parallels sodium clearance; sodium depletion can cause toxic lithium levels; low therapeutic index; can cause leukocytosis; baseline EKG changes may include specifically flattening, isoelectricity, or inversion of T-waves. Also has been reported to be arrhythmogenic, as well as causing various conduction defects (speculation that lithium may substitute for intracellular potassium); may have antipsychotic

TABLE 22–30.   **DOSAGES OF ANTIDEPRESSANT DRUGS**

Class/Drug	Typical Therapeutic Dose (mg/day)
TRICYCLICS	
Amitriptyline (Elavil)	150–300
Desipramine (Norpramin)	150–300
Doxepin (Sinequan)	150–300
Imipramine (Tofranil)	150–300
Protriptyline (Vivactil)	15–30
Nortriptyline (Pamelor)	75–150
Trimipramine (Surmontil)	75–300
HETEROCYCLICS	
Amoxapine(Asendin)	200–300
Maprotiline (Ludiomil)	100–225
Trazodone (Desyrel)	300–600
SEROTONERGIC AGENTS	
Fluoxetine (Prozac)	20–80
*Clomipramine (Anafranil)	25–250
DOPAMINE REUPTAKE BLOCKER	
Bupropion (Wellbutrin)	300–450
MONOAMINE OXIDASE INHIBITORS	
Isocarboxazid (Marplan)	10–30
Phenelzine (Nardil)	30–90
Tranylcypromine (Parnate)	10–60

*Approved for treatment of obsessive-compulsive disorder.

activity; often used with antipsychotics for treatment of acute mania with psychotic features; direct antimanic effect may take up to 10–14 days.

1. **Lithium levels.** Draw sample 8–12 hours after last dose, usually in morning after bedtime dose; must measure level at least 2 times/week while stabilizing patient; half-life—22 hours, excreted in urine (95%).

2. **Therapeutic range.** 0.6–1.2 mEq/L for maintenance; 1.0–1.5 mEq/L for acute mania. (Some patients may respond at lower levels, whereas others may require higher levels—true therapeutic range may be wider, but a response at a level below 0.4 mEq/L is probably placebo).

B. **Other antimanic drugs.** Major new developments are the apparent usefulness of anticonvulsants and calcium channel blockers. The alpha-2 agonist clonidine (Catapres) has also been used.

1. **Anticonvulsants.** In general, anticonvulsants should be considered for use under the following circumstances: (1) inadequate response or intolerance with antipsychotics or lithium, (2) manic symptoms, (3) rapid cycling, (4) EEG abnormalities, and (5) head trauma.

2. The three most commonly used anticonvulsants are carbamazapine, valproic acid, and clonazepam.

   a. **Carbamazepine (Tegretol)** — structurally similar to the tricyclic antidepressants; FDA approved for use in treating complex partial seizures, tonic clonic seizures, and paroxysmal pain syndromes, such as trigeminal neuralgia and phantom limb pain.

      i. **Psychiatric uses.** (1) acute mania, (2) depression, (3) psychiatric symptoms secondary to seizure disorders, (4) acute exacerbations of schizophrenia (additive benefits with antipsychotics), (5) schizoaffective disorders, and (6) episodic dyscontrol syndromes.

ii. **Factors potentially predictive of antimanic response to carbamazepine:** (1) lithium nonresponders; (2) rapid cycling (more than four episodes/year; (3) more severely manic, depressed, anxious, or dysphoric patients; (4) more severely ill patients; (5) schizoaffective/psychotic features; (6) evidence of organic brain damage; and (7) subgroup with primarily manic episodes, no family history, or early onset.

iii. **Pharmacology.** Half-life—initially 3 days—12 hours or less at steady state; peak levels reached 6 hours after intake.

Metabolized almost exclusively by liver (90%) through P450 cytochrome system. Starting dose usually 200 mg BID—increased by 200 mg every few days as needed.

Therapeutic level 8–12 μg/mL.

iv. **Drug interactions**

(a) With all drugs also metabolized by P450 system.

(b) Phenytoin (Dilantin), phenobarbital, theophylline—decrease level of carbamazepine.

(c) Erythromycin, lithium, verapamil, INH, diltrazem, propoxyphene, cimetidine (Tagamet)—increase level of carbamazepine.

(d) Carbamazepine—decreases blood levels of clonazepam, haloperidol, tricyclic antidepressants, tetracycline, valproic acid, Warfarin (Coumadin), ethosuximide (Zarontin), octacalcium phosphates; increases blood levels of clomipramine, digitalis.

v. **Preliminary workup.** physical examination, CBC with differential if WBC is less than 4,000; liver function tests (LFTs); renal function tests; for first month, weekly CBCs; afterwards, every 3 months.

vi. **Contraindications.** WBC is less than 3,000; hematocrit less than 32%; red blood cells less than 4,000,000/cu mm; platelets less than 100,000/cu mm; hemoglobin less than 11 gm/100 mL.

vii. **Common side effects.** (1) mild leukopenia, (2) nausea and vomiting, (3) rash (about 10%), (4) diplopia, (5) sedation, (6) dizziness, and (7) ataxia.

viii. **Rare side effects.** (1) Stevens Johnson exfoliative dermatitis, (2) hepatitis, (3) aplastic anemia, (4) agranulocytosis, and (5) thrombocytopenia.

ix. **Other important interactions/side effects.** (1) lithium and carbamazepine—neurotoxicity; (2) slows intracardiac conduction and may worsen preexisting cardiac conduction disease; (3) antidiuretic properties—stimulates antidiuretic hormone (ADH) receptor function; (4) suppresses circulating levels of T_3 and T_4.

b. **Valproic acid (Depakene)** — FDA approved for use in treatment of (1) absence seizures, (2) myoclonic seizures, and (3) generalized tonic clonic seizures.

    i. **Uses in psychiatry.** (1) bipolar disorder and (2) schizoaffective disorder.

    ii. **Pharmacology.** Half-life about 8 hours; peak levels 1–4 hours after intake; metabolized by liver.

    iii. **Dose.** Starting dose about 250 mg 2 or 3 times/day; can increase every 2–3 days by 250 mg; usual dose range 750–3,800 mg; therapeutic level about 40–150 mg/mL.

    iv. **Common side effects.** Nausea (5%), sedation (5%), hand tremor, weight gain; asymptomatic transient dose dependent increase in LFTs.

    v. **Rare side effects.** Fatal hepatitis—showing an unclear relation to hepatic enzymes; seen in children on phenobarbitol with mental retardation/seizure disorder; rare disease in platelets or platelet dysfunction.

  c. **Clonazepam (Klonopin)** — FDA approved for treatment of (1) akinetic seizures, (2) myoclonic seizures, and (3) atypical absence seizures; also for infantile spasms.

    i. **Psychiatric uses.** (1) acute mania—doses of about 2–16 mg/day; (2) panic attacks—doses 3–6 mg/day; (3) drug withdrawal and detoxification from benzodiazepines; (4) Tourette's disorder; (5) unconfirmed antidepressant effects.

    ii. **Mechanism of action.** Unknown, but hypothesized to have three possible mechanisms: (1) potentiates serotonin synthesis, (2) potentiates γ-aminobutyric acid (GABA)ergic transmission, and (3) mimics neurotransmitter glycine.

    iii. **Pharmacology.** A 7 nitrobenzodiazepine derivative (in same class as diazepam); half-life—79 hours; peak levels—1–3 hours after intake.

       Starting doses about 0.5 mg 2 times/day; can increase by 0.5 mg every 3 days to usual maximum of 3–6 mg/day (higher in acute mania); metabolized by liver.

    iv. **Side effects.** (1) ataxia, (2) paradoxical behavior changes including disinhibition, and (3) drowsiness; less common—sexual dysfunction.

  d. **Verapamil (Calan, Isoptin)**

    i. **FDA approved** for treatment of (1) angina pectoris, (2) hypertension, and (3) some supraventricular tachyarrhythmias.

    ii. **(not FDA approved) Nonpsychiatriatric uses.** (1) migraines, (2) hypertropic cardiomyopathies, (3) dysmenorrhea, (4) Raynaud's disease, (5) insulinomas, (6) cerebral vasospasm following intracerebral bleed, and (7) premature labor.

    iii. **Other possible uses in psychiatry**

       (a) Depression—no controlled studies.

       (b) Anxiety—one anecdotal report.

       (c) Schizophrenia—one report.

    iv. **Pharmacology.** Half-life—5 hours; peak concentration—1–2 hours

after intake; metabolized by liver; need to decrease dose by 1/3 in patients with liver dysfunction.
   v. **Dose.** Starting dose 80 mg BID. Can increase by 80 mg every other day to range of approximately 320–480 mg (maximum) or until therapeutic benefit.
   vi. **Side effects.** (1) hypotension, (2) bradycardia, (3) dizziness, (4) nausea, and (5) headache.
   vii. **Contraindications.** (1) severe liver dysfunction, (2) less than 90 mm Hg systolic, (3) sick sinus syndrome, and (4) 2°, 3° A-V block.
   viii. **Interactions.** Decreased lithium level; studies show may be additively cardiotoxic with lithium; increases carbamazepine levels.

VI. Other drugs
A. **Beta blockers.** These medications have had many applications in other medical areas. The different agents have different degrees of action on beta-1 and beta-2 adrenergic receptors. They also have different degrees of lipid solubility that affect their centrally mediated effects, as well as side effects (most significantly, depression). Propranolol (Inderal), the most widely studied beta blocker, blocks both beta-1 and beta-2 receptors and is highly lipid soluble. Always be cautious in prescribing beta blockers to patients with asthma or cardiac disease.
   1. **Pharmacology**
   2. **FDA approved indications.** (1) hypertension, (2) angina, (3) some tachyarrhythmias, (4) symptoms of thyrotoxicosis, (5) glaucoma, and (6) prevention of migraine.
   3. **Psychiatric uses (not FDA approved)**
      a. Performance anxiety—stage fright—best effects with peripherally acting (less lipophilic) beta blockers (atenolol, nadolol).
      b. Treatment of lithium tremor.
      c. Neuroleptic-induced akathisia—usual doses of about 20–80 mg/day of propranolol or equivalent.
      d. Ethanol withdrawal (plus benzodiazepine)—control tremor, improve vital signs.
      e. Impulsive violence in patients with organic mental syndrome.
      f. Generalized anxiety and panic disorders—autonomic symptoms only—doses 40–320 mg/day of propranolol or equivalent.
   4. **Side effects**—hypotension, bradycardia, dizziness, depression, fatigue, nausea, and diarrhea.
B. **Clonidine (Catapres).** A centrally acting alpha-2 agonist; causes decreased central adrenergic output; used for hypertension.
   1. **Possible uses in psychiatry (not FDA approved)**
      a. **Opioid withdrawal**—suppresses autonomic symptoms; not effective in suppressing craving. Useful during withdrawal from methadone. Doses 0.1 mg BID or TID; taper with completion of withdrawal.
      b. **Tourette's disorder**—characterized by multiple motor and vocal tics developing in childhood.

Clonidine—alternative to haloperidol; may take 2–3 months for response; start at 0.5 mg/day.

c. **Mania**—for patients refractory to other more conventional treatments; doses 0.2–0.4 mg BID.

d. **Anxiety disorders**—inconclusive results.

e. **Neuroleptic induced akathesia**—doses 0.2–0.8 mg/day.

2. **Pharmacology.** Half-life—9 hours, given BID; peak concentration 1–3 hours after intake; very lipophilic—readily crosses blood-brain barrier; 50% metabolized in liver, 50% excreted unchanged by kidneys; slow taper to prevent rebound hypertensive crisis.

3. **Side effects.** Dry mouth, sedation, dizziness, nausea, impotence, fluid retention, synergistic with alcohol, vivid dreams and nightmares, insomnia, restlessness, depression, anxiety.

4. **Interactions.** With tricyclic antidepressants—decreased antihypertensive effect.

VII. Electroconvulsive therapy. ECT may be safer than tricyclic antidepressants for some patients. Usually reserved for patients who have failed other therapeutic attempts or for patients who are so acutely dangerous or suicidal that a course of pharmacotherapy might be too slow.

A. **Indications**

1. Major depression (any type).
2. Bipolar disorder—depressed.
3. Bipolar disorder—manic (only after a medication failure or if acutely dangerous).
4. Schizophrenia (this remains controversial)—nonchronic, acute, especially paranoid, catatonic, or with prominent affective symptoms.
5. Pregnancy—ECT often is the treatment of choice in pregnant patients who should not receive psychotropic drugs.

B. **Course.** ECT usually is given 3 times/week. Depressed patients usually require 6-10 treatments. Schizophrenic patients usually require 10-20 treatments. Each patient must be reassessed between treatments, and ECT should be stopped when there is no evidence of additional benefit from continuation.

1. ECT does not cure any illness but can induce remissions in an acute episode.
2. ECT should be combined with other treatments, e.g., medications and psychotherapy after a course of ECT has been completed.
3. ECT also may be used prophylactically to prevent recurrence.

C. **Side effects**

1. **Cardiac.** PVCs (through vagal hyperactivity); sympathetically mediated ventricular arrhythmias; side effects of succinylcholine (Anectidine)—hyperkalemia, direct cardiotoxicity of succinylcholine.

2. **Central nervous system.** Transient memory impairment—retrograde and anterograde (usually resolves in 1–2 weeks); headaches; prolonged seizures (these can be treated initially with an increased dose of anesthetic; if this fails, then treat as if status epilepticus); prolonged memory impairment—usually limited to events around the time of ECT, but may be

worse, especially in patients with preexisting cognitive deficits; brain herniation—may occur as a result of increased intracranial pressure from seizures in a patient with an undiagnosed brain tumor.

D. Medical workup. CBC, urinalysis, serum chemistry profile, chest x-ray, spinal x-rays (to document preexisting fractures or other abnormalities), EKG, optional computed tomography (CT) scan of head.

E. Pertinent history

1. Hypertension—antihypertensive patients may require dosage adjustments to compensate for elevated blood pressure during seizure. Nitroglycerine or propranolol often is given prophylactically in hypertensive patients.
2. Musculoskeletal injuries—require more muscle relaxants.
3. Taking reserpine or anticholinesterases—must stop for 1 week.
4. Lithium—some reports of increased cognitive impairment in patients treated with ECT while on lithium, so lithium is usually discontinued.
5. Tricyclic antidepressants—usually discontinued because of cardiovascular side effects.
6. Antipsychotics—usually continued because they decrease the seizure threshold and have few complicating effects.
7. MAOIs—no general consensus.
8. Drugs that raise the seizure threshold should be discontinued, e.g., anticonvulsants, benzodiazepines, lidocaine.

F. Preparing the patient

1. Informed consent.
2. Alternative treatments.
3. Side effects.
4. Convalescent period (usually 1–3 weeks under close supervision until cognitive deficits resolve).

G. Procedure. No food after midnight, may have liquid breakfast if ECT scheduled for after noon. Must have area prepared for cardioplumonary resuscitation and advanced cardiac life support. Should usually have an anesthesiologist or anesthetist. Must have someone adept at endotracheal intubation. Requires suction, EKG monitoring, and usually electroencephalogram (EEG) monitoring.

1. Anticholingerics. Atropine 0.5 mg IV until pulse increases by 10% (may also give IM 1/2 hour before treatment). Decreases risk of arrhythmias and aspiration.

2. Anesthesia. Usually use barbiturates, and dosage should be adjusted to minimum effective amount because higher dosages will increase the seizure threshold and prolong apneic period. Frequently used are:

a. Thiopental (Pentothal) 100–300 mg—has longer half-life than methohexital and may cause a desired postictal sedation.

b. Methohexital (Brevital) 30–160 mg—rapid, less cardiotoxic than thiopental.

c. Ketamine (Ketalar) can be used if seizures are too brief or if no seizure occurs when device is on maximum setting.

3. Muscle relaxants

a. Succinylcholine (Anectine) 40–80 mg—a competitive muscarinic agonist, which is displaced from the receptor slowly. Causes fasciculations initially and paralysis later. Half-life is increased by some antibiotics, quinidine, lithium, and phenelzine. A tourniquet applied to an extremity can be used to prevent distribution of muscle relaxant and allow the seizure to be observed in that extremity (especially if EEG monitoring is not available).

   b. Curare—a muscarinic antagonist, may be added if the patient complains of muscle pain. Curare will eliminate the fasciculations caused by succinylcholine.

4. Types of electrical stimuli
   a. Sine wave—delivers more energy and may cause more neurologic and cognitive side effects.
   b. Brief pulse—requires longer duration of stimulation but delivers less actual energy to brain tissue.

5. Electrode placement
   a. Bilateral—1–1.5 inches above midpoint between lateral canthus of eye and upper tragus of ear (estimate).
   b. Nondominant unilateral—same as bilateral for first electrode on nondominant side. Second electrode is placed slightly lateral to vertex, leaving 4–5 inches between electrodes.

TABLE 22–31.   **BILATERAL VERSUS UNILATERAL NONDOMINANT**

	Bilateral	Unilateral
Clinical response	Probably equal	
Number of treatments needed	Maybe less	Maybe more
Amnesia	Greater	Less
Persistent cognitive deficits	More likely	Less likely

Note: Always shave the area, remove debris and skin oil, and use an abrasive to improve skin adhesion. Also check electrode impedance to make sure it is as low as possible before administering stimulus. High impedance will require a larger stimulus and may cause skin burns.

6. Administering the stimulus
   a. Check vital signs (temperature, cardiac rhythm, blood pressure, pulse).
   b. Apply electrodes and make sure treatment bed is not grounded.
   c. Clear patient's mouth, remove hearing aids.
   d. Begin anesthesia (before muscle relaxants).
   e. Muscle relaxants.
   f. Ventilation.
   g. Apply bite block.
   h. Apply electrical stimulus.
   i. Induce a seizure between 35–80 seconds' duration (if direct EEG monitoring and the tourniquet test are not available, use seizure-induced tachycardia as a rough estimate).

   If three attempts are made during one period of anesthesia without an adequate seizure, stop and try again on the next scheduled day (usually

3 times/week) to avoid side effects of prolonged anesthesia and muscle relaxants.

7. **Relative contraindications.** (1) fever, (2) signifiicant arrhythmias, (3) extreme hypertension, (4) coronary ischemia.

8. **Monitoring**

a. EKG—expect sinus tachycardia, increased T-wave amplitude during seizure (also increased blood pressure).

b. EEG—anesthetic effect (increased amplitude slow and fast waves), epileptic recruiting rhythm, tonic phase (high-frequency polyspike), clonic phase (repetitive polyspike and wave), termination period.

VIII. Psychosurgery. Neurosurgical intervention to treat severe or incurable mental disorder. Frontothalamic tracts are severed. Reported to be useful in deteriorated schizophrenic patients or intractable obsession-compulsive disorders. Not a recommended treatment and rarely used in the United States today.

For more detailed discussion of this topic, see Grebb JA: Introduction and Overview, Sec. 31.1, pp 1574–1578; Gorman JM, Davis JM: Antianxiety Drugs, Sec. 31.2, pp 1579–1591; Davis JM, Barter JT, Kane JM: Antipsychotic Drugs, Sec. 31.3, pp 1591–1626; Davis JM, Glassman AH: Antidepressant Drugs, Sec. 31.4, pp 1627–1655; Jefferson JW, Griest JH: Lithium Therapy, Sec. 31.5, pp 1655–1662; Davis JM, Dysken MW: The Pharmacology of Psychotropic Drugs and Drug-Drug Interactions, Sec. 31.6, pp 1662–1670; Weiner RD: Electroconvulsive Therapy, Sec. 31.7, pp 1670–1678, in *CTP/V*.

23
Legal Issues

I. **General introduction.** From the perspective of the law, the clinical psychiatrist functions in two distinct contexts: (1) the treatment of the patient and (2) the performance of certain legal evaluations.

The treatment of the patient involves a relationship of trust that places specific duties and responsibilities on the treating psychiatrist, such as the duty to maintain confidentiality and to obtain informed consent.

Psychiatrists also are called on to perform evaluations for legal purposes, such as evaluations for involuntary commitment, evaluations related to various types of mental competency, and evaluations in the criminal justice system. In this respect, the psychiatrist acts as an expert consultant to the legal process.

A word of caution: The laws and regulations applicable to a specific psychiatric situation usually are determined by the cases and legislation in that particular state. These laws and regulations can change rapidly as new legislation is passed or new cases are decided. It is therefore strongly recommended that practitioners seek legal advice when there is uncertainty in psychiatric situations that raise legal issues.

II. **Legal issues in psychiatric practice**
   A. **Informed consent.** The doctrine of informed consent embodies respect for the patient's autonomy and arises whenever psychiatric treatment of any sort is being considered.

   Proper informed consent requires that the patient be informed about the particular treatment, alternative treatments, and their potential risks and benefits; that the patient understands this information; and that the patient freely and knowingly gives consent. The psychiatrist should document the patient's consent (preferably) with a signed form.

   There are a number of exceptions to the rules of informed consent:
   1. **Emergencies.** Usually defined in terms of imminent physical danger to the patient or others.
   2. **Therapeutic privilege.** Information that in the opinion of the psychiatrist would harm the patient or be antitherapeutic, may be withheld.
   B. **Confidentiality.** The therapeutic relationship itself gives rise to a legal and ethical duty of confidentiality. These derive from the Hippocratic Oath, which binds the physician to hold secret all information given to him/her by a patient. Breach of the legal duty of confidentiality can result in an action for damages for defamation, invasion of privacy, or breach of contract.

   A number of exceptions to the duty of confidentiality include the requirements to report (1) contagious diseases, (2) gun and knife wounds, and (3) child abuse.
   1. **The duty to warn.** For psychiatrists, the most important exception is the duty to warn, which was first created by the Tarasoff case (California, 1974). This case

requires psychotherapists to warn potential victims of their patient's expressed intention to harm the victim. In 1976, the Tarasoff II ruling required the therapist to take some action in the face of the threat of harm to another (the duty to protect).

2. **Release of information.** Consent by the patient for disclosure of information in a patient's record is required before the psychiatrist can release that information. The actual physical record is the legal property of the psychiatrist or the institution; however, the patient has the legal right to his/her psychiatric records. The psychiatrist may claim therapeutic privilege as noted above, but in this case, disclosure must be made to a representative of the patient, according to the particular law of the state, usually the patient's lawyer or advocate.

3. **Testimonial privilege.** Historically, the following relationships have given rise to testimonial privilege: (1) attorney—client, (2) priest—penitent, (3) husband—wife, and (4) physician—patient.

    Testimonial privilege protects the patient's right to privacy and belongs to the patient. The psychiatrist may not reveal information about patients against their will.

    Some exceptions to the doctrine of testimonial privilege are (1) hospitalization proceedings, (2) court-ordered examinations (military or civilian), (3) child custody hearings, and (4) malpractice claims.

C. Laws governing hospitalization

1. The power of the state (society) to confine an individual (legally known as commitment) is based on two separate concepts: (1) the police power of the state, to protect society for society's benefit. The issue here is the dangerousness of the individual. (2) the *parens patriae* power of the state, in which the needs of the individual are of concern. The issue here is the need for treatment.

2. **Types of admissions procedures.** Patients may be admitted to a psychiatric hospital in one of four ways:

    a. **Informal.** Entry into and release from the hospital may be requested orally. The patient may leave at any time, even against medical advice.

    b. **Voluntary.** Written application for admission with limitations placed on release—to allow for conversion into involuntary.

    c. **Involuntary.** Invokes profound limitations on patient's autonomy—strict limitations in procedures and patient rights. Patient may be danger to self (suicidal) or to others (homicidal).

    d. **Emergency.** A form of involuntary civil commitment, but usually an easier process. Patient cannot be hospitalized against his/her will for more than 15 days.

3. **Criteria for commitment.** Although specific criteria for commitment under the various categories differ across states, all require mental illness, in addition to dangerousness to self or others, need for care and treatment, or lack of judgment to care for themselves.

4. **Procedural safeguards.** Similarly, the requirements governing specific procedural safeguards that have been instituted to meet due process vary among states. These include (1) application requirements, (2) physician's evaluation, (3) patient's advocate, (4) judicial review, (5) limits on retention, and (6) notice of rights.

5. **Level of proof.** The level of proof required in commitment proceedings had been in dispute. Although the usual level of proof in civil cases, a "mere preponderance of the evidence," had been the rule, those wishing to limit the extent of involuntary civil commitment sought to have the criminal law level of proof, "beyond a reasonable doubt," applied. In *Addington v. Texas* (1979), the Supreme Court settled on an intermediary level, stating that the evidence supporting involuntary commitment had to be "clear and convincing."

6. **The right to treatment.** The right of an involuntarily committed patient to active

treatment has been enunciated by lower federal courts and enacted in some state statutes.

The principle case, *Wyatt v. Stickney*, was litigated (1972–1976) in the federal courts in Alabama and set the pattern of reform by requiring specific changes in the operations of institutions and their programs, including changes in the physical conditions, staffing, and quality of treatment provided.

The 1975 Supreme Court case of *Donaldson v. O'Connor* also is relevant. Rather than supporting a right to treatment, however, this case set forth what could be termed a right to freedom for involuntarily committed patients. It held than an individual involuntarily committed who is not dangerous and is capable of surviving by himself/herself or with help must be released from the hospital.

7. **The right to refuse treatment.** One of the most controversial legal issues in the practice of psychiatry today is the right to refuse treatment. To put this subject into perspective, most persons take the right to refuse treatment for granted. The question of a right to refuse treatment arises in the practice of psychiatry when the patient is of questionable competence to make the necessary decisions.

   a. **Status of the patient.** Only involuntary patients may be treated against their will.
   b. **Types of treatments.** Controversies exist in regard to medication and electro-convulsive therapy (ECT). Variables to be considered include the intrusiveness of the treatment, its irreversibility, its dangerousness, and its side effects.
   c. **Who decides?** In the past, the treating psychiatrist had the prerogative simply to order treatment, e.g., medication, in the face of a patient's objection. Subsequently, procedures were developed to obtain a second or third opinion of psychiatrists in the facility (a so-called administrative review). This is still the extent of the process in many states. Other patterns of decision making are emerging. For example:
      i. New Jersey requires that the opinion of an outside psychiatrist be obtained (*Rennie v. Klein*, 1979).
      ii. In Massachusetts, the court must appoint a guardian to consent to treatment (*Rogers v. Okin*, 1980).
      iii. New York requires a full judicial hearing after which the judge decides (*Rivers v. Katz*, 1987).
8. **Involuntary outpatient commitment.** This procedure, which has been adopted in a number of states, permits the immediate hsopitalization of an outpatient who becomes noncompliant with medications. As such, it has been found to be a useful adjunct to hospitalization and treatment in the community.

D. Malpractice

1. **Definition.** Literally denotes bad professional activity. More broadly, malpractice can be defined as occurrences in a professional practice that result in injury to the patient, which are the consequence of the psychiatrist's lack of care or skill.
2. A special type of legal negligence (there need not be an intention to hurt the patient).
3. Four elements must be proved in a malpractice case (known as the four Ds):
   a. **Duty.** A standard of care; a requirement to exercise a particular degree of skill and care. This duty is predicated on the existence of a professional, i.e., therapist-patient, relationship. There is no duty to cure. The standard of care is usually a national standard rather than a local one.
   b. **Dereliction.** A failure to exercise this care, i.e., a breach of this duty. Dereliction may be due to carelessness, incompetence, inappropriate treatment, or failure to obtain the proper consent.
   c. **Direct causation.** A direct, or proximate, causal relationship between the dereliction of duty and the damage to the patient. Sometimes phrased as "but for" the dereliction of the duty, the damage would not have occurred.

d. Damages. Some specific damage or injury to the patient must be proved.

4. Some common causes of malpractice lawsuits in psychiatry:

a. Suicide. The suicide of a psychiatric patient almost automatically raises the question of malpractice and is the most common basis of malpractice lawsuits in psychiatry. It is for this reason that careful documentation of the treatment of a suicidal patient is necessary.

b. Improper somatic therapy. The negligent administration of medications or ECT is the second largest source of malpractice lawsuits in psychiatry. Tardive dyskinesia and fractures, respectively, are the concerns.

c. Negligent diagnosis. Although this is a relatively rare basis for a lawsuit, there are signs that it may be used when there is a failure to properly assess a patient's dangerousness.

d. Sexual activity with patient. An area of increasing concern, it is now a crime in a number of states. Sexual activity with a patient has been deemed unethical in the American Psychiatric Association (APA) ethical annotations and has been found to be a breach of contract as well as malpractice.

e. Informed consent. The alleged failure of the psychiatrist to obtain proper informed consent is often the underlying basis of the malpractice lawsuit.

III. Legal issues in psychiatry and civil law

A. General introduction

1. Criminal law and civil law. As the guarantor of public safety, the criminal law pits the state against the individual. Fairness in the criminal law requires that the individual's rights become a focus of attention.

In civil law matters, in which individuals are arrayed against each other, the law's concern with fairness relates to maintaining the relative equality of parties before the law.

2. Mental competency. Psychiatrists often are called on to give an opinion about an individual's psychological capacity or competency to perform certain civil, legal functions, e.g., to make a will, to manage one's financial affairs.

Competency is context related, i.e., the ability to perform a certain function for a particular legal purpose. It is especially important to emphasize that incompetency in one area does not imply incompetency in any or all other areas.

B. Contracts.

When a party to an otherwise legal contract is seriously mentally ill at the time the contract was made, and this condition directly and adversely affected the person's ability to "understand what he/she was doing," (his/her "contractual capacity"), the law may void the contract.

In other words, if the person's competency (his/her "capacity to consent") was adversely affected by his/her mental illness, the law may provide relief from the requirements of the contract.

The psychiatrist must evaluate the condition of the party seeking to void the contract at the time that the contract was supposedly entered into. The psychiatrist must then render an opinion whether the psychological condition of the party caused the incapacity to understand the important aspects or ramifications of the contract.

C. Wills.

The criteria concerning wills, termed testamentary capacity, are whether at the time of the making of the will, the testator was capable of knowing, without prompting, (1) the nature of the act he/she is making,

(2) the nature and extent of his/her property, and (3) the natural objects of his/her bounty and their claims on him/her, e.g., heirs, relatives, family members.

The mental health of the testator also will indicate whether he/she was in such a condition as to be subject to undue influence.

D. Marriage. Marital capacity in the eyes of the law is similar to contractual capacity. A marriage may be void or voidable if one of the parties was incapacitated due to mental illness such that he/she could not make a legal marriage contract in that he/she was "unable to understand, in a reasonable manner, the nature and consequences of the transaction, i.e., consent to the marriage."

E. Guardianship. Guardianship, an area that will become increasingly important, also may be regarded as an aspect of contractual capacity. It involves a court proceeding for the appointment of a guardian if there is a formal adjudication of incompetence. The criteria are whether, by reason of mental illness, the individual can manage his/her own affairs.

IV. Legal issues in child and adolescent psychiatry

A. Involuntary commitment of minors. In a landmark decision, *Parham v. J.R.* (1979), the U.S. Supreme Court held that minors may be "voluntarily" committed to a psychiatric facility by their parents or guardians. Parents, the Supreme Court said, should "retain a substantial if not dominant role" in the commitment decision.

However, while minors may be "voluntarily" committed to a psychiatric facility by their parents or guardians, such civil commitment of juveniles now requires various procedural safeguards. In *Kremens v. Bartley* (1977), the Supreme Court held that civil commitment of juveniles requires the constitution's safeguards, including the right to counsel.

Once committed, housing and treatment must be adequate, and in *Morales v. Turman* (1977), the Supreme Court added that inadequate housing or lack of treatment for committed juveniles is unconstitutional.

B. Consent of minors. The principles of informed consent noted above apply, except that the issue of competency turns on the state's legal definition of minority for the particular issue involved.

An emancipated minor is usually one who is married or financially independent. For particular situations, usually related to contracts, the emancipated minor is treated as an adult.

Controversy surrounds matters of abortion and contraceptive services. At what age is the young woman entitled to contraceptive and/or abortion services without the knowledge or consent of her parents? The Supreme Court seems to support the right of parents to know about abortion.

C. Custody. The increasing divorce rate has led to a substantial increase in number of cases of contested custody.

Recently, it has become almost universally accepted that in cases of disputed custody, the criterion is "the best interests of the child." In this context, the task of the psychiatrist is to provide an expert opinion and supporting data as to which party by being granted custody will best serve the interests of the child.

The mental disability of a parent can lead to the transfer of custody to the other parent or to a public agency. When the mental disability is chronic and the parent is incapacitated, a procedure for the termination of parental rights may result. This also is the case when evidence of child abuse is pervasive.

Matters relating to juveniles often are determined in Family Court. In the Gault decision (1967), the Supreme Court held that a juvenile also has constitutional rights to due process and procedural safeguards, such as counsel, jury, and trials.

V. Legal issues in psychiatry and the criminal law

A. Competency to stand trial. At any point in the criminal justice process, the psychiatrist may be called on to assess a defendant's present competency: to be arraigned, to be tried, to take a plea, to be sentenced, even to be executed. The criteria for competency to be tried are whether, in the presence of a mental disorder, the defendant (1) understands the charges against him/her and (2) can assist in his/her defense. The principles underlying these requirements relate to the striving for fairness (in the prohibition against trials in absentia) and the dignity of the judicial process.

The U.S. Supreme Court has set out a number of further standards. In the case of *Dusky v. U.S.* (1960), the court held that the criteria for competency to stand trial require more than a mere orientation and some recall of the event. The defendant must be able to consult with his/her lawyer "with a reasonable degree of rational understanding" and have a "rational as well as factual understanding of the proceedings against him." In *Pate v. Robinson* (1966), it held that the psychiatric examination for competency to stand trial is a constitutional right. Finally, in *Jackson v. Indiana* (1972), the court held that a permanently incompetent individual (in this case, a retarded deaf mute) must be discharged from the criminal justice system.

B. Criminal responsibility (the insanity defense). The legal issues of competency to stand trial and criminal responsibility (the insanity defense) are different in a number of respects and must not be confused. In contrast to competency to stand trial, the question of criminal responsibility involves a time in the past during which the criminal act was committed. The outcomes are different: finding of incompetency to stand trial usually only delays the legal proceedings, whereas a successful insanity plea results in exculpation in the form of a verdict of "not guilty by reason of insanity." The underlying philosophical principles are different: competency to stand trial involves the integrity of the judicial process, whereas criminal responsibility relates to moral blameworthiness. In contrast to the criteria for competency to stand trial, the criteria for criminal responsibility involve two separate aspects: whether, at the time of the act, as a consequence of mental disorder, the defendant (1) did not know what he/she was doing or that it was wrong (a cognitive test) or (2) could not conform his/her conduct to the requirements of the law (a volitional test).

Because states vary concerning the criteria used, and some are attempting to abolish the insanity defense altogether, it is especially important to determine the rule in each particular state.

The most famous set of criteria for the insanity defense were developed by the House of Lords after the defendant was exculpated in the M'Naghten case (England, 1843) for killing Sir Robert Peel. The M'Naghten rule states that the defendant is to be acquitted if "at the time of the committing of the act, the party accused was laboring under such a defect of reason, from disease of the mind, as not to know the nature and quality of the act he was doing, or, if he did know it, that he did not know he was doing what was wrong." The M'Naghten rule, therefore, also is a cognitive test.

Dissatisfaction with the limitations of the M'Naghten rule led Judge D. Bazelon of the Federal District Court in Washington, D.C., to enunciate the so-called product test in the case of *Durham v. U.S.* (U.S. Federal Court, 1954). The product test states that "an accused is not criminally responsible if his unlawful conduct was the product of mental disease or defect." Because this test placed too much power in the hands of the testifying psychiatrist, it never gained popularity and eventually was overruled.

Dissatisfaction with the limits of the cognitive test also gave rise to the irresistible impulse test, which eventually was embodied in the volitional test of the American Law Institutes (ALI) Penal Code. The ALI rule has been adopted in a substantial number of states. The criteria for legal insanity set out in this rule is that "a person is not responsible for criminal conduct if at the time of such conduct he lacks substantial capacity either to appreciate the criminality (wrongfulness) of his conduct [this section is known as the 'cognitive' prong of the ALI test] or to conform his conduct to the requirements of the law." This section is known as the "volitional" prong of the ALI test.

To prevent the inclusion of the psychopath (known today as the antisocial personality disorder), the ALI rule adds: "As used in this article, the terms, 'mental disease or defect' do not include an abnormality manifested only by repeated criminal or otherwise antisocial conduct."

The ALI rule was used in the *John Hinckley case* (U.S. Federal Court, 1983). Hinckley's acquittal raised a storm of protest. It seemed clear that the jury had decided that although Hinckley knew what he was doing when he attempted to murder President Reagan, he could not control himself, so they acquitted him by means of the volitional prong of the test. In response to powerful political demands, both the APA and the American Bar Association recommended a return to the M'Naghten rule, i.e., the cognitive test only. The American Medical Association went so far as to recommend abolishing the insanity defense altogether.

C. Correctional psychiatry.   The psychiatrist providing treatment in a jail or a prison is subject to the same legal and ethical duties as his/her colleagues. However, in what usually are oppressive surroundings and overcrowded conditions with scarce resources, providing adequate psychiatric care is a challenge.

Correctional psychiatry presents special problems in relation to divided loyalties, confidentiality, and countertransference.

VI. Conclusion.   Implicit in this brief summary of the legal issues in the practice of psychiatry is that when dealing with such matters, the psychiatrist is playing on the legal court—on the lawyer's turf, so to speak. Care and caution are required and, again, when there is any doubt, seek a consultation.

For more detailed discussion of this topic, see Gutheil TG: Legal Issues in Psychiatry, Sec. 49.1, pp 2107–2124; Winslade WJ: Ethics in Psychiatry, Sec. 49.2, pp 2124–2131, in *CTP/V*.

24

Laboratory Tests in Psychiatry

I. General introduction. No psychiatric diagnosis can be made exclusively on the basis of a laboratory test. Laboratory tests are used to (1) screen for medical illnesses, (2) assist in making diagnoses, (3) determine whether a treatment can be given, and (4) evaluate toxic and therapeutic effects of a treatment.

Occult medical problems may present initially as psychiatric syndromes. For example, thyroid disease and other endocrinopathies may present as a mood disorder or psychosis; cancer may present as depression; and infection and connective tissue diseases may present as acute changes in mental status. In addition, a range of organic mental or neurologic conditions may present initially to the psychiatrist. These include multiple sclerosis, Parkinson's disease, Alzheimer's disease, Huntington's chorea, acquired immune deficiency syndrome (AIDS) dementia, and temporal lobe epilepsy, among others. Any suspected medical/neurologic condition should be thoroughly evaluated with appropriate laboratory tests and consultation.

The initial evaluation must always include a thorough assessment of prescribed and over-the-counter medications that the patient is taking. Many psychiatric syndromes can be iatrogenically caused by medications—for example, depression due to antihypertensives, delirium due to anticholinergics, and psychosis due to steroids. Often, if clinically possible, a washout of medications may help in diagnosis. Below are three tables of medications and/or conditions associated with depression or psychosis.

II. Screening tests for medical illnesses (Tables 24–1, 24–2, and 24–3).

TABLE 24–1. **MAJOR MEDICAL CAUSES OF PSYCHOSIS**

Endocrinopathy	Drug-Related
Thyroid	Adrenergic psychosis
Hypothyroidism	Sympathomimetic drugs
Thyrotoxicosis	Sedative-hypnotic drug withdrawal
Corticosteroid	Anticholinergic psychosis
Cushing's disease	Hallucinogen-induced
Addison's disease	Iatrogenic
Iatrogenic	Expected side effect
	Dose-related effect
Alcohol-Related	Idiosyncratic drug reaction
Intoxication states	
Withdrawal states	
Chronic alcoholism organicity	

Table from Sternberg DE: Testing for physical illness in psychiatric patients. J Clin Psych 47:3, supplement, 1986, with permission.

TABLE 24–2. **MEDICAL DISEASES ASSOCIATED WITH DEPRESSION**

Endocrinopathies and Metabolic Disorders Hyperthyroidism Hypothyroidism Addison's disease Cushing's disease Diabetes Hyperparathyroidism Hypoglycemia	Cancer Carcinoma of the head and pancreas Central Nervous System disorders Parkinson's disease Cerebral arteriosclerosis Senile dementia Normal pressure hydrocephalus Focal lesions of the nondominant lobe Subarachnoid hemorrhage
Viral infections Influenza Hepatitis Viral pneumonias	Disabling Diseases of All Kinds Postsurgical Procedures
Rheumatoid Arthritis Systemic Lupus Erythomatosus	Metal Intoxications Thallium Mercury

Table from Sternberg DE: Testing for physical illness in psychiatric patients. J Clin Psych 47:3, supplement, 1986, with permission.

TABLE 24–3. **DRUGS COMMONLY ASSOCIATED WITH DEPRESSION**

Class and Generic Name	Trade Name
Antihypertensives	
Reserpine	Serpasil, Ser-Ap-Es, Sandril
Methyldopa	Aldomet
Propranolol hydrochloride	Inderal
Guanethidine sulfate	Ismelin sulfate
Hydralazine hydrochloride	Apresoline hydrochloride
Clonidine hydrochloride	Catapres
Antiparkinsonian Agents	
Levodopa	Dopar, Laradopa
Levodopa and carbidopa	Sinemet
Amantadine hydrochloride	Symmetrel
Hormones	
Estrogen	Evax, Menrium
Progesterone	Lipo-Lutin, Prolution
Corticosteroids	
Cortisone acetate	Cortone acetate
Antituberculosis	
Cycloserine	Seromycin
Anticancer	
Vincristine sulfate	Oncovin
Vinblastine sulfate	Verban

Table from Sternberg DE: Testing for physical illness in psychiatric patients. J Clin Psych 47:3, supplement, 1986, with permission.

A. **Outpatients.** For routine outpatient psychotherapy, no specific tests are needed, but obtain a good medical history and order tests if indicated. Suspected organicity warrants a neurologic consultation. For medications, see below.

B. **Inpatients.** Rule out organic causes for the psychiatric disorder. A thorough screening battery of laboratory tests given on admission may detect a significant amount of morbidity.

1. Routine admission workup
  a. Complete blood count (CBC) with differential.
  b. Complete blood chemistries (including electrolytes, glucose, calcium, magnesium, hepatic and renal function tests).
  c. Thyroid function tests (TFTs).
  d. Rapid plasma reagin (RPR) or Venereal Disease Research Laboratory (VDRL).
  e. Urinanalysis.
  f. Urine toxicology screen.
  g. Electrocardiogram (EKG).
  h. Chest x-ray (for patients over 35).
  i. Plasma levels of any drugs being taken, if appropriate.

III. Medications. Before prescribing any psychotropic medication, take a detailed medical history, noting a previous response to specific drugs, family response to specific drugs, allergic reactions, renal or hepatic disease, and glaucoma (for any drugs that have anticholinergic activity).

A. Benzodiazepines. No special tests needed before prescribing benzodiazepines, although liver function tests (LFTs) are often useful. These drugs are metabolized in liver by either oxidation or conjugation. Impaired hepatic function will increase the elimination half-life of benzodiazepines that are oxidized, but it will have less effect on benzodiazepines that are conjugated (oxazepam [Serax], lorazepam [Ativan], and temazepam [Restoril]). Benzodiazepines also can precipitate porphyria.

B. Antipsychotics. No special tests needed, although it is good to have baseline LFTs and CBC. Antipsychotics are metabolized primarily in the liver, with metabolites excreted primarily in urine. Many metabolites are active. Peak plasma level usually 2–3 hours after oral dose. Elimination half-life is 12–30 hours, but may be much longer. Steady state requires at least 1 week at a constant dose (months at a constant dose of depot antipsychotics). With the exception of clozapine (Clozaril), all antipsychotics acutely cause elevation in serum prolactin (due to tuberoinfundibular activity). A normal prolactin level often indicates either noncompliance or nonabsorption.

Side effects include leukocytosis, leukopenia, impaired platelet functioning, mild anemia (both aplastic and hemolytic), and agranulocytosis. Bone marrow and blood element side effects can occur abruptly even when dosage has remained constant. Low-potency antipsychotics are most likely to cause agranulocytosis, which is the most common bone marrow side effect. They also can cause EKG changes (not as frequently as with tricyclic antidepressants), including prolonged QT interval; flattened, inverted, or bifid T-waves; and U-waves. Large differences among patients in dose/plasma level relationships. High plasma levels probably offer no clinical benefit and increase risk of side effects.

Side effects include hypotension, sedation, lowering of the seizure threshold, anticholinergic effects, tremor, dystonia, cogwheel rigidity, rigidity without cogwheeling, akathisia, akinesia, rabbit syndrome, and tardive dyskinesia.

C. Cyclic antidepressants. Must have baseline EKG and at least annual follow-up EKGs—heart block is a relative contraindication. Baseline LFTs and CBC are useful. TFTs also necessary because thyroid disease may present as depression. Also, antidepressants can have synergistic effects with thyroxine. Side effects include bone marrow depression, neurologic (anticholinergic, in particular), hepatic, gastrointestinal, dermatologic, platelet dysfunction and other blood element side effects, and lowering of the seizure threshold. Orthostatic hypotension—a very common and possibly dangerous side effect—no tolerance develops to this. Nortriptyline (Pamelor, Aventyl) less likely to cause hypotension than imipramine (Tofranil), desipramine (Norpramin), and amitriptyline (Elavil). Congestive heart failure considerably increases risk of hypotension. Patients with congestive heart failure who develop hypotension from tricyclic antidepressants should be treated with nortriptyline. Toxic EKG changes include prolonged PR interval ($>$ .2 sec.), prolonged QRS interval ($>$ .12 sec.), prolonged QT interval ($>$ ⅓ of R-R), sinus tachycardia (often due to hypotension), and heart block (of all kinds—more likely in patients with preexisting conduction defects—site of effect thought to be intraventricular bundle). At therapeutic levels, tricyclic antidepressants usually suppress arrhythmias, including premature ventricular contractions (PVCs), bigeminy, and ventricular tachycardia (V-tach) by quinidine-like effect.

Note: Trazodone (Desyrel), an antidepressant unrelated to the cyclic antidepressants, has been reported to cause ventricular arrhythmias, particularly in patients with underlying cardiac disease. Trazodone also has been associated with priapism, mild leukopenia, and neutropenia.

D. Monoamine oxidase inhibitors (MAOIs). Must record normal blood pressure (BP) and follow BP during treatment because MAOIs can cause hypertensive crisis if tyramine-restricted diet is not followed. MAOIs also often cause orthostatic hypotension (direct drug side effect unrelated to diet). Recommend baseline TFTs. Relatively devoid of other side effects, although some patients may have insomnia or become irritable. May induce mania.

E. Lithium.
1. Must have baseline TFTs, CBC, electrolytes, serum blood urea nitrogen/creatinine (BUN/Cr).
2. If serum BUN/Cr are abnormal, progress to 2-hour creatinine clearance and then to 24-hour creatinine clearance.
3. Must follow with regular serum lithium levels, electrolytes, especially in patients also on diuretics.
4. Must monitor thyroid and renal status—lithium can cause renal insufficiency, hypothyroidism, and rarely hyperthyroidism.
5. Renal clearance parallels serum sodium (Na^+).
6. Sodium depletion can cause toxic lithium levels.
7. Low therapeutic index.
8. Can cause leukocytosis.
9. Baseline EKG recommended. Lithium can cause reversible acute EKG changes, specifically flattening, isoelectricity, or inversion of T-waves. Also has been reported to be arrhythmogenic as well as causing various conduction defects (speculation that lithium may substitute for intracellular potassium).

10. May have antipsychotic activity.
11. Often used with antipsychotics for treatment of acute mania with psychotic features.
12. Direct antimanic effect may take up to 10–14 days.
13. Lithium levels
    a. Draw sample 8–12 hours after last dose usually in AM after bedtime dose.
    b. Must measure level at least 2 times/week while stabilizing patient.
    c. Half-life = 22 hours, excreted in urine (95%).
14. Therapeutic range
    a. 0.6–1.2 mEq/L for maintenance.
    b. 1.0–1.5 mEq/L for acute mania. (Some patients may respond at lower levels, others may require higher levels—true therapeutic range may be wider, but a response at a level below 0.4 mEq/L is probably placebo response).

IV. Laboratory Tests
A. Dexamethasone suppression test (DST)
1. Procedure
   a. Give dexamethasone 1 mg orally at 11 PM.
   b. Measure plasma cortisol at 4 PM and 11 PM the next day (may also take 8 AM sample).
   c. Any plasma cortisol > 5 mcg/dL is abnormal (although normal range should be adjusted according to the local assay so that 95% of normals are within the normal range).
   d. Baseline plasma cortisol may be helpful.
2. Indications
   a. To help confirm diagnostic impression of major depression. If a patient is clinically depressed and has an abnormal DST, then somatic treatment is required.
   b. To follow a depressed nonsuppressor through treatment of depression.
   c. To differentiate major depression from minor dysphoria.
   d. Some evidence that depressed nonsuppressors are more likely to have positive response to treatment with electroconvulsive therapy (ECT) or tricyclic antidepressants.
   e. Proposed utility in predicting outcome of treatment, but DST may normalize before depression resolves.
   f. Proposed utility in predicting relapse in patients who are persistent nonsuppressors or whose DSTs revert to abnormal.
   g. Possible utility in differentiating delusional from nondelusional depression.
   h. Highly abnormal plasma cortisol results (>10 mcg/dL) are more significant than mildly elevated levels.
   i. False-positives—dementia, anorexia nervosa, bulimia nervosa, alcohol or barbiturate use, anticonvulsant treatment (particularly carbamazepine [Tegretol]), tricyclic antidepressant withdrawal, benzodiazepine withdrawal, recent weight loss, acute psychosis, diabetes mellitus, advanced age.

   j. Sensitivity of DST—45% in major depression; 70% in psychotic mood disorders.
   k. Specificity of DST—90% compared with controls; 77% compared with other psychiatric diagnoses overall.

B. Thyrotropin releasing hormone (TRH) stimulation test. Used to help diagnose hypothyroidism.
1. Procedure.
   a. At 8 AM after an overnight fast, have patient lie down and explain that the patient may feel urge to urinate after the injection.
   b. Measure baseline thyroid stimulating hormone (TSH) and T_3, T_4, T_3 resin uptake.
   c. Inject 500 mcg of TRH intravenously.
   d. Measure TSH at 15, 30, 60, and 90 minutes.
2. Indications
   a. Marginally abnormal thyroid tests or suspicion of subclinical hypothyroidism.
   b. Suspected lithium-induced hypothyroidism.
   c. Detection of patient who may require T_3 and tricyclic antidepressant.
   d. Can often detect incipient hypothyroidism of which depression is often the first symptom.
   e. 8% of all depressed patients have some thyroid illness.
3. Results
   a. If TSH changes by:
      i. more than 35 mIU/mL → Positive
      ii. between 20–35 mIU/mL → Early hypothyroidism
      iii. less than 7 mIU/mL → Blunted (may correlate with diagnosis of depression).
   b. Peak TSH should reach about double the baseline value in normals, i.e., 7–20 mIU/mL.
   c. Does not distinguish well between hypothalamic and pituitary disease.

C. Polysomnography
1. Measures many aspects of sleep: EKG, electroencephalogram (EEG), electrooculography (EOG), electromyography (EMG), chest expansion, penile tumescence, blood oxygen saturation, body movement, body temperature, galvanic skin response (GSR), gastric acid.
2. Indications—to assist in the diagnosis of
   a. Sleep disorders—insomnias, hypersomnias, parasomnias, sleep apnea, nocturnal myoclonus, and bruxism.
   b. Childhood sleep-related disorders—functional enuresis, somnambulism (sleepwalking), and sleep terror disorder (pavor nocturnus).
   c. Other disorders—impotence, seizure disorders, migraine and other vascular headaches, drug abuse, gastroesophageal reflux, and major depression.
   d. Comments
      i. Correlation between decreased rapid eye movement (REM) latency and major depression, with degree of decreased REM latency correlating with degree of depression.

ii. Shortened REM latency as a diagnostic test for major depression seems to be slightly more sensitive than DST.

iii. Use with DST and/or TRH stimulation test can improve sensitivity. Preliminary data indicate that depressed DST nonsuppressors show extremely high rate of having shortened REM latency.

3. Polysomnographic findings in major depression
   a. Most depressed patients (80–85%) show hyposomnia.
   b. Depressed patients have decreased slow wave (delta wave) sleep and shorter sleep stages 3 and 4.
   c. Depressed patients have a shortened time between onset of sleep and onset of the first REM period (REM latency).
   d. Depressed patients have a greater percentage of their REM sleep early in the night (the opposite is true for nondepressed controls).
   e. Depressed patients have been found to have more REMs over the entire night (REM density) than nondepressed controls.

D. Electroencephalography (EEG)

1. First clinical application was by the psychiatrist Hans Berger in 1929.
2. Measures voltages between electrodes placed on skin.
3. Gives gross description of electrical activity of central nervous system (CNS) neurons.
4. Each individual's EEG is unique, like a fingerprint.
5. For decades, researchers have attempted to correlate specific psychiatric conditions with characteristic EEG changes but have been unsuccessful.
6. Changes with age.
7. Normal EEG does not rule out seizure disorder or organic disease; yield is higher with sleep-deprived studies and also with nasopharyngeal leads.
8. Uses
   a. General organic mental syndrome (OMS) workup.
   b. Part of routine workup for any first-break psychosis.
   c. Can diagnose specific seizure disorders.
   d. Helpful in diagnosing CNS lesions—space-occupying lesions, vascular lesions, and encephalopathies, among others.
   e. Characteristic changes caused by specific drugs.
   f. EEG is exquisitely sensitive to drug changes.
   g. Diagnose brain death.
9. EEG Waves
   a. Beta 14–30 Hz. (cycles per second)
   b. Alpha 8–13 Hz.
   c. Theta 4–7 Hz.
   d. Delta 0.5–3 Hz.
10. Grand mal seizures. Onset characterized by epileptic recruiting rhythm of rhythmic synchronous high-amplitude spikes between 8–12 Hz. After 15–30 seconds, spikes may become grouped and may be separated by slow waves (correlates with clonic phase). Finally, a quiescent phase of low amplitude delta (slow) waves.
11. Petit mal seizures. Sudden onset of bilaterally synchronous generalized spike and wave pattern with high amplitude and characteristic 3 Hz frequency.

E. Lactate provocation of panic attacks

1. Indications
   a. Possible diagnosis of panic disorder.
   b. Lactate-provoked panic confirms presence of panic attacks.
   c. Up to 72% of panic patients will have a lactate-provoked attack.
   d. Has been used to induce flashbacks in patients with post-traumatic stress disorder.
2. Procedure
   a. Inject a 5% dextrose in water solution intravenously slowly for 28 minutes, then rapidly for 2 minutes.
   b. Infuse 0.5 M racemic sodium lactate (total 10 mL/kg of body weight) over a 20-minute period or until panic occurs.
3. Physiologic changes from lactate infusion include hemodilution, metabolic alkalosis (metabolized to bicarbonate), hypocalcemia (Ca bound to lactate), and hypophosphatemia (due to increased glomerular filtration rate [GFR]).
4. Comments
   a. Effect is a direct response to lactate or its metabolism and occurs peripherally.
   b. Simple hyperventilation has not been as sensitive in inducing panic attacks.
   c. Lactate-induced panic is not blocked by peripheral beta blockers, but is blocked by alprazolam (Xanax) and by tricyclic antidepressants.
   d. CO_2 inhalation precipitates panic attacks, but mechanism is thought to be central and related to CNS concentrations of CO_2, possibly as a locus ceruleus stimulant (CO_2 crosses blood-brain barrier [BBB] while bicarbonate does not).
   e. Lactate crosses BBB via an easily saturated active transport system.
   f. L-lactate is metabolized to pyruvate.

F. Amytal interview   (amobarbital—a medium half-life barbiturate with a half-life of 8–42 hours).

1. Diagnostic indications—catatonia; hysterical stupor; unexplained muteness; differentiating functional and organic stupors (organic conditions should worsen, and functional conditions should improve because of decreased anxiety).
2. Therapeutic indications (as an interview aid for disorders of repression and dissociation):
   a. Abreaction of post-traumatic stress disorder.
   b. Recovery of memory in psychogenic amnesia and fugue.
   c. Recovery of function in conversion disorder.
3. Procedure
   a. Have patient recline in an environment in which cardiopulmonary resuscitation is readily available should hypotension or respiratory depression develop.
   b. Explain to patient medication should help him/her to relax and feel like talking.
   c. Insert narrow-bore needle into peripheral vein.
   d. Inject 5% solution of sodium amytal (500 mg dissolved in 10 cc of sterile water) at a rate no faster than 1 cc/minute (50 mg/minute).

    e. Conduct interview using frequent suggestion and beginning with neutral topics. Often helpful to prompt patient with known facts about his/her life.

    f. Continue infusion until either sustained lateral nystagmus or drowsiness is noted.

    g. To maintain level of narcosis, continue infusion at a rate of 0.5–1.0 cc/ 5 minutes (25–50 mg/5 minutes).

    h. Have patient remain in reclining position for at least 15 minutes after interview is terminated and until patient can walk without supervision.

    i. Use the same method every time to avoid dosage errors.

  4. Contraindications

    a. Presence of upper respiratory infection or inflammation.

    b. Severe hepatic or renal impairment.

    c. Hypotension.

    d. History of porphyria.

    e. Barbiturate addiction.

G. Tricyclic levels. Should be routine when using imipramine, desipramine, or nortriptyline in the treatment of depression. Levels must also include measurement of active metabolites:

$$\text{imipramine} \rightarrow \text{desipramine}$$
$$\text{amitriptyline} \rightarrow \text{nortriptyline}$$

These assays are difficult and are measuring extremely low concentrations. Active metabolites could contaminate results. Reported data collected only on inpatients with nondelusional endogenous depression.

  1. All tricyclics show complete gastrointestinal absorption, high degree of tissue and plasma protein binding, large volume of distribution, hepatic metabolism with prominent first-pass effect, plasma level directly correlated to brain level when at steady-state.

    a. Imipramine (Tofranil)

      i. Favorable response correlates with plasma level in a linear manner between 200–250 ng/mL.

      ii. Some patients may respond at a lower level.

      iii. At levels >250 ng/mL, there is no improved favorable response and side effects increase.

    b. Nortriptyline (Pamelor)

      i. Therapeutic window (therapeutic range) between 50–150 ng/mL.

      ii. Decreased response rate at levels over 150 ng/mL.

    c. Desipramine (Norpramin)

      i. Levels >125 ng/mL correlate with higher percentage of favorable response.

    d. Amitriptyline (Elavil)

      i. Different studies with conflicting results.

  2. Some patients are unusually poor metabolizers of tricyclic antidepressants and may have levels as high as 2,000 ng/mL while taking normal dosages. These patients may show a favorable response only at these extremely high levels, but must be monitored very closely for cardiac side effects. Other patients have been reported with extremely high plasma levels at normal dose who did not respond until the level was maintained somewhere between the usual therapeutic dose and their extremely high levels.

3. Procedure. Draw blood specimen 10–14 hours after most recent dose. Usually, this is in the morning after a bedtime dose. Patient must have been on a stable daily dose for at least 5 days. Use an appropriate specimen container.

4. Indications
   a. Routine for patients receiving imipramine, desipramine, or nortriptyline.
   b. Poor response at a normal dose.
   c. High-risk patient for whom you want to maintain the lowest possible therapeutic level.

H. Antipsychotic levels

1. In general, plasma level does not correlate with clinical response.
2. Possible correlation between high plasma levels and toxic side effects (especially with chlorpromazine [Thorazine] and haloperidol [Haldol]).
3. Minimum therapeutic levels may be determined in the future but have been difficult to establish because of wide individual variation.
4. Radioreceptor assays measure serum dopamine blockade activity and can account for active metabolites, but correlation with brain dopamine blockade is unclear.
5. No known relationship between antipsychotic levels and tardive dyskinesia.
6. Conclusions
   a. Generally only useful to detect noncompliance or nonabsorption (but prolactin levels can also help).
   b. May be useful in identifying the nonresponder.
   Table 24–4 lists therapeutic and toxic blood levels for various drugs.

TABLE 24–4. **THERAPEUTIC AND TOXIC BLOOD LEVELS**

Drug	Therapeutic Level	Toxic Level
Amitriptyline	>120 ng/mL	500 ng/mL
Bromide	20–120 mg/dL	150 mg/dL
Carbamazepine	8–12 μg/mL	15 μg/mL
Desipramine	>125 ng/mL	500 ng/mL
Imipramine	200–250 ng/mL	500 ng/mL
Lithium	0.6–1.5 mEq/L	2.0 mEq/L
Meprobamate	10–20 μg/mL	30–70 μg/mL
Nortriptyline	50–150 ng/mL	500 ng/mL
Phenobarbital	15–30 μg/mL	40 μg/mL
Phenytoin	10–20 μg/mL	30 μg/mL
Primidone	5–12 μg/mL	15 μg/mL
Propranolol	40–85 ng/mL	>200 ng/mL
Valproic acid	50–100 μg/mL	200 μg/mL

I. Brain Imaging

1. **Computed Tomography (CT) Scan** (formerly computerized axial tomography [CAT] scan)
   a. Clinical indications—dementia/depression, general OMS workup, and routine workup for any first break psychosis.
   b. Research
      i. Differentiating subtypes of Alzheimer's disease.

ii. Cerebral atrophy in alcohol abusers.

iii. Cerebral atrophy in benzodiazepine abusers.

iv. Cortical and cerebellar atrophy in schizophrenia.

v. Increased ventricle size in schizophrenia.

2. **Magnetic resonance imaging (MRI)** (formerly nuclear magnetic resonance)

a. Measures radiofrequencies emitted by different elements in the brain following application of an external magnetic field and produces slice images.

b. Measures structure, not function.

c. Technique has been available to other sciences for 30 years.

d. Much higher resolution than CT scan, particularly in grey matter.

e. No radiation involved; minimal or no risk to patients from strong magnetic fields.

f. Can image deep midline structures well.

g. Does not actually measure tissue density; measures density of particular nucleus being studied.

h. A major problem is time needed to make a scan (5–40 minutes).

i. May offer information about cell function in the future, but stronger magnetic fields are needed.

j. The ideal technique for evaluating multiple sclerosis and other demyelinating diseases.

3. **Positron emission tomography (PET) scan**

a. Positron emitters, e.g., carbon-11 or fluorine-18, are used to label glucose, amino acids, neûrotransmitter precursors, and many other molecules—particularly high-affinity ligands, e.g., N-methylspiperone—which are used to measure receptor densities.

b. Can follow the distribution and fate of these molecules.

c. Produces slice images like CT scan.

d. Labeled antipsychotics, e.g., N-methylspiperone, can map out location and density of dopamine receptors.

e. It has been shown that dopamine receptors decrease with age (through PET scans).

f. Can assess regional brain function and blood flow.

g. 2-Deoxyglucose (a glucose analog) is absorbed into cells as easily as glucose, but is not metabolized. Can be used to measure regional glucose uptake.

h. Measures brain function and physiology.

i. Potential for developing understanding of brain functioning and sites of action of drugs.

j. Research

i. Usually compare laterality, antero-posterior gradients, and cortical-subcortical gradients.

ii. Findings reported in schizophrenia

(a) Cortical hypofrontality (was also found in depressed patients).

(b) Steeper subcortical to cortical gradient.

(c) Decreased uptake in left compared with right cortex.

    (d) Higher activity in left temporal lobe.

    (e) Lower metabolism in left basal ganglia.

    (f) Higher density of dopamine receptors (only one study, which was not replicated).

    (g) Higher increase in metabolism in anterior brain regions in response to unpleasant stimuli, but this finding not specific to patients with schizophrenia.

4. Brain electrical activity mapping (BEAM)

  a. Topographic imaging of EEG and evoked potentials (EPs).

  b. Shows areas of varying electrical activity in the brain through scalp electrodes.

  c. New data processing techniques produce new ways of visualizing massive quantities of data produced by EEG and EP.

  d. Each point on the map is given a numerical value representing its electrical activity.

  e. Each value is computed by linear interpolation among the three nearest electrodes.

  f. Some preliminary results show differences in schizophrenic patients. EPs differ spatially and temporally; increased asymmetric beta wave activity in certain regions; increased delta wave activity, most prominent in frontal lobes.

5. Regional cerebral blood flow (rCBF)

  a. Yields a two-dimensional cortical image, which represents blood flow to different brain areas.

  b. Blood flow believed to correlate directly with neuronal activity.

  c. Xenon-133 (low energy gamma-ray emitting radioisotope) is inhaled—crosses BBB freely but is inert.

  d. Detectors measure rate at which Xenon-133 is cleared from specific brain areas and compare to calculated control yielding a mean transit time for the tracer.

    i. Gray matter—clears quickly.

    ii. White matter—clears slowly.

  e. rCBF may have great potential in studying diseases that have a decrease in the amount of brain tissue, e.g., dementia, ischemia, atrophy.

  f. Highly susceptible to transient artifacts, e.g., anxiety → hyperventilation → low pCO_2 → high CBF.

  g. Test is fast, equipment relatively inexpensive ($140,000).

  h. Low radiation.

  i. Compared with PET, has less spatial resolution but better temporal resolution.

  j. Preliminary data show that schizophrenic patients may have decreased dorsolateral frontal lobe and increased left hemisphere CBF when activated, e.g., Wisconsin Card-Sorting Test.

  k. No differences found in resting schizophrenic patients.

  l. Still under development.

6. Single photon emission computed tomography (SPECT)

  a. Adaptation of rCBF techniques to obtain slice tomograms rather than two-dimensional surface images.

b. Presently can get tomograms at 2, 6, and 10 cm above and parallel to the canthomeatal line.

V. Other laboratory tests. Laboratory tests listed in Table 24–5 have application for clinical and research psychiatry. The reader is directed to a standard textbook of medicine to determine laboratory values. Always know the normal values of the particular laboratory performing the test, because those values vary from one laboratory to another. Two types of measurements currently are in use—the conventional and the Système International (SI) units. The latter, now the more commonly accepted, is an international language of measurement calculated by multiplying the conventional unit by a number factor being adopted by many laboratories. The SI measurement system uses *moles* as the basic unit for the amount of a substance, *kilograms* for its mass, and *meters* for its length. Conversion factors are listed on Table 24–6. Drugs of abuse that can be tested in urine are listed in Table 24–7.

TABLE 24–5. **OTHER LABORATORY TESTS**

Test	Major Psychiatric Indications	Comments
Acid phosphatase	Organic workup	Increased in prostate cancer, benign prostatic hyperplasia, excessive platelet destruction, bone disease
Adrenocorticotropic hormone (ACTH)	Organic workup	May be increased in seizures, psychoses, Cushing's disease or in response to stress. Decreased in Addison's disease
Alanine aminotransferase (ALT) (formerly called serum glutamic pyruvic transaminase [SGPT])	Organic workup	Increased in hepatitis, cirrhosis, liver metastases Decreased in pyridoxine (vitamin B_6) deficiency
Albumin	Organic workup	Increased in dehydration Decreased in malnutrition, hepatic failure, burns, multiple myeloma, carcinomas
Aldolase	Eating disorders Schizophrenia	Increased in patients who abuse ipecac, e.g., bulimic patients (secondary to myopathy), schizophrenia (60–80%)
Alkaline phosphatase	Organic workup Use of psychotropic medications	Increased in Paget's disease, hyperparathyroidism, hepatic disease, hepatic metastases, heart failure, phenothiazine use Decreased in pernicious anemia (vitamin B_{12} deficiency)
Serum amylase	Eating disorders	May be increased in bulimia nervosa, pancreatitis
Aspartate aminotransferase (AST) (formerly SGOT)	Organic workup	Increased in heart failure, hepatic disease, pancreatitis, eclampsia, cerebral damage, alcoholism Decreased in pyridoxine (vitamin B_6) deficiency or terminal stages of liver disease
Serum bicarbonate	Panic disorder Eating disorders	Decreased in hyperventilation syndrome and panic disorder May be elevated in patients with bulimia nervosa, in laxative abuse, and in psychogenic vomiting
Bilirubin	Organic workup	Increased in hepatic disease
Blood urea nitrogen (BUN)	Delirium Use of psychotropic medications	Elevations associated with lethargy, delirium. If elevated, can increase toxic potential of psychiatric medications, especially lithium and amantadine
Serum bromide	Dementia Psychosis	Bromide intoxication can cause psychosis, hallucinations, delirium. Part of dementia workup, especially when serum chloride is elevated
Serum caffeine levels	Anxiety	Evaluation of patients with suspected caffeinism

TABLE 24–5. OTHER LABORATORY TESTS (Continued)

Test	Major Psychiatric Indications	Comments
Serum calcium (Ca)	Organic workup Mood disorders Psychosis Eating disorders	Increased in hyperparathyroidism, bone metastases Increase associated with delirium, depression, psychosis Decreased in hypoparathyroidism, renal failure. Decrease associated with depression, irritability, delirium, chronic laxative abuse
Carotid ultrasound	Dementia	Occasionally included in dementia workup, especially to rule out multi-infarct dementia. Primary value is in search for possible infarct etiologies
Cerebrospinal fluid (CSF)	Organic workup	Increased protein and cells in infection, positive VDRL in neurosyphilis, bloody CSF in hemorrhage conditions
Serum chloride (CL)	Eating disorders Panic disorder	Decreased in patients with bulimia and psychogenic vomiting Mild elevation in hyperventilation syndrome and panic disorder
Cholecystokinin (CCK)	Eating disorders	Compared with controls, blunted in bulimic patients after eating meal (may normalize after treatment with antidepressants)
CO_2 inhalation Sodium bicarbonate infusion	Anxiety, panic disorder	Panic attacks produced in subgroup of patients
Direct and indirect Coombs test	Hemolytic anemias secondary to psychotropic medications	Evaluation of drug-induced hemolytic anemias, such as those secondary to chlorpromazine, phenytoin, levodopa, and methyldopa
Serum ceruloplasmin Serum copper	Organic workup	Low in Wilson's disease (hepatolenticular disease)
Urine copper	Organic workup	Elevated in Wilson's disease
Cortisol (hydrocortisone) (see DST)	Organic workup Mood disorders	Excessive level may indicate Cushing's disease, anxiety, depression, and a variety of other conditions
Creatinine phosphokinase (CPK)	Use of antipsychotics Use of restraints Substance abuse	Increased in neuroleptic malignant syndrome, intramuscular injection, rhabdomyolysis (secondary to substance abuse), patients in restraints, patients experiencing dystonic reactions; asymptomatic elevations seen with use of antipsychotics
Creatinine	Organic workup Substance abuse Lithium use	Increased in renal failure, dehydration; rhabdomyolysis secondary to substance abuse (cocaine, heroin, phencyclidine [PCP]). Part of pretreatment workup for lithium
Dopamine (DA) (L-dopa stimulation of dopamine)	Depression	DA inhibits prolactin. Test used to assess functional integrity of dopaminergic system, which is impaired in Parkinson's disease, depression

TABLE 24–5. OTHER LABORATORY TESTS (Continued)

Test	Major Psychiatric Indications	Comments
Doppler ultrasound	Impotence Organic workup	Carotid occlusion in OMS/transient ischemic attack (TIA), reduced penile blood flow in impotence
Nocturnal penile tumescence tests (NPTs)	Impotence	Quantification of penile circumference changes, penile rigidity, frequency of penile tumescence Evaluation of erectile function during sleep. Erections associated with REM sleep. Helpful in differentiation between organic and functional causes of impotence
Echocardiogram	Panic disorder	10–40% of patients with panic disorder show mitral valve prolapse.
Electroencephalogram (EEG)	Organic workup	Seizures, e.g., petit mal, brain death, lesions; shortened REM latency in depression. High-voltage activity in stupor; low-voltage fast activity in excitement; in functional nonorganic cases, e.g., dissociative states, alpha activity is present in the background, which responds to auditory and visual stimuli. Biphasic or triphasic slow bursts seen in dementia of Creutzfeldt-Jakob disease
Epstein-Barr virus (EBV) Cytomegalovirus (CMV)	Organic workup Chronic fatigue Mood disorders	Part of herpes virus group. EBV is causative agent for infectious mononucleosis, which can present with depression and personality change. CMV can produce anxiety, confusion, mood disorders. EBV associated with chronic mononucleosis-like syndrome associated with chronic depression and fatigue. May be association between EBV and major depression
Erythrocyte sedimentation rate (ESR)	Organic workup	An increase in ESR represents a nonspecific test of infectious, inflammatory, autoimmune, or malignant disease
Serum folate (folic acid)	Alcohol abuse Use of specific medications	Usually measured with vitamin B_{12} deficiencies associated with psychosis, paranoia, fatigue, agitation, dementia, and delirium. Associated with alcoholism, use of phenytoin, oral contraceptives, and estrogen
Follicle stimulating hormone (FSH)	Depression	High normal in anorexia nervosa; higher values in postmenopausal women; low in patients with panhypopituitarism
Serum glutamyl transaminase	Alcohol abuse Organic workup	Increase in alcohol abuse, cirrhosis, liver disease
Fasting blood glucose (FBS)	Panic attacks Anxiety Delirium Depression	Very high FBS associated with delirium. Very low FBS associated with delirium, agitation, panic attacks, anxiety, depression

TABLE 24–5. **OTHER LABORATORY TESTS (Continued)**

Test	Major Psychiatric Indications	Comments
Growth hormone (GH) test	Depression Schizophrenia	Blunted GH responses to insulin-induced hypoglycemia in depressed patients. Increased GH responses to dopamine agonist challenge in schizophrenic patients
Hematocrit (HCT) Hemoglobin (HG)	Organic workup	Assessment of anemia (anemia may be associated with depression and psychosis)
Hepatitis A viral antigen (HAAg)	Mood disorders Organic workup	Less severe, better prognosis that hepatitis B—may present with anorexia, depression
Hepatitis B surface antigen (HBsAg) Hepatitis Bc antigen (HBcAg)	Mood disorders Organic workup	Active hepatitis B infection indicates greater degree of infectivity and of progression to chronic liver diease. May present with depression
Holter monitor	Panic disorder	Evaluation of panic disordered patients with palpitations and other cardiac symptoms
17-Hydroxycorticosteroids	Depression	Deviations detect hyperadrenocorticism, which can be associated with major depression
17-Ketosteroids	Depression	(see above)
5-Hydroxyindoleacetic acid (5-HIAA)	Depression Suicide Violence	Decrease in CSF in aggressive or violent patients with suicidal or homicidal impulses; may be indicator of decreased impulse control and predictor of suicide
Serum ferritin	Organic workup	Most sensitive test for iron deficiency
Serum iron	Organic workup	Iron deficiency anemia
Human immunodeficiency virus (HIV)	Organic workup	CNS involvement: AIDS dementia, organic personality disorder, organic mood disorder, acute psychosis
Lactate dehydrogenase (LDH)	Organic workup	Increased in myocardial infarction, pulmonary infarction, hepatic disease, renal infarction, seizures, cerebral damage, megaloblastic (pernicious) anemia, factitious elevations secondary to rough handling of blood specimen tube
Lupus erythematosis (LE) Test Antinuclear antibody test (ANA) AntiDNA antibodies	Depression Psychosis Delirium Dementia	Positive test associated with Systemic LE which may present with various psychiatric disturbances, such as psychosis, depression, delirium, and dementia
Lupus anticoagulant (LA)	Use of phenothiazines	An antiphospholipid antibody, which has been described in some patients using phenothiazines, especially chlorpromazine
Lutenizing hormone (LH)	Depression	Lower in patients with panhypopituitarism; decrease associated with depression

TABLE 24–5.　OTHER LABORATORY TESTS (Continued)

Test	Major Psychiatric Indications	Comments
Serum magnesium	Alcohol abuse Organic workup	Decreased in alcoholism; low levels associated with agitation, delirium, seizures
Platelet MAO	Depression	Low in depression
MCV (mean corpuscular volume) = (average volume of a red blood cell)	Alcohol abuse	Elevated in alcoholism
3-Methoxy-4-hydroxyphenyglycol (MHPG); Breakdown product of norepinephrine	Depression Anxiety	Most useful in research; decreases in urine may indicate decreases centrally
Heavy metal intoxication, serum or urinary	Organic workup	Lead—apathy, irritability, anorexia, confusion Mercury—psychosis, fatigue, apathy, decreased memory, emotional lability, "mad hatter" Manganese—"Manganese madness" Aluminum—dementia Arsenic—fatigue, blackouts, hair loss
Urine myoglobin	Phenothiazine use Substance abuse Use of restraints	Increased in neuroleptic malignant syndrome, in PCP, cocaine, or lysergic acid diethylamide (LSD) intoxication, and in patients in restraints
Parathyroid (parathormon) hormone test	Anxiety Organic workup	Low level causes hypocalcemia and anxiety. Dysregulation associated with wide variety of organic mental disorders
Serum phosphorous	Organic workup Panic disorder	Increased in renal failure, diabetic acidosis, hypoparathyroidism, hypervitamin D; decreased in cirrhosis, hypokalemia, hyperparathyroidism, panic attack, hyperventilation syndrome
Platelet count	Use of psychotropic medications	Decreased by certain psychotropic medications (carbamazepine, clozapine, phenothiazines)
Serum potassium (K)	Organic workup Eating disorders	Increased in hyperkalemic acidosis; increase is associated with anxiety in cardiac arrhythymia Decreased in cirrhosis, metabolic alkalosis, laxative abuse, diuretic abuse; decrease is common in bulimic patients and in psychogenic vomiting
Porphyria synthesizing enzyme test	Psychosis Organic workup	Acute panic attack or OMS can occur in acute porphyria attacks which may be precipitated by barbiturates, imipramine, benzodiazepines
Porphobilinogen (PBG)	Organic workup	Increased in acute porphyria

Test	Indication	Description
Serum prolactin	Use of antipsychotic medications	Antipsychotics, by decreasing dopamine, increase prolactin synthesis and release, especially in women
	Cocaine use	Elevated prolactin levels may be seen secondary to cocaine withdrawal
	Pseudoseizures	Lack of prolactin rise after seizure suggests pseudoseizure
Serum protein, total	Organic workup	Increased in multiple myeloma, myxedema, lupus. Decreased in cirrhosis, malnutrition, overhydration
	Use of psychotropic medications	Low serum protein can result in greater sensitivity to conventional doses of protein-bound meds (lithium is not protein-bound)
Prothrombin time (PT)	Organic workup	Elevated in significant liver damage (cirrhosis)
Reticulocyte count (estimate of red blood cell production in bone marrow)	Organic workup	Low in megaloblastic or iron deficiency anemia, as well as anemia of chronic disease
Serum salicylate	Organic hallucinosis	Toxic levels may be seen in suicide attempts and may cause organic hallucinosis
	Suicide attempts	
Serum sodium (Na^+)	Organic workup	Increased with excessive salt ingestion. Decreased in hypoadrenalism, myxedema, congestive heart failure, diarrhea, polydypsia, use of carbamazepine
	Use of lithium	Low levels associated with greater sensitivity to conventional dose of lithium
Serum testosterone	Impotence	May be decreased in organic workup of impotence
	Inhibited sexual desire	Decrease may be seen with inhibited sexual desire
Urinalysis	Organic workup	Provides clues to etiology of various OMSs (assessing general appearance, pH, specific gravity, bilirubin, glucose, blood, ketones, protein, etc.)
Venereal Disease Research laboratory (VDRL)	Syphilis	Positive (high titers) in secondary syphilis (may be positive or negative in primary syphilis). Lower titers (or negative) in tertiary syphilis
Serum vitamin A	Depression	Hypervitaminosis A is associated with variety of mental status changes
	Delirium	
Serum vitamin B_{12}	Organic workup	Part of workup of megaloblastic anemia and dementia. B_{12} deficiency associated with psychosis, paranoia, fatigue, agitation, dementia, delirium.
	Dementia	Associated often with chronic alcohol abuse
White blood cell (WBC)	Use of psychotropic medications	Leukopenia and agranulocytosis associated with certain psychotropic medications, such as phenothiazines and carbamazepine. Leukocytosis associated with lithium and neuroleptic malignant syndrome

TABLE 24–6. **CONVERSION FACTORS**

1 gram	=	1,000 milligrams (mg)
1 milligram (mg)	=	1,000 micrograms (μg)
1 microgram (μg)	=	1,000 nanograms (ng)
Blood levels:		
1 microgram per mL	=	100 micrograms per dL
	=	1 milligram per liter
	=	1,000 nanograms per mL
100 mg per dL	=	0.1 gram per dL
	=	1,000 mg (1 gram) per liter
	=	1.0 mg per mL

TABLE 24–7. **DRUGS OF ABUSE THAT CAN BE TESTED IN URINE**

Drug	Length of Time Detected in Urine
Alcohol	7–12 hours
Amphetamine	48 hours
Barbiturate	24 hours (short acting)
	3 weeks (long acting)
Benzodiazepine	3 days
Cocaine	6–8 hours (metabolites 2–4 days)
Codeine	48 hours
Heroin	36–72 hours
Marijuana (THC)	3 days–4 weeks (depending on use)
Methadone	3 days
Methaqualone	7 days
Morphine	48–72 hours
Phencyclidine (PCP)	8 days
Propoxyphene	6–48 hours

For more detailed discussion of this topic, see Kirch DG: Medical Assessment and Laboratory Testing in Psychiatry, Sec. 9.7, pp 525–533, in *CTP/V*.

25
Acquired Immune Deficiency Syndrome (AIDS)

I. General considerations. AIDS was first reported in 1981. In the United States, over 100,000 active cases of AIDS have already been diagnosed. The human immunodeficiency virus type 1 (HIV-1) has been implicated as the causal agent of AIDS. Estimates place the number of Americans infected with this virus at 1–2 million, with most of these persons predicted to develop the full-blown disease of AIDS. The AIDS virus is transmitted between individuals by means of bodily fluids, such as blood and semen, and can be transmitted through sexual activity, through intravenous use of contaminated syringes and blood transfusions, and from mother to fetus during pregnancy.

Recent data strongly suggest that treatment of asymptomatic HIV-positive patients, i.e., patients who have not yet developed full-blown AIDS, with such drugs as azidothymidine (AZT) acts to decrease the emergence of symptoms of AIDS. Therefore, early screening is crucial. Possible indications for HIV testing are outlined in Table 25–1.

TABLE 25–1. **POSSIBLE INDICATIONS FOR HUMAN IMMUNODEFICIENCY VIRUS (HIV) TESTING**

1. Patients who belong to a high-risk group: 1) men who have had sex with another man since 1977; 2) intravenous drug abusers since 1977; 3) hemophiliacs or other patients who have received since 1977 blood or blood product transfusions not screened for HIV; 4) sexual partners of people from any of these groups; 5) sexual partners of people with known HIV exposure—people with cuts, wounds, sores, or needlesticks whose lesions have had direct contact with HIV-infected blood.

2. Patients who request testing. Note that not all patients will admit to the presence of risk factors (e.g., because of shame, fear).

3. Patients with symptoms of AIDS or ARC.

4. Women belonging to a high-risk group who are planning pregnancy or who are pregnant.

5. Blood, semen, or organ donors.

6. Patients with dementia in a high-risk group.

Note. ARC = AIDS-related complex. Table from Rosse RB, Giese AA, Deutsch SI, Morihisa JM: *Laboratory & Diagnostic Testing in Psychiatry.* American Psychiatric Press, Washington, DC, 1989, p 54, with permission.

Some patients are so concerned about the possibility of having contracted the AIDS virus that the patient and physician may feel it necessary to perform the test even if no apparent risk factors are present.

HIV testing must be accompanied by informed pre- and posttest counseling. Physicians must be cognizant that tremendous psychologic stress can accompany HIV testing. Some of the major issues involved in pretest counseling are listed in Table 25–2.

Pretest counseling anticipates the potential reactions patients will have on receiving the results of their test. Patients should be informed that testing centers

TABLE 25–2. **PRETEST HIV COUNSELING**

1. Discuss meaning of a positive result and clarify distortions (e.g., the test detects exposure to the AIDS virus; it is not a test for AIDS).

2. Discuss the meaning of a negative result (e.g., seroconversion requires time, recent high-risk behavior might require follow-up testing).

3. Be available to discuss the patient's fears and concerns (unrealistic fears might require appropriate psychological intervention).

4. Discuss why the test is necessary. (Remember, not all patients will admit to high-risk behaviors).

5. Explore the patient's potential reactions to a positive result (e.g., "I'll kill myself if I'm positive.") Take appropriate necessary steps to intervene in a potentially catastrophic reaction.

6. Explore past reactions to severe stresses.

7. Discuss the confidentiality issues relevant to the testing situation (e.g., is it an anonymous or nonanonymous setting). Inform the patient of other possible testing options where the counseling and testing can be done completely anonymously (e.g., where the result would not be made a permanent part of a hospital chart). Discuss who might have access to the test results.

8. Discuss with the patient how being seropositive can potentially affect social status (e.g., health and life insurance coverage, employment, housing).

9. Explore high-risk behaviors and recommend risk-reducing interventions.

10. Document discussions in chart.

11. Allow the patient time to ask questions.

Table from Rosse RB, Giese AA, Deutsch SI, Morihisa JM: *Laboratory & Diagnostic Testing in Psychiatry.* American Psychiatric Press, Washington, DC, 1989, p 55, with permission.

exist where only the patient knows the result, and physicians should be aware that the medical record is not always confidential. Records can be subpoenaed and become a part of public record; insurance companies can occasionally gain access to a patient's file. The patient should be informed prior to testing whether the testing center requires the physician to inform sexual partners of positive test results.

Some of the issues involved in the posttest counseling, when a patient who has been HIV tested is informed of the result, are described in Table 25–3.

TABLE 25–3. **POSTTEST HIV COUNSELING**

1. Interpretation of test result:
   - *Clarify distortion* (e.g., "a negative test still means you could contact the virus at a future time—it does not mean you are immune from AIDS").
   - Ask questions of the patient about his or her understanding and emotional reaction to test result.

2. Recommendations for prevention of transmission (careful discussion of high-risk behaviors and guidelines for prevention of transmission).

3. Recommendations on the follow-up of sexual partners and/or needle contacts.

4. If test is positive, recommendations against donating blood, sperm, or organs and against sharing razors, toothbrushes, or anything else that might have blood on it.

5. Referral for appropriate psychological support:
   - HIV-positive individuals often need to have available a mental health team (assess need for inpatient versus outpatient care; consider individual or group supportive therapy). Common themes include shock of diagnosis, fear of death and social consequences, grief over potential losses, and dashed hope for good news. Also look for depression, hopelessness, anger, frustration, guilt, and obsessional themes.
   - Activate supports available to patient (e.g., family, friends, community services).

Table from Rosse RB, Giese AA, Deutsch SI, Morihisa JM: *Laboratory & Diagnostic Testing in Psychiatry.* American Psychiatric Press, Washington, DC, 1989, p 58, with permission.

Safe Sex. A common question that physicians should be prepared to answer is, "What is safe and unsafe sex?" Patients should be advised that if they are HIV-positive or if a new sexual partner's history is unknown to them and there is any reason for concern, the guidelines listed in Table 25–4 should be followed:

TABLE 25–4. **AIDS SAFE SEX GUIDELINES**

Remember: ANY activity that allows for exchange of body fluids of one person and the mouth, anus, vagina, bloodstream, cuts, or sores of another person is considered UNSAFE at this time.

Safe-Sex Practices
- Massage, hugging, body-to-body rubbing.
- Dry social kissing
- Masturbation
- Acting out sexual fantasies (that do not include any unsafe sex practices)
- Using vibrators or other instruments (provided they are not shared)

Low-Risk Sex Practices
These activities are not considered completely safe.
- French (wet) kissing (without mouth sores)
- Mutual masturbation
- Vaginal and anal intercourse using a condom
- Oral sex, male (fellatio) using a condom
- Oral sex, female (cunnilingus), with barrier
- External contact with semen or urine provided there are no breaks in the skin

Unsafe-Sex Practices
- Vaginal or anal intercourse without a condom
- Semen, urine, or feces in the mouth or vagina
- Unprotected oral sex (fellatio or cunnilingus)
- Blood contact of any kind
- Sharing sex instruments or needles

Table from Moffatt B, Spiegel J, Parrish S, Helquist M: *AIDS: A Self-Care Manual.* IBS Press, Santa Monica, CA, 1987, p 125, with permission.

II. Central nervous system clinical manifestations.   HIV-infected patients are commonly reported to have central nervous system involvement, even in the absence of other signs or symptoms of AIDS. When AIDS is present, approximately 60% of patients exhibit neurologic symptoms; neuropathologic changes are reported in 80–90% of patients at autopsy.

Organic mental disorders associated with HIV infection include AIDS dementia, organic mood disorder, and organic personality disorder. Psychiatric conditions associated with HIV infection include depression, acute psychosis, and mania. Diseases that occasionally cause dementia in patients with AIDS include cerebral toxoplasmosis, cryptococcal meningitis, and primary brain lymphoma. A distinct neurologic entity, AIDS encephalopathy (also known as AIDS dementia complex) is the most common neurologic problem in AIDS. HIV-1 is believed to be the direct cause of this syndrome. The major clinical manifestations of AIDS dementia complex are outlined in Table 25–5.

Evidence suggests that signs and symptoms of the AIDS dementia complex may occur before the diagnosis of AIDS is made. Clinicians initially may mistake the patient's social withdrawal, apathy, psychiatric retardation, and deficits in concentration or memory as depression. AIDS dementia complex may present acutely after the use of psychoactive drugs or other stress, although careful questioning of the patient's family or friends usually reveals that the onset was not as acute as it appeared. The prognosis of AIDS dementia is poor.

TABLE 25–5.   CLINICAL MANIFESTATIONS OF THE AIDS DEMENTIA COMPLEX

Common manifestations
  Decreased memory
  Inability to concentrate
  Apathy
  Social withdrawal
  Psychomotor retardation
  Abulia (loss of will)
  Mild headache

Occasional manifestations
  Motor deficits
  Seizures
  Psychiatric problems

Uncommon manifestations
  Decreased level of consciousness
  Aphasia
  Apraxia

Table from Bredesen DE: Clinical features. In Ho DD, moderator. The acquired immunodeficiency syndrome (AIDS) dementia complex. Ann Intern Med, *111*:401, 1989, with permission.

A. **Medical therapy.**   Treatment of medical complications should be vigorous and involve a broad range of agents (Table 25–6). In addition, agents with activity against HIV should be instituted (Table 25–7).

B. **Pharmacotherapy.**   When CNS involvement occurs, especially symptoms of an organic mental disorder, such as anxiety, psychosis, or depression, appropriate psychotropic medications are indicated. Antipsychotics (e.g., tri-fluoperazine [Stelazine], haloperidol [Haldol]) in small doses may be useful in controlling agitation. Antidepressants, particularly those with few anti-cholinergic side effects, are of benefit in treating depression. If brain damage is present, drugs with anticholinergic effect must be used cautiously to prevent an atropine pyschosis. Some clinicians have had postitive results treating de-pressed AIDS patients with small doses of amphetamine. Benzodiazepines often are useful for anxiety or insomnia, although they may exacerbate cog-nitive symptoms. Small doses of sedating antipsychotics (e.g., 25 mg of thior-idazine [Mellaril]) or an antihistamine may then be used. Lithium may be useful in persons with manic symptoms, but renal function and lithium con-centrations must be carefully monitored if there is renal impairment from the illness. Suicidal depression is common in advanced cases; antidepressant med-ication and close supervision of the patient, including psychiatric hospitali-zation with suicidal precautions, may be necessary. Approximately 60 percent of AIDS patients develop some type of organic mental syndrome, and the usual measures of medical, environmental, and social support should be in-stituted in those situations (Table 25–8).

C. **Psychotherapy.**   The role of psychotherapy, both individual and group, is important. The psychiatrist can help patients deal with feelings of guilt re-garding behavior that contributed to developing AIDS that is disapproved of by other segments of society. Many AIDS patients feel they are being punished for a deviant life-style. Difficult health care decisions (e.g., whether to par-ticipate in an experimental drug trial), as well as terminal care and life support systems, should be explored. In addition, all infected persons must be educated

TABLE 25–6. **TREATMENT OF OPPORTUNISTIC INFECTIONS**[a]

Infection	Treatment	Dosage[*]
Pneumocystis carinii	Sulfamethoxazole-trimethoprim	20 mg/kg/day of trimethoprim 100 mg/kg/day of sulfamethoxazole
	or	
Cryptococcal meningitis	Pentamidine isethionate	4 mg/kg/day IV
	Amphotericin B	0.4–0.6 mg/kg/day IV
	and	
Toxoplasmosis	Flucytosine	100 mg/kg/day
	Sulfadiazine sodium	4 g/day p.o.
	and	
	Pyrimethamine	25–50 mg/day p.o.
Mycobacterium avium-intracellulare	No clearly active agent	
Cryptosporidiosis	No clearly active agent	
Oral candidiasis	Clotrimazole troche	5 troches/day
	or	
	Nystatin swish	5,000 U q.i.d.
	or	
Esophageal candidiasis	Ketoconazole	200–400 mg b.i.d.
Cytomegalovirus	Ketoconazole	200 mg b.i.d.
	9-(2-hydroxy-1-[hydroxymethyl] ethoxymethyl) guanine	Dose not full established (investigational)
Herpes simplex	Acyclovir sodium	200 mg five times daily
Herpes zoster (disseminated)	Acyclovir sodium	10 mg/kg/day IV
		800 mg five times daily p.o.

Table from Kaplan LD, Wofsy C, Volberding P: Treatment of patients with acquired immunodeficiency syndrome and associated manifestations. JAMA, 257:1367, 1987, with permission.
[*]IV indicates administered intravenously; p.o., by mouth, q.i.d. four times daily; U, units.
[a]A syndrome called AIDS-related complex (ARC) has been described in patients who do not have an opportunistic infection. Such patients are seropositive and present with weight loss, fever, night sweats, generalized lymphadenopathy, chronic fatigue, and depression.

TABLE 25-7. **AGENTS WITH ACTIVITY AGAINST HIV**

Agent	Mechanism of Action	Major Toxicity
Suramin sodium	Inhibits reverse transcriptase	Fever, rash, fatigue, adrenal insufficiency, renal insufficiency, hepatic failure
Ribavirin	Guanosine analogue interferes with 5' capping of viral mRNA	Hemolytic anemia
HPA-23	Inhibits reverse transcriptase	Thrombocytopenia
Phosphonoformate	Inhibits reverse transcriptase	Renal failure
Azidothymidine	Inhibits reverse transcriptase, DNA chain terminator	Headache, leukopenia, macrocytic anemia
α-interferon	Interferes with assembly of viral proteins	Flu-like symptoms, fatigue, weight loss, neutropenia
AL721	Extracts cholesterol from cellular membranes	No data
2', 3'-Dideoxynucleosides	Chain terminators of DNA synthesis	No data

Table from Kaplan LD, Wofsy C, Volberding P: Treatment of patients with acquired immunodeficiency syndrome and associated manifestations. JAMA 257:1367, 1987, with permission.

TABLE 25–8. **SOMATIC TREATMENT OF PSYCHIATRIC SIGNS AND SYMPTOMS ASSOCIATED WITH AIDS**

Psychiatric Signs and Symptoms	Treatment	Comment
Anxiety Insomnia	Anxiolytics Antihistamines	Benzodiazepines are useful but may exacerbate cognitive symptoms; low doses of sedating antipsychotics, e.g., thioridazine (Mellaril), or antihistamines (diphenhydramine [Benadryl]) may be helpful.
Severe anxiety Organic mental syndromes with agitation Psychotic episode	Antipsychotics	Chlorpromazine (Thorazine) equivalents of 50–200 mg/day (may need lower doses than generally used due to presence of brain damage).
Major depression	Antidepressants	Those drugs with few anticholinergic side effects are favored to decrease possibility of atropine psychosis; low-dose amphetamines have been used.
Mania	Lithium	Renal function must be carefully monitored.

concerning safe sexual practices. Treatment of homosexuals and bisexuals with AIDS often involves helping the patient "come out" to his family and dealing with the possible issues of rejection, guilt, shame, and anger. Involvement of a homosexual patient's lover in the couple's therapy is warranted in many cases.

Treatment of intravenous drug users involves discussing the patient's continued use of intravenous drugs. The possible ill effects of drug abuse on a patient's health needs to be weighed against the effect of adding drug withdrawal to an AIDS patient's existing problems. Educating patients about the danger of sharing contaminated needles is of utmost importance.

A subgroup of patients termed the "worried well" comprises persons in high-risk groups who, although they are seronegative and disease-free, develop anxiety or an obsession about contracting the virus or AIDS. Some patients are reassured by a negative enzyme-linked immunosorbent assay (ELISA), the serum test used to detect HIV. Others, however, obsess about the possible long incubation period and cannot be reassured; they can have an underlying somatoform disorder. Supportive or insight-oriented psychotherapy is indicated in these cases. Often, there are unconscious feelings of guilt about forbidden sexual activities, and patients punish themselves with obsessive thoughts or fantasies. ARC patients especially benefit from group therapy composed of similar patients, as do persons who are at risk on the basis of past sexual activity or current practices.

For more detailed discussion of this topic, see Wolcott DL, Dilley JW, Mitsuyasu RT: Psychiatric Aspects of Acquired Immune Deficiency Syndrome, Sec. 26.2, pp 1297–1316, in *CTP/V*.

Index

Note: Page numbers followed by t indicate tables.

A

Abstraction, definition, 15
Abuse. *See* Child abuse; Sexual abuse
Academic problem, 6
Academic skills disorder, 192
Acetaminophen, in pain control, 154t
Acetophenazine, 241t, 246–247
  therapeutic doses, 242t
Acid phosphatase, laboratory evaluation of,
  290t
Acquired immune deficiency syndrome, 24, 37,
  277, 297–303
  central nervous system clinical
    manifestations, 299
  in children and adolescents, 207
  common medical symptoms, 148t
  diagnostic problems, 148t
  impaired performance and behavior in, 148t
  neurologic symptoms, 299
  psychiatric signs and symptoms associated
    with, 148t
    somatic treatment of, 303t
  sex and age prevalence, 148t
  treatment, 300–303
Actomal. *See* Mebanazine
Addington v. Texas, 271
Addisonian anemia
  common medical symptoms, 149t
  diagnostic problems, 149t
  impaired performance and behavior in, 149t
  psychiatric symptoms and complaints, 149t
  sex and age prevalence, 149t
Addison's disease
  common medical symptoms, 148t
  diagnostic problems, 148t
  impaired performance and behavior in, 148t
  psychiatric symptoms and complaints, 148t
  sex and age prevalence, 148t
ADHD. *See* Attention-deficit hyperactivity
  disorder
Adjustment disorder(s)
  with anxious mood, vs. anxiety disorders,
    102
  biologic factors, 141
  in childhood, 206
  course, 141
  definition, 5, 141
  with depressed mood, 84
  differential diagnosis, 141
  epidemiology, 141

  etiology, 141
  genetics, 141
  prognosis, 141
  psychosocial factors, 141
  signs and symptoms, 141
  treatment, 141–142
Adolescent(s). *See also* Child and adolescent;
  Child and adolescent disorders
  substance abuse problems, 36
Adolescent mania, 86
Adrenal cortical insufficiency
  common medical symptoms, 148t
  diagnostic problems, 148t
  impaired performance and behavior in, 148t
  psychiatric symptoms and complaints, 148t
  sex and age prevalence, 148t
Adrenocorticotropic hormone, laboratory
  evaluation of, 290t
Adrenogenital syndrome, 200
Affect
  assessment of, 10
  definition, 16
  in depression, 81
  in mania, 85
  in schizophrenia, 57
Affective disorder(s). *See* Mood (affective)
  disorder(s)
Aggression, definition, 16
Aggressive patient, interview for, 9t
Aging
  CNS neurochemical changes in, 211
  cognitive changes in, 212–215
  epidemiology of, 208
  functional loss in, order and time course of,
    217t
  morbidity in, 208
  mortality in, 208
  normal, vs. dementia, 25
  physiologic changes of, 208
  sleep and, 133
Agitation
  consultation-liaison for, 151t
  definition, 16
Agoraphobia, 96, 103, 168
  definition, 4
  psychoanalytic theory of, 101
  psychodynamics, 102t
AIDS. *See* Acquired immune deficiency
  syndrome
AIDS dementia complex, 299
  clinical manifestations of, 300t

U

Ulcerative colitis, 146t
Uncomplicated bereavement. *See* Bereavement
Undifferentiated attention-deficit disorder, 206
Undoing (or restitution), definition, 20t
Unipolar depression, 83
Urecholine. *See* Bethanechol
Urinalysis, 295t
Urine, drugs of abuse that can be tested in, 296t
Urophilia, 131t
Urticaria, 147t
Uvulopharyngopalatoplasty, for obstructive sleep apnea, 137

V

Vaginismus, 123t, 128
    DSM-III-R diagnostic criteria for, 128t
    treatment, 131
Valium. *See* Diazepam
Valproic acid
    for bipolar disorder, 94
    dose, 264
    drug interactions, 263
    pharmacology, 264
    side effects, 264
    therapeutic level, 286t
    toxic level, 286t
    uses in psychiatry, 264
Venereal Disease Research Laboratory test, 295t
Verapamil
    approved uses, 264–265
    for bipolar disorder, 94
    contraindications, 265
    dose, 265
    drug interactions, 263, 265
    nonpsychiatric uses, 264
    pharmacology, 265
    side effects, 265
Verban. *See* Vinblastine sulfate
Verbigeration, definition, 20
Versed. *See* Midazolam
Vesprin. *See* Triflupromazine
Vinblastine sulfate, depression caused by, 278t
Vincristine sulfate, depression caused by, 278t
Violence, 172
    impending, signs of, 174
    management of, 174–175

prevention of, 174–175
    risk of, assessment of, 174
    and schizophrenia, 66–67
Vistaril. *See* Hydroxyzine
Vitamin A, serum, laboratory evaluation of, 295t
Vitamin B$_{12}$, serum, laboratory evaluation of, 295t
Vivactil. *See* Protriptyline
Volatile hydrocarbons
    abuse, treatment, 47t
    behavioral effects, 47t
    lab findings with, 47t
    physical effects, 47t
Volition, altered, in schizophrenia, 57
Volitional test, of insanity defense, 276
Vomiting, in somatization disorder, 112
Voyeurism, 131t
    definition, 5

W

Warfarin, drug interactions, 250t, 264
Waxy flexibility, definition, 16
Wellbutrin. *See* Bupropion
Wernicke-Korsakoff syndrome, 3
Wernicke's encephalopathy, 3, 50, 56, 175
White blood cell count, 295t
Wills, 273–274
Wilson's disease, 31
    common medical symptoms, 149t
    diagnostic problems, 149t
    impaired performance and behavior in, 149t
    psychiatric symptoms and complaints, 149t
    sex and age prevalence, 149t
Withdrawal, definition, 37
Withdrawal delirium, 3
Withdrawal syndromes, 176
Withdrawn patient, interview for, 9t
Word salad, definition, 20
Work shift changes, 138
Wyatt v. Stickney, 272

X

Xanax. *See* Alprazolam

Z

Zinc deficiency, 200
Zoophilia, 131t
Zung Self-Rating Scale, 9

PSYCHOTIC DISORDERS NOT ELSEWHERE CLASSIFIED

298.80 Brief reactive psychosis
295.40 Schizophreniform disorder
        Specify: without good prognostic features or with good prognostic features
295.70 Schizoaffective disorder
        Specify: bipolar type or depressive type
297.30 Induced psychotic disorder
298.90 Psychotic disorder NOS (Atypical psychosis)

MOOD DISORDERS

Code current state of Major Depression and Bipolar Disorder in fifth digit:
  1 = mild
  2 = moderate
  3 = severe, without psychotic features
  4 = with psychotic features (*specify* mood-congruent or mood-incongruent)
  5 = in partial remission
  6 = in full remission
  0 = unspecified

For major depressive episodes, *specify* if chronic and *specify* if melancholic type.

For Bipolar Disorder, Bipolar Disorder NOS, Recurrent Major Depression, and Depressive Disorder NOS, *specify* if seasonal pattern.

Bipolar Disorders

Bipolar disorder,
296.6x mixed, _____
296.4x manic, _____
296.5x depressed, _____
301.13 Cyclothymia
296.70 Bipolar disorder NOS

Depressive Disorders

Major Depression,
296.2x single episode, _____

296.3x recurrent, _____
300.40 Dysthymia (or Depressive neurosis)
        Specify: primary or secondary type
        Specify: early or late onset
311.00 Depressive disorder NOS

ANXIETY DISORDERS (or Anxiety and Phobic Neuroses)

Panic disorder
300.21 with agoraphobia
        Specify current severity of agoraphobic avoidance
        Specify current severity of panic attacks
300.01 without agoraphobia
        Specify current severity of panic attacks
300.22 Agoraphobia without history of panic disorder
        Specify with or without limited symptom attacks
300.23 Social phobia
        Specify if generalized type
300.29 Simple phobia
300.30 Obsessive-compulsive disorder (or Obsessive-compulsive neurosis)
309.89 Post-traumatic stress disorder
        Specify if delayed onset
300.02 Generalized anxiety disorder
300.00 Anxiety disorder NOS

SOMATOFORM DISORDERS

300.70* Body dysmorphic disorder
300.11   Conversion disorder (or Hysterical neurosis, conversion type)
         Specify: single episode or recurrent
300.70* Hypochondriasis (or Hypochondriacal neurosis)
300.81   Somatization disorder
307.80   Somatoform pain disorder
300.70* Undifferentiated somatoform disorder
300.70* Somatoform disorder NOS

DISSOCIATIVE DISORDERS (or Hysterical Neuroses, Dissociative Type)

300.14 Multiple personality disorder
300.13 Psychogenic fugue
300.12 Psychogenic amnesia
300.60 Depersonalization disorder (or Depersonalization neurosis)
300.15 Dissociative disorder NOS

SEXUAL DISORDERS

Paraphilias

302.40 Exhibitionism
302.81 Fetishism
302.89 Frotteurism
302.20 Pedophilia
        Specify: same sex, opposite sex, same and opposite sex
        Specify if limited to incest
        Specify: exclusive type or nonexclusive type
302.83 Sexual masochism
302.84 Sexual sadism
302.30 Transvestic fetishism
302.82 Voyeurism
302.90* Paraphilia NOS

Sexual Dysfunctions

Specify: psychogenic only, or psychogenic and biogenic (Note: If biogenic only, code on Axis III)
Specify: lifelong or acquired
Specify: generalized or situational

Sexual desire disorders
302.71 Hypoactive sexual desire disorder
302.79 Sexual aversion disorder

Sexual arousal disorders
302.72* Female sexual arousal disorder
302.72* Male erectile disorder

Orgasm disorders
302.73 Inhibited female orgasm
302.74 Inhibited male orgasm
302.75 Premature ejaculation

Sexual pain disorders
302.76 Dyspareunia
306.51 Vaginismus

302.70 Sexual dysfunctions NOS

Other Sexual Disorders

302.90* Sexual disorder NOS

SLEEP DISORDERS

Dyssomnias

Insomnia disorder
307.42* related to another mental disorder (nonorganic)
780.50* related to known organic factor
307.42* Primary insomnia

Hypersomnia disorder
307.44 related to another mental disorder (nonorganic)
780.50* related to a known organic factor

780.54	Primary hypersomnia
307.45	Sleep-wake schedule disorder
	Specify: advanced or delayed phase type, disorganized type, frequently changing type
	Other dyssomnias
307.40*	Dyssomnia NOS

Parasomnias

307.47	Dream anxiety disorder (Nightmare disorder)
307.46*	Sleep terror disorder
307.46*	Sleepwalking disorder
307.40*	Parasomnia NOS

FACTITIOUS DISORDERS

	Factitious disorder
301.51	with physical symptoms
300.16	with psychological symptoms
300.19	Factitious disorder NOS

IMPULSE CONTROL DISORDERS NOT ELSEWHERE CLASSIFIED

312.34	Intermittent explosive disorder
312.32	Kleptomania
312.31	Pathological gambling
312.33	Pyromania
312.39*	Trichotillomania
312.39*	Impulse control disorder NOS

ADJUSTMENT DISORDER

	Adjustment disorder
309.24	with anxious mood
309.00	with depressed mood
309.30	with disturbance of conduct
309.40	with mixed disturbance of emotions and conduct
309.28	with mixed emotional features
309.82	with physical complaints
309.83	with withdrawal

| 309.23 | with work (or academic) inhibition |
| 309.90 | Adjustment disorder NOS |

PSYCHOLOGICAL FACTORS AFFECTING PHYSICAL CONDITION

| 316.00 | Psychological factors affecting physical condition |
| | *Specify* physical condition on Axis III |

PERSONALITY DISORDER
Note: These are coded on Axis II.

Cluster A

301.00	Paranoid
301.20	Schizoid
301.22	Schizotypal

Cluster B

301.70	Antisocial
301.83	Borderline
301.50	Histrionic
301.81	Narcissistic

Cluster C

301.82	Avoidant
301.60	Dependent
301.40	Obsessive-compulsive
301.84	Passive aggressive
301.90	Personality disorder NOS

V CODES FOR CONDITIONS NOT ATTRIBUTABLE TO A MENTAL DISORDER THAT ARE A FOCUS OF ATTENTION OR TREATMENT

| V62.30 | Academic problem |
| V71.01 | Adult antisocial behavior |

| V40.00 | Borderline intellectual functioning (Note: This is coded on Axis II.) |

V71.02	Childhood or adolescent antisocial behavior
V65.20	Malingering
V61.10	Marital problem
V15.81	Noncompliance with medical treatment
V62.20	Occupational problem
V61.20	Parent-child problem
V62.81	Other interpersonal problem
V61.80	Other specified family circumstances
V62.89	Phase of life problem or other life circumstance problem
V62.82	Uncomplicated bereavement

ADDITIONAL CODES

300.90	Unspecified mental disorder (nonpsychotic)
V71.09*	No diagnosis or condition on Axis I
799.90*	Diagnosis or condition deferred on Axis I

| V71.09* | No diagnosis or condition on Axis II |
| 799.90* | Diagnosis or condition deferred on Axis II |

MULTIAXIAL SYSTEM

Axis I	Clinical Syndromes V Codes
Axis II	Developmental Disorders Personality Disorders
Axis III	Physical Disorders and Conditions
Axis IV	Severity of Psychosocial Stressors
Axis V	Global Assessment of Functioning